Women's Health Care Nurse Practitioner Certification Review Guide

Editor

Susan B. Moskosky, M.S., R.N.C.
Nurse Consultant
Former Director Women's Health Care
Advanced Nurse Practitioner Program
University of Texas
Southwestern Medical Center
Dallas, Texas

Health Leadership Associates, Inc.
Potomac, Maryland

Family Nurse Practitioner Set
by
Health Leadership Associates, Inc.

Adult Nurse Practitioner Certification Review Guide

Pediatric Nurse Practitioner Certification Review Guide

Women's Health Care Nurse Practitioner Certification Review Guide

Summary of Changes

The following is a revision made to the First Edition, second printing of the Woman's Health Care Nurse Practitioner Certification Review Guide.

Page	Location	Change
34	3. d. (1) (c) & (d)	Revised (Description of location of auscultation sites)

Health Leadership Associates, Inc.

Production Manager: Martha M. Pounsberry
Manuscript Editor: Virginia Millonig
Cover and Design: Port City Press, Inc.
Production: Port City Press, Inc.

Printed in the United States of America

Health Leadership Associates, Inc. • P.O. Box 59153 • Potomac, Maryland 20859

Library of Congress Cataloging-in-Publication Data

Women's health care nurse practitioner certification review guide /
   editor, Susan B. Moskosky.
       p.   cm. — (Family nurse practitioner set)
    ISBN 1-878028-13-8 (alk. paper). — ISBN 1-878028-14-6 (set : alk. paper)
     1. Nurse practitioners—Examinations, questions, etc.   2. Women—
Diseases—Examinations, questions, etc.   3. Women—Health and
hygiene—Examinations, questions, etc.   4. Gynecologic nursing—
Examinations, questions, etc.   5. Maternity nursing—Examinations,
questions, etc.   I. Moskosky, Susan B.   II. Series,
   [DNLM: 1. Nurse Practitioners—examination questions.   2. Women's
Health—examination questions.   3. Genital Diseases, Female—
nursing—examination questions.   4. Obstetrical Nursing—
examination questions.   WY 18.2 W872 1995]
RT82.8.W66   1995
610.73'06'92—dc20
DNLM/DLC
for Library of Congress   95-33625
                                         CIP

10 9 8 7 6 5 4 3 2

Second printing July 1996

Contributing Authors

TEST TAKING STRATEGIES AND TECHNIQUES

Susan B. Moskosky, M.S., R.N.C.
Nurse Consultant
Former Director Women's Health Care
Advanced Nurse Practitioner Program
University of Texas
Southwestern Medical Center
Dallas, Texas

Nancy Dickenson Hazard, M.S.N., C.P.N.P., F.A.A.N.
Executive Officer
Sigma Theta Tau International
Indianapolis, Indiana

GENERAL ASSESSMENT

Jacki S. Witt, J.D., M.S.N., R.N.C.
Region VII
Chlamydia Control Project Coordinator
Clinical Instructor
School of Nursing
University of Missouri
Kansas City, Missouri

NON-GYN DISORDERS

Mary C. Knutson, M.N., R.N.C.
Nursing Care Consultant
Family Planning and Reproductive Health
Washington State Department of Health
Olympia, Washington

NORMAL WOMEN'S HEALTH

Carolyn M. Sutton, M.S., R.N.C.
Associate Director for Clinical Services
Division of Maternal Health and Family Planning
Department of Obstetrics and Gynecology
University of Texas
Southwestern Medical Center
Dallas, Texas

GYNECOLOGIC DISORDERS

Carolyn M. Sutton, M.S., R.N.C.
Associate Director for Clinical Services
Division of Maternal Health and Family Planning
Department of Obstetrics and Gynecology
University of Texas
Southwestern Medical Center
Dallas, Texas

PREGNANCY

Barbara Peterson Sinclair, M.N., R.N.C., O.G.N.P., F.A.A.N.
Professor
Department of Nursing
California State University, Los Angeles
Los Angeles, California

Jane G. Conner, M.S., R.N.C., O.G.N.P.
Women's Health Care Nurse Practitioner
Lecturer
Department of Nursing
California State University
Los Angeles, California

Jane Heath, B.S.N., R.N.C., O.G.N.P.
Nurse Practitioner
Department of Obstetrics and Gynecology
Kaiser Permanente, Orange County
South Laguna, California

PROFESSIONAL ISSUES

Judith Grandin, Ed.D., M.S.N., R.N.C.S.
Assistant Professor
Coordinator
Family Nurse Practitioner Program
School of Nursing
Georgetown University
Washington, D.C.

Reviewers

Marcia S. Davis, M.S., M.S.Ed., R.N.C.
Adult Nurse Practitioner
Women's Health Care Nurse Practitioner
Department of Maternal Child Nursing
Nurse Practitioner Program
Medical College of Virginia
Virginia Commonwealth University
Richmond, Virginia

Susan Rawlins, M.S., R.N.C.
Director
Women's Health Care Advanced Nurse Practitioner Program
Division of Maternal Health and Family Planning
Department of Obstetrics and Gynecology
University of Texas
Southwestern Medical Center
Dallas, Texas

Sharon B. Schnare, M.S.N., R.N.C.
Family Nurse Practitioner
Nurse Midwife
Ob/Gyn Nurse Practitioner
Clinician, Consultant, Educator
Seattle, Washington

Joan Ann Swiatek, M.S., R.N.C.S.
Adult Nurse Practitioner
Healthy Alternatives
Women's Health/Sexual Medicine
Chicago, Illinois

Preface

The Women's Health Care Nurse Practitioner Certification Review Guide has been developed as a comprehensive review of the specific knowledge nurses need to practice as providers of women's health care. This book will replace the *Ob-Gyn Nurse Practitioner Certification Review Guide*. The title has been changed to reflect the more comprehensive content on women's health care throughout the life cycle. The text has been written for Health Leadership Associates, Inc. by experts in the field of women's health nursing, with the specific goal of assisting women's health care and family nurse practitioners preparing for national certification examinations.

This book differs substantially from the *Ob-Gyn Nurse Practitioner Certification Review Guide* in many respects. Each section has been significantly expanded and updated. The number of test questions has been expanded and the bibliographies for each section have been enhanced. Additionally, a chapter has been added on Non-Gynecologic Disorders that will assist with review of primary care content needed to provide comprehensive women's health services.

The purpose of the book is twofold. First, the book will assist individuals engaged in self study preparation for Certification Examinations, and may also be used as a brief reference guide in the practice setting. Second, this is one of three books that comprises the "Family Nurse Practitioner Set," the others being the Pediatric Nurse Practitioner Certification Review Guide and the Adult Nurse Practitioner Certification Review Guide.

Many nurses preparing for certification examinations find that reviewing an extensive body of scientific knowledge requires a very difficult search of many sources that must be synthesized to provide a review base for the examination. The purpose of this publication is to provide a succinct, yet comprehensive review of the core material.

The book has been organized to provide the reader with test taking and study strategies first. This is followed by chapters on health assessment, non-gynecologic disorders, and specific women's health content throughout the life cycle, from adolescence through postmenopause. Common disorders are presented in summary form, including definitions, etiology, signs and symptoms, physical findings, differential diagnoses, diagnostic tests/findings and management/treatment. The final chapter addresses professional issues that directly impact the nurse practitioner, including nursing research, nurse practitioner role, ethical issues, health policy/legislative issues, and legal aspects of nurse practitioner practice.

Following each chapter are test questions, which are intended to serve as an introduction to the testing arena. Questions may be followed by three or four answer choices, to reflect different certification examinations that may include question formats of either type. In addition, a bibliography is included at the completion of each chapter for those who need a more in depth discussion of the subject matter in each chapter. These references can serve as additional instructional material for the reader.

The editor and contributing authors are certified nurse practitioners who are respected experts in the field of women's health care nursing. They have designed this book to assist potential examinees to prepare for success in the certification examination process.

It is assumed that the reader of this review guide has completed a course of study in either a women's health care or family nurse practitioner program. The *Women's Health Care Nurse Practitioner Certification Review Guide* is not intended to be a basic learning tool.

Certification is a process that is gaining recognition both within and outside the profession. For the professional, it is a means of gaining special recognition as a certified nurse practitioner, which not only demonstrates a level of competency, but may also enhance professional opportunities and advancement. For the consumer, it means that a certified nurse has met certain predetermined standards set by the profession.

Acknowledgements

Special acknowledgements go to the authors and reviewers of this book, all of whom are practicing professionals, who believed in this project, and gave unselfishly of their time and talents. Also, thank you to the many nurse practitioners throughout the country who have provided suggestions and direction in the development of this Review Guide.

Finally, the editor wishes to express her appreciation to Virginia L. Millonig and the staff at Health Leadership Associates, Inc., who were always available to provide encouragement and support, moral and otherwise, throughout the development of this work.

CONTENTS

4 **Normal Women's Health Care** *Carolyn Sutton*

5 **Gynecologic Disorders** *Carolyn Sutton*

6 **Pregnancy** *B. Peterson-Sinclair, J. Conner, J. Heath*

7 **Professional Issues** *Judith Grandin*

Test Taking Strategies and Techniques

Nancy A. Dickenson Hazard
Susan B. Moskosky

We all respond to testing situations in different ways. What separates the successful test taker from the unsuccessful one is knowing how to prepare for and take a test. Preparing yourself to be a successful test taker is as important as studying for the test. Each person needs to assess and develop individual test taking strategies and skills. The primary goal of this chapter is to assist potential examinees in knowing how to study for and take a test.

STRATEGY #1 Know Yourself

When faced with an examination, do you feel threatened, experience butterflies or sweaty palms, have trouble keeping your mind focused on studying or on test questions? These common symptoms of test anxiety plague many of us, but can be used advantageously if understood and handled correctly (Divine & Kylen, 1979). Over the years of test taking, each of us has developed certain testing behaviors, some of which are beneficial, while others present obstacles to successful test taking. You can take control of the test taking situation by identifying the undesirable behaviors, maintaining the desirable ones and developing skills to improve test performance.

Technique #1:   From the following descriptions of test taking personalities, find yourself (Table 1). Write down those characteristics which describe you even if they are from different personality types. Carefully review the problem list associated with your test taking personality characteristics. Write down the problems which are most troublesome. Then make a list of how you can remedy these problems from the improvement strategies list. Be sure to use these strategies as you prepare for and take examinations.

STRATEGY #2 Develop Your Thinking Skills

Understanding Thought Process: In order to improve your thinking skills and subsequent test performance, it is best to understand the types of thinking as well as the techniques to enhance the thought process.

Everyone has a personal learning style, but we all must proceed through the same process to think.

Thinking occurs on two levels—the lower level of memory and comprehension and the higher level of application and analysis (ABP, 1989). Memory is the ability to recall facts. Without adequate retrieval of facts, progression through the higher levels of thinking cannot occur easily. Comprehension is the ability to understand memorized facts. To be effective, comprehension skills must allow the person to translate recalled information from one context to another. Application, or the process of using information to know why something occurs, is a higher form of learning. Effective application relies on the use of understood, memorized facts to verify intended action. Analysis is the ability to use abstract or logical forms of thought to show relationships and to distinguish the cause and effect between the variables in a situation.

Table 1

Test Taker Profile

Type	Characteristics	Pitfalls	Improvement Strategies
The Rusher	• Rushes to complete the test before the studied facts are forgotten	• Unable to read question and situation completely	• Practice progressive relaxation techniques
	• Arrives at test site early and waits anxiously	• At high risk for misreading, misinterpreting and mistakes	• Develop a study plan with sufficient time to review important content
	• Mumbles studied facts	• Difficult items heighten anxiety	• Avoid cramming and last minute studying
	• Tense body posture	• Likely to make quick, not well-thought-out guesses	• Take practice tests focusing on slowing down and reading and answering each option carefully
	• Accelerated pulse, respiration and neuromuscular excitement		• Read instructions and questions slowly
	• Answers questions rapidly and is generally one of the first to complete		
	• Experiences exhaustion once test is over		
The Turtle	• Moves slowly, methodically, deliberately through each question	• Last to finish; often does not complete the exam	• Take practice tests focusing on time spent per item
	• Repeated rereading, underlining and checking	• Has to quickly complete questions in last part of exam, increasing errors	• Place watch in front of examination paper to keep track of time
	• Takes 60 to 90 seconds per question versus an average of 45 to 60 seconds	• Has difficulty completing timed examinations	• Mark answer sheet for where one should be halfway through exam based on total number of questions and total amount of time for exam
			• Study concepts not details
			• Attempt to answer each question as you progress through the exam

Type	Characteristics	Pitfalls	Improvement Strategies
The Personalizer	• Mature person who has personal knowledge and insight from life experiences	• Risk in relying on what has been learned through observation and experience since one may develop false understandings and stereotypes	• Focus on principles and standards that support nursing practice
		• Personal beliefs and experiences are frequently not the norm or standard tested	• Avoid making connections between patients in exam clinical situations and personal clinical experience
		• Has difficulty identifying expected standards measured by standardized examination	• Focus on generalities not experiences
The Squisher	• View exams as threat, rather than an expected event in education	• Procrastinates studying for exams	• Establish a plan of progressive, disciplined study
	• Preoccupied with grades and personal accomplishment	• Unable to study effectively since waits until last minute	• Use defined time frames for studying content and taking practice exams
	• Attempts to avoid responsibility and accountability associated with testing in order to reduce anxiety	• Increased anxiety over test since procrastinating study impairs ability to learn and perform	• Use relaxation techniques • Return to difficult items • Read carefully
The Philosopher	• Academically successful person who is well disciplined and structured in study habits	• Over analysis causes loss of sight of actual intent of question	• Focus on questions as they are written
	• Displays great intensity and concentration during exam	• Reads information into questions answering with own added information rather than answering the actual intent of question	• Work on self confidence and not on question. Initial response is usually correct
	• Searches questions for hidden or unintended meaning		• Avoid multiple rereadings of questions
	• Experiences anxiety over not knowing everything		• Avoid adding own information and unintended meanings
			• Practice, practice, practice with sample tests
The Second Guesser	• Answers questions twice, first as an examinee, second as an examiner	• Altering an initial response frequently results in an incorrect answer	• Reread only the few items of which one is unsure. Avoid changing initial responses

Type	Characteristics	Pitfalls	Improvement Strategies
The Lawyer	• Believes second look will allow one to find and correct errors	• Frequently changes answers because the pattern of response appears incorrect (i.e., too many "true" or too many correct responses)	• Take exam carefully and progressively first time, allowing little or no time for rereading • Study facts • Avoid reading into questions
	• Frequently changes initial responses (i.e., grades own test)		
	• Attempts to place words or ideas into the question (leads the witness)	• Veers from the obvious answer and provides response from own point of view	• Focus on distinguishing what patient is saying in question and not on what is read into question
	• Occurs most frequently with psychosocial or communication questions which ask for the most appropriate response	• Reads a question, jumps to a conclusion then finds a response that leads to predetermined conclusion	• Avoid formulating responses aimed at obtaining certain information
			• Choose responses that allow patient to express feelings which encourage hope, not catastrophe, those which are intended to clarify, which identify feeling tone of patient or which avoid negating or confronting patient feelings
			• Carefully read entire question before selecting a response

From: "Making the grades as a test-taker," by N. Dickenson-Hazard, (1989) *Pediatric Nursing, 15,* p. 303. Adapted from: *Nurse's guide to successful test-taking* by M. B. Sides and N. B. Cailles, 1989. Philadelphia: J. B. Lippincott, Co., pp 59–70, 199–203. Copyright 1989 by A. J. Jannetti, Inc. Reprinted by permission.

As related to testing situations, the thought process from memory to analysis occurs quite quickly. Some examination items are designed to test memory and comprehension while others test application and analysis. An example of a memory question is as follows:

Non insulin dependent diabetes results from dysfunction of the:

- a) liver
- b) *pancreas*
- c) adrenal glands
- d) kidneys
- e) pituitary gland

To answer this question correctly, the individual has to retrieve a memorized fact.

Understanding the fact, knowing why it is important or analyzing what should be done in this situation is not needed. An example of a question which tests comprehension is as follows:

> You are taking a history on a 47 year-old white female during a routine health assessment visit. She reports that in the past month she has experienced increased thirst and needs to urinate frequently. She reports recurrent episodes of vaginitis and is concerned about an abrasion on her leg which will not heal. You note that her blood pressure is recorded at 150/90 and that she is overweight. You would most likely suspect which of the following?
>
> a) Urinary tract infection
> b) Hyperthyroidism
> c) Type I diabetes mellitus
> d) Essential hypertension
> e) *Type II diabetes mellitus*

To answer this question correctly, an individual must retrieve facts about the physiology of diabetes mellitus in order to understand and differentiate the presenting symptoms.

In answering an examination question that requires a higher level of thought, an individual must be able to recall a fact, understand that fact in the context of the question, and apply this understanding to determine why one answer is correct, after analyzing possible answer choices as they relate to the situation (Sides & Korchek, 1994). An example of an application analysis question is as follows:

> A 48 year-old diabetic woman wants to enroll in a low-impact aerobics class. Her diabetes is being well managed with twice daily insulin injections. Your best advice is to:
>
> a) Increase daily doses of insulin
> b) *Have an extra snack before exercise class*
> c) Administer a dose of regular insulin after exercise is completed
> d) Tell her participating in the class is not advisable

To answer this question correctly, the individual must recall physiologic facts of insulin dependent diabetes, understand what is happening in this situation, consider each option and how it applies to the patient's condition and analyze why each advice option works or doesn't work for this patient. Application/analysis questions require the examinee to use logical rationale, based on a well defined principle or fact. Problem solving ability becomes important as the examinee must think through each question option, determining its relevance and importance to the situation in the question.

Building your thinking skills: Effective memorization is the cornerstone to learning and building thinking skills (Olney, 1989). We have all experienced "memory power outages" at some time, due in part to trying to memorize too much, too fast, too ineffectively. Developing skills to improve memorization is important to increasing the effectiveness of your thinking and subsequent test performance.

Technique #1: Quantity is NOT quality, so concentrate on learning important content. For example, it is important to know the various pharmacologic agents appropriate for the management of sexually transmitted diseases (STDs), not the specific dosages for each medication.

Technique #2: Memory from repetition, or saying something over and over again to remember it, usually fades. Developing memory skills which trigger retrieval of needed facts is more useful. Such skills are as follows:

Acronyms: These are mental crutches which facilitate recall. Some are already established such as PERRL (pupils equal, round, reactive to light), CHF for (congestive heart failure), or TIA for (transient ischemic attack). Developing your own acronyms can be particularly useful since they are your own word association arrangements in a singular word. Nonsense words or funny, unusual ones are often more useful since they attract your attention.

Acrostics: This mental tool arranges words into catchy phrases. The first letter of each word stands for something which is recalled as the phrase is said. Your own acrostics are most valuable in triggering recall of learned information since they are your individual situation associations. An example of an acrostic is as follows:

Sam **E**xercises **B**y **W**eight-lifting and **R**unning stands for the aspects of non-drug therapy/management for hypertension: **S**alt restriction, **E**xercise, **B**iofeedback, **W**eight reduction, and **R**elaxation techniques.

ABCs: This technique facilitates information retrieval by using the alphabet as a crutch. Each letter stands for a symptom, which when put together creates a picture of the clinical presentation of the disease. For example, the characteristics of peptic ulcer disease using the ABC technique is as follows:

a) Antacids relieve pain
b) Burning epigastric pain
c) Cycle of pain two hours after eating
d) Discomfort awakens at night
e) Experiences weight loss
f) Food sometimes aggravates pain

Imaging: This technique can be used in two ways. The first is to develop a nickname for a clinical problem which when said produces a mental picture. For example, "PID shuffle" might be used to visualize a woman with severe lower abdominal pain caused by acute pelvic inflammatory disease, making it necessary for her to walk in a stooped position, sliding her feet in a "shuffling" fashion to avoid "jostling" her lower body. A second form of imaging is to visualize a specific patient while you are trying to understand or solve a clinical problem when studying or answering a question. For example, imagine a young woman who is experiencing an acute asthma attack. You are trying to analyze the situation and place her in a position which maximizes respiratory effort. In your mind you visualize her in various positions of sidelying, angular and forward, imaging what will happen to the woman and her respiratory effort in each position.

Rhymes, music & links: The absurd is easier to remember than the most common. Rhymes, music or links can add absurdity and humor to learning and remembering (Olney, 1989). These retrieval tools are developed by the individual for specific content. For example, making up a rhyme about diabetes may be helpful in remembering the predominant female incidence, origin of disease, primary symptoms and management as illustrated by:

> There once was a woman
>   whose beta cells failed
> She grew quite thirsty
>   and her glucose levels sailed
> Her lack of insulin caused her to
>   increase her intake
> And her increased urinary output
>   was certainly not fake
> So she learned to watch her diet
>   and administer injections
> That kept her healthy, growing
>   and free of complications.

Setting content to music is sometimes useful to remembering. Melodies which are repetitious jog the memory by the ups and downs of the notes and the rhythm of the music.

Links connect key words from the content by using them in a story. An example given by Olney (1989) for remembering the parts of an eye is IRIS watched a PUPIL through the LENS of a RED TIN telescope while eating CORN-EA on the cob.

Additional memory aids may also include the use of color or drawing for improving recall. Use different colored pens or paper to accentuate the material being learned. For example, highlight or make notes in blue for content about respiratory problems and in red for cardiovascular content. Drawing assists with visualizing content as well. This is particularly helpful for remembering the pathophysiology of the specific health problem.

The important thing to remember about remembering is to use good recall techniques.

Technique #3: Improving higher level thinking skills involves exercising the application and analysis of memorized facts. Small group review is particularly useful for enhancing these high level skills. Small group interaction allows verbalization of thought processes and receipt of input about content and thought process from others (Sides & Korchek, 1994). Individuals not only hear how they think, but how others think as well. This interaction allows individuals to identify flaws in their thought process as well as to strengthen their positive points.

Taking practice tests are also helpful in developing application/analysis thinking skills. Practice tests permit the individual to analyze thinking patterns as well as the cause and effect relationships between the question and its options. The problem solving skills needed to answer application/analysis questions are tested, giving the individual more experience through practice (Dickenson-Hazard, 1990).

STRATEGY #3 Know The Content

Your ability to study is directly influenced by organization and concentration (Dickenson-Hazard, 1990). If effort is spent on both of these aspects of exam preparation, examination success can be increased.

Preparation for studying: Getting organized. Study habits are developed early in our education experiences. Some of our habits enhance learning while others do not. To increase study effectiveness, organization of study materials and time is essential.

Organization decreases frustration, allows for easy resumption of study and increases concentrated study time.

Technique #1: Create your own study space. Select a study area that is yours alone, free from distractions, comfortable and well lighted. The ventilation and room temperature should be comfortable since a cold room makes it difficult to concentrate and a warm room may make you sleepy (Burkle & Marshak, 1989). All study materials should be left in a specific study space. The basic premise of a study space is that it facilitates a mind set that you are there to study. When study is interrupted, it is best to leave study materials just as they are. Don't close books or put away notes as they will have to be relocated, wasting valuable time, when study is resumed.

Technique #2: Define and organize the content. Secure an outline or the content parameters which are to be examined from the examining body. If outline is sketchy, develop a more detailed one for yourself using the recommended text as a guideline. Next, identify available study resources: class notes, old exams, handouts, textbooks, review courses, or study groups. For national standardized exams, such as initial licensing or certification, it is best to identify one or two study resources which cover the content being tested and stick to them. Attempting to review all available resources is not only mind boggling, but increases anxiety and frustration as well. Make your selections and stay with them.

Technique #3: Conduct a content assessment. Using a simple rating scale of:

   1 = requires no review
   2 = requires minimal review
   3 = requires intensive review
   4 = start from the beginning

Read through the content outline and rate each content area (Dickenson-Hazard, 1990). Table 2 provides a sample exam content assessment. Be honest with your assessment. It is far better to recognize your content weaknesses when you can study and remedy them, rather than wishing during the exam that you had studied more. Likewise with content strengths: If you know the material, don't waste time studying it.

Technique #4: Develop a study plan. Coordinate the content which needs to be studied with the time available (Sides & Korchek, 1994). Prioritize your study needs, starting with weak areas first. Allow for a general review at the end of the study plan. Finally, establish an overall goal for yourself; something that will motivate you when brought to mind.

Table 3 illustrates a study plan developed on the basis of the exam content assessment in Table 2. Conducting an assessment and developing a study plan should require no more than 50 minutes. It is a wise investment of time with potential payoffs of reduced study stress and exam success.

Technique #5: Begin now and use your time wisely. The smart test taker begins the study process early (Olney, 1989). Sit down, conduct the content assessment and develop a study plan as soon as you know about the exam. DON'T PROCRASTINATE!

Getting Down To Business—The Actual Studying: There is no better way to prepare for an examination than individual study (Dickenson-Hazard, 1989). The responsibility to achieve the goal you set for this exam lies with you alone. The means you employ to achieve this goal do vary and should begin with identifying your peak study times and using techniques to maximize them.

Table 2

Sample Content Assessment

Exam Content: Non-Gyn Medical Problems	
Category: Provided by Examining Body	*Rating: Provided by Examinee*

I. Respiratory
    A. Allergies
        1. Etiology 1
        2. Pathophysiology 2
        3. Symptomatology 2
        4. Differential Diagnosis 2
        5. Diagnostic Tests 3
        6. Management/Treatment 2

    B. Pneumonia
        1. Etiology 2
        2. Pathophysiology 2
        3. Symptomatology 1
        4. Differential Diagnosis 2
        5. Diagnostic Tests 2
        6. Management/Treatment 2

    C. Asthma
        1. Etiology 1
        2. Pathophysiology 2
        3. Symptomatology 2
        4. Differential Diagnosis 2
        5. Diagnostic Tests 2
        6. Management/Treatment 2

Table 3

Sample Study Plan
Goal: Master content on Non-Gyn Medical Problems.
Time Available for Content: 4 days.

Objective	Activity	Date Accomplished
Master content on allergies	Read Chapter 11. Take notes on chapter content according to outline.	August 5,1 hour
	Review class notes combined with chapter notes.	August 5, 1 hour
	Review sample test questions.	August 5, 1 hour
Know content on pneumonia	Read Chapter 12. Take notes on chapter content according to outline.	August 6, 1 hour
	Review class notes combined with chapter notes.	August 6, 1 hour
	Review sample test questions.	August 6, 30 minutes
Know content on asthma	Read Chapter 13. Take notes on chapter content according to outline.	August 7, 1 hour
	Review class notes combined with chapter notes.	August 7, 1 hour
	Review sample test questions	August 7, 30 minutes
Demonstrate understanding of all material	Review with another person.	August 8, 1 hour
	Review all notes.	August 8, 1 hour
	Take sample test.	August 8, 30 minutes

Technique #1:   Study in short bursts. Each of us have our own biologic clock which dictates when we are at our peak during the day. If you are a morning person, you are generally active and alert early in the day, slowing down and becoming drowsy by evening. If you are an evening person, you don't completely wake up until late morning and hit your peak in the afternoon and evening. Each person generally has several peaks during the day. It is best to study during those times when your alertness is at its peak (Dickenson-Hazard, 1990).

During our concentration peaks, there are mini peaks, or bursts of alertness (Olney, 1989). These alertness (''mini'') peaks occur during a concentration peak because levels of concentration are at their highest during the first part and last part of a study period. These bursts can vary from ten minutes to one hour depending on the extent of concentration. If studying is sustained for one hour there are only two mini peaks; one at the beginning and one at the end. There are eight mini peaks if that same hour is divided into four, 10-minute intervals. Hence it is more helpful to study in short bursts (Olney, 1989). More can be learned in less time.

Technique #2:   Cramming can be useful. Since concentration ability is highly variable, some individuals can sustain their mini peaks for 15, 20 or even 30 minutes at a time. Pushing your concentration beyond its peak is fruitless and verges on cramming, which in general is a poor study technique. There are, however, times when cramming, a short term memory tool, is useful. Short term memory generally is at its best in the morning. A quick review or cram of content in the morning can be useful the day of the exam (Olney, 1989). Most studying, however, is best accomplished in the afternoon or evening when long term memory functions at its peak.

Technique #3: Give your brain breaks. Regular times during study to rest and absorb the content is needed by the brain. The best approach to breaks is to plan them and give yourself a conscious break (Dickenson-Hazard, 1990). This approach eliminates the "day dreaming" or "wandering thought" approach to breaks that many of us use. It is better to get up, leave the study area and do something non-study related for longer breaks. For shorter breaks of five minutes or so, leave your desk, gaze out the window or do some stretching exercises. When your brain says to give it a rest, accommodate it! You'll learn more in less stress free time.

Technique #4: Study the correct content. It is easy for all of us to become bogged down in the detail of the content we are studying. However, it is best to focus on the major concepts or the "state of the art" content. Leave the details, the suppositions and the experience at the door of your study area. Concentrate on the major textbook facts and concepts which revolve around the subject matter being tested.

Technique #5: Fit your studying to the test type. The best way to prepare for an objective test is to study facts, particularly anything printed in italics. Memory enhancing techniques are particularly useful when preparing for an objective test. If preparing for an essay test, study generalities, examples and concepts. Application techniques are helpful when studying for this type of an exam (Burkle & Marshak, 1989).

Technique #6: Use your study plan wisely. Your study plan is meant to be a guide, not a rigid schedule. You should take your time with studying. Don't rush through the content just to remain on schedule. Occasionally study plans need revision. If you take more or less time than planned, readjust the plan for the time gained or lost. The plan can guide you, but you must go at your own pace.

Technique #7: Actively study. Being an active participant in study rather than trying to absorb the printed word is also helpful. Ways to be active include: taking notes on the content as you study; constructing questions and answering them; taking practice tests and discussing the content with yourself. Also, using your individual study quirks is encouraged. Some people stand, others walk around and some play background music. Whatever helps you to concentrate and study better, you should use.

Technique #8: Use study aids. While there is no substitute for individual studying, several resources, if available, are useful in facilitating learning. Review courses are an excellent means for organizing or summarizing your individual study. They generally provide the content parameters and the major concepts of the content which you need to know. Review courses also provide an opportunity to clarify not-well-understood content, as well as to review known material (Dickenson-Hazard, 1990). Study guides are useful for organizing study. They provide detail on the content which is important to the exam. Study groups are an excellent resource for summarizing and refining content. They provide an opportunity for thinking through your knowledge base, with the advantage of hearing another person's point of view. Each of these study aids increases understanding of content and when used correctly, increases effectiveness of knowledge application.

Technique #9: Know when to quit. It is best to stop studying when your concentration ebbs. It is unproductive and frustrating to force yourself to study. It is far better to rest or unwind, then resume at a later point in the day. Avoid studying outside your A.M. or P.M. concentration peaks and focus your study energy on your right time of day or evening.

STRATEGY #4 Become Test-wise

Most nursing examinations are composed of multiple choice questions (MCQs). This type of question requires the examinee to select the best response(s) for a specific circumstance or condition. Successful test taking is dependent not only on content knowledge but on test taking skill as well. If you are unable to impart your knowledge through the vehicle used for its conveyance, i.e., the MCQ, your test taking success is in jeopardy.

Technique #1: Recognize the purpose of a test question. Most test questions are developed to examine knowledge at two separate levels: memory (or recall) and comprehension (or application). A memory question requires the examinee to recall facts from their knowledge base while an application question requires the examinee to use and apply the knowledge (ABP, 1989). Memory questions test recall while application questions test synthesis and problem-solving skills. When taking a test, you need to be aware when you are being asked to recall a fact, and when you are being asked to use that fact.

Technique #2: Recognize the components of a test question. Multiple choice questions may include the basic components of a background statement, a stem and a list of options. The background statement presents information which facilitates the examinee in answering the question. The stem asks or states the intent of the question. The options are 3 to 5 possible responses to the question. The correct option is called the keyed response and all other options are called distractors (ABP, 1989). Knowing the components of a test question helps you sift through the information presented and focus on the question's intent (see Table 4).

Technique #3: Identify the key word(s) in a test question. Key words are generally included in the stem of a test question, whereas key concepts or conditions appear in the background statement. You should pay particular attention to the key words in the stem and their impact on the intent of the question (See Table 5).

Technique #4: Recognize the item types. Basically two styles of MCQs are used for examinations. One requires the examinee to select the one best answer; the other requires selection of multiple correct answers. Among the one best answer styles there are three types. The A type requires the selection of the best response among those offered. The B type requires the examinee to match the options with the appropriate statement. C type items require the examinee to compare or contrast two related conditions. The X type asks the examinee to respond either true or false to each option (ABP, 1989). Table 6 illustrates these item types.

Technique #5: Read the directions to the questions carefully. Since an examination may have several types of questions, it is imperative to read the directions carefully. If different item types are used on an exam, they are generally grouped together by type and marked clearly with directions. Be on the lookout for changing item types and be sure you understand how you are to answer before you begin reading the question.

Table 4

Anatomy Of A Test Question

Background Statement:	A 32 year-old black female is being seen for a complaint of sores in the vaginal area. She has been experiencing a low-grade fever, headache and malaise over the past five days. Physical examination reveals inguinal lymphadenopathy, vaginal erythema and multiple labial and vaginal vesicular lesions.
Stem:	Which of the following causative organisms would you most likely suspect?
Options:	(A) *Herpes simplex virus 2* (B) Condylomata lata (C) Herpes simplex virus 1 (D) Treponema pallidum

Table 5

Test Question Key Words And Phrases

First	Priority	True Statements
Best	Advice	Correct Statements
Most	Approach	Contributing to
Initial	Consideration	Of the following
Important	Management	Which of the following
Major	Expectation	Each of the following
Common	Intervention	
Least	Assessment	
Except	Contraindication	
Not	Evaluation	
Greatest	Counseling	
Earliest	Facilitative	
Useful	Indicative	
Leading	Suggestive	
Significant	Appropriate	
Immediate	Accurately	
Helpful	Likely	
Closely	Characteristics	

From "Anatomy of a test question" by N. Dickenson-Hazard, 1989, *Pediatric Nursing 15*, p. 395. Copyright 1989 by A. J. Jannetti, Inc. Reprinted by permission.

Technique #6: Apply the basic rules of test taking. Examination candidates can avert many problems associated with test taking if they give thought to the mechanics of sitting down, reading the question and noting their answers. Timing yourself to avoid spending too much time on a question, returning to difficult questions, and not changing your answers are all techniques that can improve performance. Table 7 provides helpful hints for the basic rules of test-taking. Review these and apply them to the testing situation.

Technique #7: Practice, practice, practice. Taking practice tests can improve performance. While they can assist in evaluation of your knowledge, their primary benefit is to assist you with test taking skills. You should use them to evaluate your thinking process, your ability to read, understand and interpret questions, and your skills in completing the mechanics of the test.

Technique #8: Be prepared for exam day. It is important to familiarize yourself with the test site, the building, the parking and travel route prior to the exam day. If you must travel, arrive early to allow time for this familiarization. It is helpful to make a list of things you need on the exam day: pencils, admission card, watch and a few pieces of hard candy as a quick energy source. On exam day allow yourself plenty of time to arrive at the site. Wear comfortable clothes and have a good breakfast that morning. The night before the exam, go to bed at a reasonable hour;

avoid last minute cramming; and avoid excessive drinking or eating (Sides & Korchek, 1994). The idea is to arrive on time at the test site, prepared and as rested as possible.

TABLE 6

Item Type Examples

A TYPE

Directions for One Best Choice Items: This item-type requires that you indicate the one best answer from the lettered alternatives offered for each item. After you have decided on the one BEST answer, completely blacken the corresponding lettered circle on the answer sheet.

  #1 A 46 year-old white female is being seen in follow-up for the treatment of migraine headaches. Your management plan would most appropriately include counseling on which of the following preventive techniques?
   a. Limiting intake of high calcium foods
   b. Encouraging additional sleep hours
   c. *Learning biofeedback techniques*
   d. Massaging posterior head and neck areas regularly
   e. Developing a rigorous exercise routine

B TYPE

Directions: Each group of questions below consists of five lettered headings followed by a list of numbered words or statements. For each numbered word or statement, select the one lettered heading that is most closely associated with it and fill in the circle beneath the corresponding letter on the answer sheet. Each lettered heading may be selected once, more than once, or not at all.

  #2-#4
  Medication Types::
   a. Anti-fungal
   b. Anti-protozoan
   c. Antiseptic
   d. Anti-viral
  Most useful for treatment of:
   2. Trichomoniasis (B)
   3. Candidiasis (A)
   4. Bacterial vaginosis (B)

C TYPE

Directions: Each set of lettered headings below is followed by a list of numbered words or phrases. For each numbered word or phrase fill in the circle on the answer sheet under A if the item is associated with (A) only, B if the item is associated with (B) only, C if the item is associated with both (A) and (B), D if the item is associated with neither (A) nor (B).
   (A) Diabetic acidosis
   (B) Insulin shock
   (C) Both
   (D) Neither

#5 — Elevated bicarbonate level in serum (D)
#6 — The duration of the condition before proper treatment is begun may influence the prognosis (C)
#7 — Deep breathing (A)
#8 — Coma (C)
#9 — Moist skin (B)

X TYPE

Directions: Each of the questions or incomplete statements below is followed by five suggested answers or completions. For EACH lettered alternative completely blacken one lettered circle in either column T or F on the answer sheet.
   Which of the following tests are useful for differentiating anemia associated with a chronic disease from iron deficiency anemia?
   a. Serum iron levels (F)
   b. Bone marrow examination (T)
   c. Reticulocyte count (F)
   d. Serum transferrin level (F)
   e. Serum ferritin level (T)

Adapted from ''Anatomy of a test question.'' by N. Dickenson-Hazard, 1989, *Pediatric Nursing 15*, p. 396. Copyright 1989 by A. J. Jannetti, Inc. Adapted by permission.

TABLE 7

Basic Rules For Test Taking

Basic Rule	Helpful Hints
Use time wisely and effectively	Allow no more than 1 minute per question —If you can't answer question, make an intelligent guess

Know the parts of a question
    Background statement: Informational
    scenario
    Stem: Specific question or intent
    statement
	Select the option that best completes question or solves the problem
	Relate options to question and balance against each other
	Consider all options

Read question carefully	Understand stem first, then look for answer Underline key words in background information and stem (i.e., first, best, initial, early, most, appropriate, except, least, not)
Identify intent of item based on information given	Don't assume any information not given Don't read in or add any information not given Actively reason through question
Answer difficult questions by eliminating obviously incorrect options first	Select the best of the viable, available options using logical thought Reread stem; select strongest option Skip difficult questions and return to them later or make an educated guess
Select responses guided by principles of communication	Choose therapeutic, respectful, communication enhancing options Avoid inappropriate, punitive responses
Know the principles of nursing practice	Select options that relate to common need or the population in general Select options that are correct without exception Select options which reflect nursing judgement
Know and use test-taking principles	Avoid changing answers without good reason Attempt every question Don't rely on flaws in test construction Be systematic and use problem-solving techniques in answering questions

From "Making the grade as a test-taker" by N. Dickenson-Hazard, 1989. *Pediatric Nursing 15*, p. 304. Adapted from *How to take tests.* (pp 15-57) by J. Millman and W. Paul, 1969, New York: McGraw-Hill Co. and from *Nurses's guide to successful test taking.* (pp 43-53) by M. B. Sides and N. B. Cailles, 1989, Philadelphia: J. B. Lippincott Co. Copyright 1989 A. J. Jannetti, Inc. Reprinted and adapted by permission.

STRATEGY #5 Psych Yourself Up: Taking tests is stressful

While a little stress can be productive, too much can incapacitate you in your studying and test taking (Divine & Kylen, 1979). Your attitude and approach to test taking and studying can influence your outcomes. Psyching yourself up can have a positive effect and make examinations a non-anxiety laden experience (Dickenson-Hazard, 1990). The following techniques are based on the principles of successful test taking as presented by Sides & Cailles (1989). Incorporation of these techniques can improve response and performance in examination situations.

Technique #1: Adopt an "I can" attitude. Believing you can succeed is the key to success. Self belief inspires and gives you the power to achieve your goals. Without a success attitude, the road to your goal is much harder. We all stand an equal chance of success in this world. It is those who believe they can who achieve it. This "I can" attitude must permeate all your efforts in test taking from studying to improving your skills, to actually writing the test.

Technique #2: Take control. By identifying your goal, deciding how to accomplish it and developing a plan for achieving it, you take control. Do not leave your success or failure to chance; control it through action and attitude.

Technique #3: Think positively. Examinations are generally based on a standard which is the same for all individuals. Everyone can potentially pass. Performance is influenced not only by knowledge and skill but attitude as well. Those individuals who regard an exam as an opportunity or challenge will be more successful.

Technique #4: Project a positive self-fulfilling prophecy. While preparing for an examination, project thoughts of the positive outcomes you will experience when you succeed. Self-talk is self-fulfilling. Expect success, not failure, of yourself.

Technique #5: Feel good about yourself. Without feeling a sense of positive self worth, passing an examination is difficult. Recognize your professional contributions and give yourself credit for your accomplishments. Think "I will pass," not "I suppose I can."

Technique #6: Know yourself. Focus exam preparation and test taking on your strengths. Try to alter your weaknesses instead of becoming hung up on them. If you tend to overanalyze, study and read test questions at face value. If you're a speed demon when taking a test, slow down and read more carefully.

Technique #7: Failure is a possibility. We all have failed at something at some point in our lives. Rather than dwelling on the failure, making excuses and believing you'll fail again, recognize your mistakes and remedy them. Failure is a time to begin again; use it as a motivator to do better. It is not the end of the world unless you allow it to be. It is best to deal with the failure and move on, otherwise it interferes with your success.

Technique #8: Persevere, persevere, persevere! Endurance must underlie all your efforts. Call forth those reserve energies when you've had all you think you can take. Rely upon yourself and your support systems to help you maintain a sense of direction and keep your goal in the forefront.

Technique #9: Motivation is muscle. Most individuals are motivated by fear or desire. The fear in an exam situation may be one of failure, the unknown or discovery of imperfection. Put your fear into perspective; realize you are not the only one with fear and that all have an equal opportunity for success. Develop strategies to reduce fear and use fear to your advantage by improving the imperfections. Desire is a powerful motivator and you should keep the rewards of your desire foremost in your mind. Whatever motivates you, use it to make you successful. Reward yourself during your exam preparation and once the exam has been completed. You alone hold the key to success; use what you have wisely.

This chapter has provided concepts, strategies and techniques for improving study and test taking skills. Your first task in improvement is to know yourself: how you study and how you take a test. You should use your strengths and remedy the weaknesses. Next you need to develop your thinking skills. Work on techniques to improve memory and reasoning. Now you need to organize your study and concentrate on using these new and used skills to be successful. Create a study space, develop a plan of action, then implement that plan during your periods of peak concentration. Before taking the exam be sure you understand the components of a test question, can identify key words and phrases and have practiced. Apply the test taking rules during the exam process. Finally, believe in yourself, your knowledge and your talent. Believing you can accomplish your goal facilitates the fact that you will.

BIBLIOGRAPHY

American Board of Pediatrics. (1989). *Developing questions and critiques.* Unpublished material.

Burke, M.M., & Walsh, M.B. (1992). *Gerontologic nursing.* St. Louis: Mosby Year Book.

Burkle, C.A., & Marshak, D. (1989). *Study program: Level 1.* Reston, VA: National Association of Secondary School Principals.

Dickenson-Hazard, N. (1989). Making the grade as a test taker. *Pediatric Nursing, 15,* 302–304.

Dickenson-Hazard, N. (1989). Anatomy of a test question. *Pediatric Nursing, 15,* 395–399.

Dickenson-Hazard, N. (1990). The psychology of successful test taking. *Pediatric Nursing, 16,* 66–67.

Dickenson-Hazard, N. (1990). Study smart. *Pediatric Nursing, 16,* 314–316.

Dickenson-Hazard, N. (1990). Study effectiveness: Are you 10 a.m. or p.m. scholar? *Pediatric Nursing,* 16, 419–420.

Dickenson-Hazard, N. (1990). Develop your thinking skills for improved test taking. *Pediatric Nursing,* 16, 480–481.

Divine, J.H., & Kylen, D.W. (1979). *How to beat test anxiety.* New York: Barrons Educational Series, Inc.

Goroll, A., May, L., & Mulley, A. (Eds.). (1988). *Primary care medicine* (2nd ed.). Philadelphia: J.B. Lippincott.

Millman, J., & Pauk, W. (1969). *How to take tests.* New York: McGraw-Hill Book Co.

Millonig, V.L. (Ed.). (1991). *The adult nurse practitioner certification review guide.* Potomac, MD: Health Leadership Associates.

Olney, C.W. (1989). *Where there's a will, there's an A.* New Jersey: Chesterbrook Educational Publishers.

Sides, M., & Cailles, N.B. (1989). *Nurse's guide to successful test taking.* Philadelphia: J.B. Lippincott Co.

Sides, M., & Korchek, N. (1994). *Nurse's guide to successful test taking* (2nd ed.). Philadelphia: J.B. Lippincott.

General Assessment

Jacki S. Witt

Health History

- Definition—the purpose of the health history is to establish rapport and collect information about the client's overall functioning, including current health status, health practices, present and past health problems, family history, mental and psychosocial status and sexual/reproductive history; goals of the health history include

  1. Collecting information regarding variables which affect health status

  2. Assessing how client's health concern(s) affect her and her support system, and identifying therapeutic and educational needs

  3. Collecting subjective information to help the nurse practitioner (NP) arrive at correct diagnoses and define therapeutic goals

- Components and Risk Factors

  1. Present illness—a summary of the client's current major health concerns

     a. If client is well, the NP describes the client's usual health and summarizes health maintenance needs and interventions

     b. If an alteration is present, a detailed, chronologic description of the current problem is collected (include client's responses to symptoms and perceptions about the problem); a systematic approach, (e.g., *OLDCART*), is helpful and ensures completeness

        (1) **O**nset

        (2) **L**ocation

        (3) **D**uration

        (4) **C**haracter

        (5) **A**ggravating/alleviating factors

        (6) **R**adiation, and **T**reatment/response

  2. Review of Systems—comprehensive review of body regions, organ systems and their functions

     a. Includes data about client's past and recent physical, social and psychological health

     b. Provides indications about client's strengths and weaknesses

    c. In acute or episodic examinations, only systems related to reason for visit or present illness are reviewed

3. Family—inquiries about diseases are made because of their genetic, familial or environmental association; a genogram, or family tree diagram, helps record information concisely

    a. Age and health, or age and cause of death of family members, with emphasis on first degree relatives; information gathered on the following conditions—alcoholism, allergies, anemia, arteriosclerosis, arthritis, cancer, coronary artery disease, diabetes, epilepsy, hypertension, kidney disease, obesity, stroke, tuberculosis, congenital anomalies, genetic diseases, mental illness

    b. Information regarding roommates, sexual partners and significant others may be relevant

4. Psychosocial/Cultural/Spiritual

    a. Nationality/ethnicity—some ethnic/cultural groups are genetically predisposed to specific diseases

        (1) Chinese—predisposed to adult lactose intolerance

        (2) African Americans—at increased risk for sickle cell anemia and hypertension

        (3) Native Americans—at increased risk for alcoholism, depression, and obesity

        (4) Hispanics—at increased risk for diabetes

        (5) Mediterraneans—at increased risk for thalassemia

    b. Religion

        (1) Beliefs

        (2) Life impact

    c. Psychosocial

        (1) Key life events

        (2) Social groups

        (3) Support systems

        (4) Personal and/or family crises coping patterns

5. Nutritional/Exercise/Lifestyle

     a. Nutrition

        (1) Diet recall for the previous 24-hour period, with comparison to food pyramid daily recommendations

        (2) Eating disorder history

     b. Exercise habits

     c. Life habits

        (1) Over the counter (OTC) medication

        (2) Alcohol

        (3) Smoking/nicotine

        (4) Drugs

        (5) Auto safety belts

     d. Hobbies/recreation

6. Medical

     a. Previous major illnesses and chronic illnesses, including psychiatric illnesses

     b. Accidents and injuries

     c. Hospitalizations, and complications

7. Surgical

     a. All procedures, including names of health care providers, hospitals or outpatient facilities, diagnoses, dates and complications

     b. Inpatient

     c. Outpatient

8. Obstetrical—all pregnancies, regardless of outcome, with dates (premature deliveries, abortions, full-term deliveries and living children)

     a. Gravidity—all pregnancies

     b. Parity—number of pregnancies reaching viability

        (1) Length of pregnancy

        (2) Type of delivery (i.e., spontaneous vaginal, Cesarean section and type of scar)

        (3) Weight and sex of infant

> (4) Length of labor
>
> (5) Complications during prenatal, intrapartum or postpartum periods
>
> (6) Infant complications

c. Stillbirths

> (1) Length of gestation
>
> (2) Cause (if known)
>
> (3) Feelings

d. Miscarriages (spontaneous abortions)

> (1) Length of gestation
>
> (2) Feelings

e. Elective abortions

> (1) Length of gestation
>
> (2) Feelings, comfort level with decision

f. Infertility evaluation or treatment

9. Menstrual

a. Age at menarche

b. Regularity, frequency and duration of menses

c. Amount of bleeding

d. Intermenstrual or postcoital bleeding

e. Dysmenorrhea (primary or secondary)

f. Premenstrual symptoms

g. Last menstrual period (date of onset and characteristics)

h. Use of medications to induce menses

i. Age at menopause, menopausal symptoms, postmenopausal bleeding

10. Sexual

a. Age at first intercourse; consensual?

b. Sexual experience in past

    c. Current sexual relationship—number of partners; interest; function; satisfaction; frequency of intercourse; sexual difficulties, including dyspareunia and inorgasmia

    d. STD/HIV risk

        (1) Number of lifetime partners

        (2) Sex for drugs or money

        (3) Sex with IV drug user

        (4) Sex with a man who has sex with men

        (5) Sex without condom

        (6) Anal or oral unprotected sex

        (7) Past sexually transmitted disease (STD) exposure—type; treatment

11. Reproductive/genital

    a. Current symptoms

        (1) Vaginal/vulvar discharge, itching, lesions, sores, blisters

        (2) Last Pap smear—date; results

        (3) Breast self-exam—any changes noted

        (4) Last mammogram—date; results

    b. Feminine hygiene habits

        (1) Pads vs tampons

        (2) Douching—type; frequency; reason

    c. Gynecologic history

        (1) DES exposure (if born before 1971, ask about maternal use during pregnancy)

        (2) Pelvic inflammatory disease (PID)

        (3) STDs

        (4) Endometriosis

        (5) Adnexal masses

        (6) Ovarian cyst

       (7)   Periods of amenorrhea

       (8)   Abnormal Pap smear, treatment, follow-up

       (9)   Infertility treatment

      (10) Hormonal therapy or hormone replacement therapy (HRT)

12. Medications

   a. Current and those used in past 6 weeks; if multiple medications are used, a survey and chronologic record of the past 24-hour use may be helpful

      (1)   Prescription drugs

      (2)   Non-prescription drugs

      (3)   Home remedies (homeopathic, herbal, "natural")

   b. Vitamin/mineral supplements

   c. Medicines borrowed from family and friends

   d. Past reactions to specific medications

   e. Past medications used for over 2 weeks

13. Contraceptive Use

   a. Current method—duration of use, success and satisfaction with use

   b. Previous methods—dates and duration of use, side effects/complications, reason(s) for discontinuation

   c. Knowledge of methods available

14. Immunizations and Allergies

   a. History of childhood illnesses (i.e., measles, mumps, chickenpox, rheumatic fever, scarlet fever)

   b. Dates and types of immunizations—tetanus (should receive every 10 years); pertussis; diphtheria (Td combination advised); polio; measles; rubella; mumps; influenza; hepatitis B; influenza; pneumonia; TB testing

   c. Overseas travel immunizations

   d. Unusual reaction, with detailed description of reaction and treatment/resolution—drugs, food, contact agents, animals

15. Violence (especially domestic violence)

   a. History of ever being emotionally or physically abused—by whom, timeframe, counseling/treatment

   b. History of physical abuse in past year—by whom, number of times, health care sought, police/legal action, counseling/treatment

   c. History of nonconsensual sexual activities—by whom, timeframe, health care sought, police/legal action, counseling/treatment

   d. Is the client now afraid of her partner or anyone named in history above?

   e. Knowledge of resources

- Risk Factor Identification—to assess client's risk status for a potential or established problem, the NP must be aware of the prevalence (existing level of disease) and incidence (rate of new disease) not only in the general population, but also in the developmental, social, cultural and geographic subgroup(s) to which the client belongs

Physical Examination

- Techniques

   1. Inspection—systematic visual examination of the body; ongoing process to observe first for general characteristics and then for specific ones

   2. Palpation—examination of tissues and organs using the sense of touch; used to assess for tenderness and warmth (light palpation) and to determine position, size, shape, consistency and mobility of organs or masses (deep palpation)

   3. Percussion—examination by tapping lightly but briskly on the body surface to produce vibrations to evaluate the density of underlying tissue and/or to elicit tenderness; sounds produced reflect size, shape, position and density of organs or tissues; heard and felt by the examiner

      a. Resonance—long, low, hollow sound heard over an intercostal space above healthy lung tissue

    b. Tympany—loud, low-pitched, drum-like sound heard over gas-filled bowel or gastric air bubble

    c. Dullness—soft, high-pitched, thudding sound heard over solid organs, e.g., liver, heart

  4. Auscultation—using a stethoscope to listen to body sounds, particularly those produced by the heart, lungs, blood vessels, stomach, and intestines

- Screening examination

  1. General appearance—concise general impression statement; purpose is to present an immediate general image of the client

    a. Mental status

    b. Body development, proportions

    c. Ambulation, posture, movement, gait

    d. Nutritional state

    e. Apparent sex and race

    f. Chronological versus apparent age

    g. Assistive devices (e.g., glasses, cane, brace)

  2. Head, neck and throat

    a. Ears

      (1) Pinna shape, position, tenderness, lesions

      (2) Mastoid tenderness (may indicate otitis media), tragus tenderness (may indicate external otitis)

      (3) Otoscopic examination

        (a) Canal

        (b) Cerumen, discharge (otorrhea), lesion, foreign body

        (c) Tympanic membrane (TM)

          i) Color (normal is pearly gray)

          ii) Three landmarks—annulus forms outer border and is paler color; malleus angles downward posteriorly from annulus to a point at center of the TM; light reflex—bright cone-shaped reflection of light in lower right aspect of TM

(4) Hearing

(a) Watch tick—gross test for high frequency sounds; patients should be able to hear ticking up to 5 inches (13 cm)

(b) Rinne—compares bone conduction to air conduction

(c) Weber—assesses bone conduction

(5) Preauricular and posterior auricular nodes—not normally palpable in healthy adults; posterior auricular lymphadenopathy may indicate ear infection

b. Eyes

(1) Brows, lashes, lid shape and position

(2) Inflammation, lesion, discharge

(3) Color conjunctiva, sclera (color varies with race, age and systemic liver disease), cornea, pupils

(4) **P**upils **E**qual, **R**ound, **R**eact to **L**ight and **A**ccommodation (PERRLA)

(5) Extraocular movements (EOM), nystagmus

(6) Snellen and confrontational visual fields

(7) Fundoscopic—red reflex, retinal vessels, disc size, shape, margins, color (general background color varies according to individual's skin color/pigmentation), macular area, lens clarity, opacities

c. Nose

(1) Patency of each nostril

(2) Septum, turbinates, mucosal color, moisture, lesions, drainage

(3) Frontal and maxillary sinuses

(a) Inspect external skin surfaces above and lateral to nose for inflammation or edema (congestion or infection)

      (b) Palpate sinuses, noting unusual warmth or tenderness (signs of infection)

  (4) Olfaction

d. Mouth and throat

  (1) Tongue surfaces—normal is moist, pink and slightly rough

  (2) Buccal mucosa—usually pink, but may be bluish-tinted or pigmentation may be patchy in dark-skinned people

  (3) Oropharynx

      (a) Uvula

      (b) Tonsils

           i) Unilateral or bilateral enlargement

           ii) Color should be same as pharyngeal mucosa

           iii) Grade tonsil size on a scale of 0 to +4, with 0 indicating normal and +4 indicating one or both tonsils extending to midline of the oropharynx

  (4) Dentition—note missing, broken or loose teeth

e. Neck and thyroid

  (1) Alignment, symmetry

  (2) Range of motion (ROM) and head movement

  (3) Jugular venous pulsation, distention

  (4) Regional lymph nodes—often nonpalpable; if palpable, should be small ($\leq$ 1 cm), smooth, firm, mobile, nontender, discrete borders

      (a) Submandibular, submental, anterior cervical and occipital

      (b) Posterior cervical nodes and spinal nerve chain

      (c) Preauricular, parotid and mastoid

      (d) Supraclavicular

      (e) Abnormalities

                i)   Inflamed nodes—enlarged, tender, mobile, blurred borders, reddened skin

               ii) Malignant nodes—enlarged, nontender, fixed, hard, nodular, irregular shape, nondiscrete borders

     (5) Thyroid

        (a) Palpate with and without swallowing

        (b) Note size, shape, consistency, tenderness

     (6) Tracheal position (deviation associated with mediastinal tumor)

3. Cardiovascular

   a. Pulse and blood pressure

   b. Precordial thrills, heaves, pulsations, lifts or retraction

   c. Point of apical impulse—formerly called point of maximum impulse (PMI)

   d. Heart sounds

     (1) Auscultate at each site

        (a) Aortic (right 2nd interspace)

        (b) Pulmonic (left 2nd interspace)

        (c) Mitral valve (left 5th interspace, midclavicular line)

        (d) Tricuspid valve (left 5th interspace, sternal border)

     (2) S_1—first heart sound; heard best in mitral and tricuspid sites (apex)

     (3) S_2—second heart sound; heard best in aortic and pulmonic sites (base)

   e. Extra heart sounds (S_3, S_4) may occur with cardiovascular disease

     (1) S_3, heard in early diastole

        (a) High-pitched

        (b) Indicates overdistension of ventricles

        (c)   Common in congestive heart failure

    (2) S_4, heard in late diastole

        (a)   Indicates resistance to ventricular filling

        (b)   Common in recent myocardial infarction (MI) and hypertension

f. Murmurs

    (1) Location—identify by auscultation site where heard loudest

    (2) Timing

        (a)   Systolic murmur—between S_1 and S_2

        (b)   Diastolic murmur—between S_2 and the next S_1

        (c)   Continuous

    (3) Pitch—high, medium or low

    (4) Quality—musical, blowing, harsh, rasping, rumbling, machine-like

    (5) Intensity—use standard grading scale, I-VI

    (6) Murmur may be innocent (nonpathologic) or pathologic

g. Bruit—continuous vibrating, blowing or rumbling sound caused by turbulent blood flow

    (1) Over carotid artery—atherosclerosis

    (2) Over abdominal aorta—aneurysm

h. Snap—very early diastolic sound, immediately after S_2; high-pitched, heard best medial to apex along lower left sternal border; results from stenotic valve (commonly mitral) attempting to open

i. Click—mid to late systole; high-pitched, heard best at apex; caused by abnormal billowing of mitral valve into left atrium; click usually precedes late systolic murmur caused by regurgitation

j. Friction rub—harsh, scratchy, scraping or squeaky sound; usually results from pericarditis

k. Pulses—carotid, brachial, radial, femoral, popliteal, posterior tibial, dorsal pedal

l. Nail/skin color—cyanosis, flushing, pallor

m. Lower extremity hair distribution

n. Lower extremity edema

o. Lower extremity lesions

4. Respiratory

a. Chest contour, dimensions, anteroposterior(AP) diameter, symmetry of movement, retractions, use of accessory muscles

b. Respiratory rate, depth, regularity, quality

c. Lung borders, respiratory excursion

d. Breath sounds—bronchial (tracheal); bronchovesicular; vesicular

e. Adventitious sounds—crackles (rales); rhonchi (rattling or snoring sound); wheezes; stridor

f. Presence of friction rub (rubbing, grating; heard on inspiration and expiration), egophony, bronchophony, whispered pectoriloquy, tactile fremitus, tenderness

5. Abdomen

a. Skin color, temperature, venous pattern, hair distribution, presence of scars

b. Shape, contour, visible aorta pulsations, fluid waves

c. Peristaltic (bowel) sounds (normal: 5–35/min.)

d. Vascular sounds are not normal (renal and aortic bruits, hums, rubs)

e. Percussion—note quality for organ size and abdominal abnormalities

(1) Liver—6-12 cm at midclavicular line

(2) Spleen—between ribs 6 and 10

f. Aorta pulsations, organ borders, organomegaly of liver, kidney, spleen

g. Masses—location, size, contour, consistency, tenderness, mobility

h. Costovertebral angle tenderness (CVAT)

i. Rigidity, guarding, rebound tenderness

j. Femoral pulses (note rate, rhythm, strength, compare side to side)

k. Inguinal lymph nodes

6. Musculoskeletal system

   a. Posture—alignment of extremities and spine, symmetry of body parts

   b. Symmetry of muscle mass, tone, flexibility, strength, presence of fasciculations, tremors

   c. Appearance of bones and joints; tenderness, masses, warmth, crepitus, ROM

   d. Spinal ROM, limitations, and presence of pain with movement

   e. Spinal contour (curvature)—examine with client standing straight and bending forward at waist

     (1) Scoliosis (lateral S curve)

     (2) Kyphosis (humpback)

     (3) Lordosis (swayback)

   f. Scapular position

   g. Feet—bony or soft tissue abnormalities related to shoes, bunions, corns

7. Neurological/mental status

   a. Mental status/cerebral function—orientation, mood/behavior, memory, knowledge/vocabulary, reasoning and calculations

   b. Speech/language

   c. Cranial nerves (CN)

     (1) Olfactory (CN I)—sensory (smell)

     (2) Optic (CN II)—sensory (vision)

(3) Oculomotor (CN III)—motor (extraocular movement, pupil constriction, upper eyelid elevation)

(4) Trochlear (CN IV)—motor (extraocular movement)

(5) Trigeminal (CN V)—sensory and motor (transmits stimuli from face and head; corneal reflex; chewing, biting, and lateral jaw movement)

(6) Abducens (CN VI)—motor (extraocular movements)

(7) Facial (CN VII)—sensory and motor (taste, facial muscle movement)

(8) Acoustic (CN VIII)—sensory (hearing and balance)

(9) Glossopharyngeal (CN IX)—sensory and motor (taste, sensations of throat)

(10) Vagus (CN X)—sensory and motor (sensations of throat, taste, swallowing movements)

(11) Accessory (CN XI)—motor (shoulder movement, head rotation)

(12) Hypoglossal (CN XII)—motor (tongue movement)

d. Cerebellar and motor function—gait, balance, Romberg, rapid alternating movements

e. Involuntary movements, sensory function

f. Deep tendon reflexes (DTRs)—grade on scale of 0 (absent) to +4 (hyperactive)

8. Skin

a. Color, texture, turgor, moisture, hygiene, scars

b. Edema, excessive perspiration, unusual odor, varicosities, hair texture and distribution, nails

c. Lesions, masses

d. Parasites, trauma, ecchymosis (bruising)

e. Moles

(1) Pattern, distribution

      (2) Warning signs (A, B, C, D, E)—**A**symmetrical; **B**orders irregular; **C**olor change or multicolor; **D**iameter changing; **E**levation

- Detailed reproductive examination

  1. Breasts

    a. Examination conducted in 5 positions to exaggerate abnormalities—sitting upright, arms at sides; arms extended over head; hands pressed on hips; standing or seated, leaning forward; supine

    b. Inspection

      (1) Size, symmetry, contour

      (2) Tanner stage

      (3) Venous pattern, skin color and texture, hair, edema, lesions, scars, rashes, retractions, dimpling, lymph nodes, supernumerary nipples

      (4) Areolar color, nipples (flat, inverted, everted), lesions, discharge, retraction

      (5) Axillary hair distribution, rashes, lesions

    c. Palpation—performed with patient upright and supine, breast tissue evenly distributed over chest wall

      (1) Masses

      (2) Tenderness

      (3) Lymph nodes (supra- and infraclavicular)

    d. Compression of nipples for discharge

  2. Pelvic examination

    a. External

      (1) Hair distribution, surface characteristics of mons pubis and labia majora

      (2) Tanner Stage

      (3) Vulvar/perineal tenderness, scarring, masses, lesions, edema, inflammation, discharge

> (4) Labia minora, clitoris, vaginal introitus, perineum
>
> (5) Bartholin's, urethra, and Skene's (BUS)

b. Internal (speculum)

> (1) Vaginal color, texture, moisture, discharge, lesions, relaxation
>
> (2) Cervical color, consistency, diameter, position, mobility, discharge, lesions, masses, edema, tenderness, inflammation, friability
>
> (3) Cervical os size, shape, erosion, ectropion, visible squamocolumnar junction, polyps, discharge

c. Bimanual

> (1) Uterine size, shape, position, consistency, contour, mobility, tenderness, cervical motion tenderness (CMT)
>
> (2) Ovarian size, shape, contour, mobility, tenderness; cul de sac bulging; tenderness; adnexal masses

d. Rectovaginal (confirms bimanual findings)

> (1) Posterior uterine segment—allows for adequate palpation of retroverted or retroflexed uterus
>
> (2) Rectovaginal septum
>
> (3) Anal sphincter and mucosa
>
> (4) Cul de sac

3. Rectal examination

a. Inspection of the sacrococcygeal and perianal areas

b. Assess sphincter tone, tenderness, induration, irregularities or nodules of rectal mucosa

c. Provides opportunity for stool check and test for occult blood, if indicated by age, history or symptoms

d. American Cancer Society advises

> (1) Annual rectal examinations from age 40 onward
>
> (2) Annual stool occult blood testing after age 50

4. Pregnancy Evaluation

a. Leopold's maneuvers—important adjunct to palpation of gravid uterus from about 28 weeks gestation on; information gained is translated into fetal lie (relationship of the long axis of fetus to mother's spine), fetal presentation and position, engagement (how far the fetal presenting part has descended into the maternal pelvis), and estimated fetal weight

   (1) First maneuver—palpate upper pole of uterine fundus to determine fetal part in fundus

   (2) Second maneuver—use palmar surfaces of hands to determine where fetal back is located

   (3) Third maneuver—use thumb and third finger over symphysis pubis to grasp presenting part and determine whether it is descending into the pelvic inlet

   (4) Fourth maneuver—attempt to determine the fetal presenting part

b. Auscultation of fetal heart rate (FHR)

   (1) Audible with doppler, or ultrasound by 12 weeks gestation

   (2) Audible with fetoscope at 17-20 weeks gestation

c. Measurement of fundal height

   (1) Early uterine enlargement may not be symmetric; most accurate sizing by bimanual in first 12-14 weeks

       (a) Nonpregnant—uterus 5.5-8 cm long, 3.5-4 cm wide

       (b) 6 weeks gestation—uterus 7.3-9.1 cm long, 3.9 cm wide

       (c) 8 weeks gestation—uterus 8.8-10.8 cm long, 5.0 cm wide

       (d) 10 weeks gestation—uterus 10.2-12.5 cm long, 6.1 cm wide

       (e) 12 weeks gestation—uterus 11.7-14.2 cm long, 7.1 cm wide and palpable just above symphysis pubis

       (f) 14 weeks gestation—uterus 13.2-15.9 cm long, 8.2 cm wide

(2) 16 weeks—uterine fundus palpable halfway between symphysis and umbilicus

(3) 20 weeks—uterine fundus is at lower border of umbilicus

(4) Between 20 and 34 weeks—measurement from top of symphysis pubis to top of uterine fundus in centimeters should roughly equal weeks of gestation

(5) After 34 weeks—fundal height measurement varies according to fetal size and position

- Infection Control

  1. Prevention of contamination

      a. Clean work surface for each client

      b. Assemble clean equipment prior to each examination

      c. Close exam table drawers before beginning examination

      d. Conduct pelvic examination using gloving style that prevents contamination to self and equipment

  2. Universal precautions

      a. Handwashing before and after every client contact

      b. Follow Centers for Disease Control and Prevention (CDC) guidelines for universal precautions whenever exposure to blood and body fluids may occur

      c. Wear gloves for any contact with blood, body fluids, discharge, mucous membranes or broken skin

      d. Dispose of needles and sharps in puncture-resistant containers; do not recap needles

      e. Ensure correct confinement and disposal of contaminated/hazardous medical waste

      f. Sterilize/disinfect durable equipment between clients

      g. Wear protective eyewear and mask for any likely splashing of eyes or mucous membranes

      h. Wear water-repellant gown when clothing could be soiled with blood or body fluids

Diagnostic Studies/Laboratory (Non-Gyn)

- Complete Blood Count—normal values

    1. Red Blood Cell Count (RBC): 4.0-5.3 million/mm³

    2. Hemoglobin (Hgb): 12-16 g/dL

        a. Hgb > 16.5—consider dehydration, diuretic use, polycythemia

        b. Hgb < 11—consider blood loss, decreased blood cell survival, decreased bone marrow production, RBC sequestration

    3. Hematocrit (Hct): 36-47%

    4. White Blood Cell Count (WBC): 4.0-11.0 million/mm³

        a. WBC 0.5-3.2 million/mm³ (decreased)—consider severe bacterial infection, influenza, infectious mononucleosis

        b. WBC 9.8-30 million/mm³ (increased)—consider physiologic reaction to stress, tissue destruction, leukemia, cancer, hemorrhage, splenectomy

    5. Differential

        a. Neutrophils (PMN): 50-70%

            (1) Elevated with physical or emotional stress, trauma, inflammatory or metabolic disorders

            (2) Decreased with aplastic anemia, viral infections, severe bacterial infections

        b. Eosinophils (PME): 2-6%—elevated with allergies, parasitic infections, leukemia and autoimmune diseases

        c. Basophils (PMB): 0-1%—elevated with leukemia; decreased in acute allergic reactions, hyperthyroidism, stress reactions

        d. Lymphocytes: 20-40%

            (1) Elevated with chronic bacterial infection, viral infection (e.g., mumps and rubella), infectious mononucleosis, infectious hepatitis

            (2) Decreased in leukemia, sepsis, immune deficiency diseases, acquired immunodeficiency syndrome, lupus erythematosus

   e. Monocytes: 0-7%

   (1) Elevated with chronic inflammatory disorders, viral infections (e.g., infectious mononucleosis), tuberculosis, chronic ulcerative colitis

   (2) Decreased with prednisone therapy

6. Blood Indices—performed to evaluate/differentiate anemias

   a. Mean corpuscular volume (MCV): 80-94 μm^3

   (1) Most important of RBC indices

   (2) Primary use is to differentiate anemias into macrocytic, normocytic or microcytic

   b. Mean corpuscular hemoglobin (MCH): 27-31 pg

   c. Mean corpuscular hemoglobin concentration (MCHC): 32-36%

7. Erythrocyte Sedimentation Rate (ESR)

   a. Women < 50 years old: 0-20 mm/hr

   b. Women 50-65 years old: 0-30 mm/hr

   c. Women > 65 years old: 0-53 mm/hr

   d. Accelerated in pregnancy, inflammatory conditions and multiple myeloma; decreased in sickle cell anemia

- Urinalysis (UA)—identifies pathology in the urinary tract and may reflect systemic metabolic abnormalities

   1. Gross examination—color; clarity

      a. Color ranges from pale yellow to amber due to presence of urochrome; indicates concentration of urine and varies with specific gravity

      b. Abnormal colors can indicate pathology or drug or food ingestion

      c. Normal urine is clear; cloudy urine may be caused by pus, RBCs or bacteria

      d. Normal urine may be cloudy due to diet (e.g., large amounts of fat)

2. Specific gravity—normal 1.001-1.035; low values suggest renal tubular dysfunction

   a. Increased with dehydration, decreased renal blood flow, glycosuria and proteinuria

   b. Decreased with overhydration, diabetes insipidus and chronic renal failure

3. pH: Fresh voided urine is generally acidic—normal pH 4.6-8; 6.0 average

4. Glucose—presence is abnormal; glycosuria associated with blood glucose level > 180 mg/dL (renal threshold)

5. Ketones—products of fat metabolism; increased in blood during periods when increased fats are being used as fuel, e.g., in starvation, uncontrolled diabetes, dehydration

6. Protein

   a. Presence is abnormal

   b. May be present with

      (1) Specimen contaminated with vaginal secretions

      (2) Pregnancy

      (3) Fever and strenuous physical exercise

      (4) Glomerulonephritis, neoplasms, infarctions, postrenal infections

7. Bilirubin—helps identify cause of jaundice; presence is abnormal

8. Urobilinogen—aids in diagnosis of extrahepatic obstruction, e.g., blockage of common bile duct, and in differential diagnosis of hepatic and hematologic disorders

9. Microscopic examination of urinary sediment

   a. RBCs

      (1) Normal: 1-2 RBCs

      (2) > 5 RBCs—microscopic hematuria; seen with glomerulonephritis, pyelonephritis and renal trauma or tumor

   b. WBCs

        (1)   Normal: 0-4 WBCs

        (2)   > 5 WBCs—UTI; culture indicated

    c. Casts (clumps of material or cells)

    d. Crystals—indicate stone formation imminent or present

    e. Bacteria—abnormal in appropriately obtained specimen; indicates UTI

10. Urine dipstick—rapid diagnostic aid

    a. Abnormalities in pH, protein, blood are nonspecific

    b. Abnormalities specifically correlated with infection

        (1)   Nitrites—generated from urinary nitrate by reductive activity of bacteria

        (2)   Leukocyte oxidase—reflects presence of WBCs

- Blood Sugar Tests

1. Differences between whole blood, serum and plasma values

    a. Venous plasma and serum glucose values are 15% higher than venous whole blood values

    b. Capillary whole blood values are 10% higher than venous whole blood

    c. Venous plasma and serum values are 5-7% higher than those found in capillary whole blood

2. Serum glucose

    a. Fasting Blood Sugar (FBS)—grossly evaluates body's ability to regulate glucose

        (1)   Normal: < 115 mg/dL

        (2)   Requires glucose tolerance test 115-140 mg/dL

        (3)   Diagnostic of diabetes: > 140 mg/dL

    b. Two-hour postprandial glucose test—demonstrates metabolism of a 100 g carbohydrate load

        (1)   Normal after 1 hour: < 170 mg/dL

        (2)   Normal after 2 hours

        (a)   In general: < 120 mg/dL

        (b)   < 50 years old: 140 mg/dL

        (c)   60-69 years old: 160 mg/dL

        (d)   70+ years old: 180 mg/dL

  c. Glucose tolerance tests (GTT)

     (1) Identifies early diabetes mellitus

     (2) Sequential blood (and rarely urine) samples taken at various intervals up to 6 hours after 75 g oral glucose load

        (a)   Fasting: Normal < 115 mg/dL

        (b)   30 minutes: < 200 mg/dL; 30-60 mg/dL over fasting level

        (c)   60 minutes: < 200 mg/dL; by end of 60 minutes, blood glucose levels begin to decline (20-50 mg/dL)

        (d)   90 minutes: < 200 mg/dL

        (e)   120 minutes: < 140 mg/dL; after 2-3 hours, blood glucose levels return to fasting level

- Blood Urea Nitrogen (BUN) and Creatinine—indicate renal function

  1. Normal renal function values

    a. BUN: 8-22 mg/dL

    b. Creatinine: 0.6-1.5 mg/dL

  2. Accurate interpretation of values requires information about

    a. Protein intake

    b. Fluid intake

    c. Conditions which increase endogenous production—muscular activity; trauma; infection/inflammation; strict dieting, starvation or fasting; intestinal obstruction, GI bleeding

- Lipid profiles

  1. Total lipids—normal: 400-1000 mg/dL

  2. Cholesterol and triglycerides—normal screening values

    a. Cholesterol: < 200 mg/dL

        (1)   200-239: Borderline risk for coronary heart disease (CHD)

        (2)   240 and above: High risk for CHD

    b. Triglycerides: 30-175 mg/dL

        (1)   Newborn to 29 years old: 10-140 mg/dL

        (2)   30–39 years old: 10-150 mg/dL

        (3)   40-49 years old: 10-160 mg/dL

        (4)   50-59 years old: 10-190 mg/dL

    c. Coronary artery disease (CAD) risk factors—male gender; smoking; family history CHD; hypertension; diabetes mellitus; severe obesity; history of vascular disease; HDL < 35 mg/dL

    d. Combined measurements essential in evaluating liver function, with decreased serum cholesterol reflecting possible hepatic disease

  3. Lipoprotein cholesterol fractionation—high density lipoproteins (HDLs), low-density lipoproteins (LDLs) and very low-density lipoproteins (VLDLs)

    a. Normal values

        (1)   HDL: > 50 mg/dL

        (2)   LDL

            (a)   < 130 mg/dL (desirable)

            (b)   130-159 (borderline risk for CHD)

            (c)   160 and above (high risk for CHD)

    b. Epidemiologic, genetic and metabolic data associate

        (1)   High LDLs to increased risk for CAD

        (2)   High HDLs and decreased risk of CHD

    c. Current recommendations—total cholesterol and LDL levels beginning at age 20 and every 5 years thereafter if normal

- Thyroid studies

  1. Thyroid-stimulating hormone (TSH) or Total Thyroxine (T_4) are initial screening tests for suspected thyroid disorders

a. TSH—normal range: 2.0-10.5 µU/mL

b. T_4—normal range: 4.5-12.5 µg/dL

2. Further testing

a. T_3 RIA—normal range: 80-200 ng/dL (adults); not reliable for distinguishing between normal and hypothyroid states; most sensitive test for thyrotoxicosis

b. TSH may help differentiate between primary and secondary hypothyroidism, particularly in milder cases

- Blood Type and Rh

1. Blood grouped according to presence or absence of

a. Antigens on the RBCs (A, B, AB, O)

b. Rh antigens on RBCs (Rh positive or Rh negative)

2. Both required to determine compatibility before whole blood or most blood components can be administered

3. Negative Rh status determines need for Rh (anti-D) globulin (RhoGAM) administration following delivery, miscarriage, or abortion to prevent Rh isoimmunization

- Infectious Disease Screening

1. Rubella (German Measles)

a. Hemagglutination Inhibition (HAI) test—detects presence of IgG and IgM antibodies of past and active infections to determine immunity to the rubella virus

b. If titer is > 1:10, client is considered immune to rubella

c. If titer is < 1:8, client is susceptible to rubella, and rubella immunization is advised if client is not pregnant

2. Human Immunodeficiency Virus (HIV) Tests

a. Enzyme-linked immunosorbent assay (ELISA) test for antibodies to HIV in serum or plasma; primary screen for HIV

b. Results

(1) Negative—sensitivity is greater than 99%, making possibility of false negative result remote (except in very early

infection when HIV antibody is undetectable, up to 6 months after exposure)

(2) Positive—specificity is good where prevalence high, but less so where low, so repeat positive test to rule out false result in low risk patient

(3) All positive ELISAs must be repeated; if ELISA is positive when repeated, confirmatory test is done

c. Western Blot—most commonly used confirmatory test for HIV; detects antibodies to several specific HIV protein antigens

(1) Greater than 99% specificity and sensitivity

(2) Indicated for repeatedly positive ELISA

(3) Results—positive or negative for HIV; positive Western Blot is conclusive evidence of HIV

(4) If ELISA repeatedly positive and Western Blot is equivocal, a second serum specimen should be tested in 2-4 months

3. Hepatitis B

a. Hepatitis: An inflammation of the liver caused by one of several common viruses—hepatitis A, hepatitis B, hepatitis C, and non A non B hepatitis virus

b. The Blood Borne Pathogen Standard (OSHA) requires that immunization for hepatitis B be offered to all workers who may come in contact with blood or body fluids in their jobs

c. Hepatitis B surface antigen (HB_sAg) test

(1) Most commonly and easily performed test for hepatitis B

(2) Surface antigen is the first indicator to become abnormal; surface antigen rises before onset of clinical symptoms, peaks with symptoms, and returns to normal by the time jaundice subsides

(3) Results—detection of HB_sAg indicates either acute or chronic infection, depending on clinical symptoms, liver enzymes, and further antibody determination, i.e., HB core IgM or IgG; if levels persist for at least 6 months, person is considered to be a carrier

    d. Hepatitis B surface antibody (HB$_s$Ab)test

        (1) Antibody appears about 4 weeks after disappearance of HB$_s$Ag and signifies end of acute infection and immunity to further infection

        (2) Indicates immunity from HBV vaccine or possibly HBIG

  4. Tuberculosis (TB)

    a. Tuberculin skin test with purified protein derivative (PPD)

    b. PPD preferred screening test for TB (CDC); unable to indicate whether infection is active or dormant

        (1) Definition of positive tuberculin test by CDC and American Thoracic Society

           (a) General population: ≥ 15 mm of induration

           (b) Household or close contacts of active cases, persons with clinical suspicion of TB, and HIV positive persons: ≥ 5 mm of induration

           (c) People with risk factors: ≥ 10 mm of induration

        (2) False positive—past vaccination with bacille Calmette-Guerin (BCG) (thought to be protective at one time)

        (3) False negative—inactive vaccine; improper placement; steroids; immune response deficiency

    c. Contraindications to test

        (1) Persons with known active TB

        (2) Persons who have received BCG

- Sickle Cell Screening

  1. Screening test detects Hgb S

    a. Normal value—no sickle cells (negative)

    b. Homozygous for Hgb S—sickle cell disease

    c. Heterozygous for Hgb S—sickle cell trait

  2. Definitive diagnosis made by hemoglobin electrophoresis—determines hemoglobin types and amounts (%)

- Liver function studies

1. Measure the ability of the liver to perform normal functions

    a. Serum albumin—a measure of protein synthesis

        (1) Normal: 4.0-6.0 g/dL

        (2) Not useful for general screening of healthy individuals

        (3) Useful in evaluating patients with edema, liver disorders, or suspected malnutrition

        (4) Elevated albumin—little or no clinical significance; commonly seen with dehydration

        (5) Decreased (< 4.0)—associated with decreased synthesis (liver insufficiency, malnutrition, malignancy); increased loss (nephrotic syndrome, excessive burns); pregnancy; inflammatory illness

    b. Serum alkaline phosphatase (ALP)—usual marker for liver diseases which are cholestatic

        (1) Normal (adults): 30-120 IU/L; pregnancy: 30-200 IU/L

        (2) Elevated (> 200)

            (a) Increased from liver—bile duct stone; biliary cancer; pancreatic cancer; pancreatitis; viral hepatitis; severe cirrhosis

            (b) Increased from osteoblastic activity—Paget's disease; osteomalacia; bony metastasis; hyperparathyroidism

            (c) Not useful screening test for asymptomatic individuals; values less than normal are of no clinical significance

    c. Aminotransferases—enzymes primarily located within hepatocytes

        (1) Normal: 0-35 IU/L

            (a) Alanine aminotransferase (ALT)—formerly serum glutamic pyruvic transaminase (SGPT)

            (b) Aspartate aminotransferase (AST)—formerly serum glutamic oxaloacetic transaminase (SGOT)

(2) Increased levels of both enzymes due to liver injury and subsequent leaking of enzymes from cells

d. Prothrombin time (PT)—measure of ability to synthesize clotting factors

(1) Useful test for monitoring anticoagulant therapy (Coumadin), and for evaluating patients with abnormal bleeding

(2) Increased PT due to—liver disease; malabsorption disorders; DIC; clotting factor deficiency; vitamin K deficiency

e. Bilirubin—measure of bile salt conjugation and excretion

(1) Levels usually proportional to level of hepatocyte injury in hepatic disease

(2) Jaundice clinically detectable only when total bilirubin > 3.0 mg/dL

(3) Normal: 0.1-1.0 mg/dL

(4) Low serum bilirubin—no clinical significance

- Stool testing for occult blood

  1. Small quantity of feces chemically tested for presence of occult blood

  2. Single positive result is not confirmatory for GI bleeding; repeat test at least 3 times while client follows meatless, high-residue diet

Health Maintenance and Risk Identification

- Disease Prevention

  1. Nutrition—critical component of overall health status; nutrition important in disease prevention and everyday functioning

     a. Identification of nutritional parameters for optimal health—Food Guide Pyramid

        (1) General outline of daily healthy diet, not rigid prescription

        (2) Emphasis on 5 food groups in larger "base" of pyramid

            (a) Bread, cereal, rice, pasta: 6-11 servings/day

            (b) Vegetables: 3-5 servings/day

        (c)   Fruits: 2-4 servings/day

        (d)   Milk, yogurt, cheese: 2-3 servings/day

        (e)   Meat, poultry, fish, dry beans, eggs, nuts: 2-3 servings/day

        (f)   Fats, sweets: Use sparingly

b. Identification of over consumption patterns, especially saturated fats, cholesterol, sugar and salt that may be linked with development of obesity, diabetes, hypertension, cardiovascular disease and cancer

c. Identification of malnutrition

d. Counseling aimed at helping clients balance consumption of nutrients

e. Normal dietary requirements

    (1) Current weight/height

    (2) Percentage of body fat and lean body weight

    (3) Dietary patterns

        (a)   Diet history (1-2 weeks)

        (b)   Dietary recall (24 hours)

    (4) Nutrient composition of diet

        (a)   Increase complex carbohydrate intake (50-55% of total caloric intake)

        (b)   Decrease fat intake ($< 30\%$ total calories/day)

            i)   Saturated fat intake: $< 10\%$ of total calories/day

           ii) Cholesterol intake: < 100 mg/1000 calories, not to exceed 300 mg daily

        (c)   Protein intake should be moderate—approximately 15% of total calories daily or < 1.6 g/kg of body weight for adults

        (d)   Increase intake of dietary fiber (5-7 grams daily)

        (e)   Limit sodium intake—reduced to approximately 1 g/1000 calories, not to exceed 6 g daily

        (f)   Adequate hydration: 8-10 glasses of water daily

  f. Counseling for specialized needs—comprehensive nutritional assessment and referral for counseling/treatment plan by clinical dietician recommended for

    (1) Weight < 80% or > 120% of ideal weight

    (2) History of unintentional weight loss > 4.5 kg (10 lb) or > 10% of usual weight

    (3) History of illnesses, symptoms, or factors that are associated with nutritional depletion or interfere with nutrient intake or absorption

2. Exercise—modern sedentary lifestyles foster unfitness and increase risk for health problems

  a. Physical fitness evaluation

    (1) Height, weight, vital signs, blood glucose and total cholesterol with fractions

    (2) Testing muscle strength and endurance

        (a)   Evaluate bent-knee sit-ups (20-26/one minute considered average for women)

        (b)   Weight resistance measurements of major muscle groups

    (3) Flexibility—toe touch (standing or sitting with legs outstretched)

    (4) Cardiovascular endurance—treadmill; bicycle; step; jump-rope

  b. Increasing physical activity

    (1) Choose activities that fit lifestyle

    (2) Set realistic goals; consider an exercise "buddy"; attend formal classes; use home videos or audiotapes

    (3) Optimal to maintain fitness: 20-30 minutes aerobic exercise 3-4 times per week

    3. Screening Techniques

       a. Periodic selective examinations determined by client's sex, age and risk factors

          (1) Pap smears—beginning with onset of sexual activity or at age 18, yearly Paps until 3 consecutive negative results, then every year to every 3 years, based on client's risk factors for cervical cancer

          (2) Pelvic exam yearly after age 40 (American Cancer Society [ACS])

          (3) Breast exam by health professional yearly; monthly self breast exam (ACS—every 3 years ages 20-40; yearly after age 40)

          (4) Mammography—baseline by age 40; every 1-2 years age 40-49; every year age 50 and over (ACS)

          (5) Stool for occult blood—every year after age 50

          (6) Sigmoidoscopy—every 3-5 years after age 50

          (7) Cholesterol and HDL—beginning at age 20, then every 5 years if normal

          (8) Blood pressure monitoring

          (9) Vision testing—every 2 years

          (10) Dental exams—every 6 months-1 year

       b. Health promotion counseling

          (1) Reduce/stop smoking

          (2) Avoid substance use/abuse

          (3) Maintain good nutritional status with special emphasis on calcium intake for women

          (4) Maintain regular exercise habits

          (5) Control stress and violent behavior

          (6) Wear safety belts

- Sexuality

    1. Sexual response cycle

a. Two principal physiological responses to sexual stimulation

   (1) Vasocongestion—tissues and vessels become engorged; corresponds to sexual excitement

   (2) Myotonia—increase in muscle tension; peaks with orgasm

b. Masters and Johnson's four phase cycle

   (1) Excitement—vagina becomes moist; nipples of breast become erect; skin becomes flushed

   (2) Plateau—clitoris swells slightly; vagina becomes longer; labia minora becomes reddened; respiratory and heart rate increase; skin becomes flushed

   (3) Orgasm—muscles of vagina and uterus contract; hips (pelvis) move in a rhythmic, forward-thrusting motion

   (4) Resolution—return to normal with slower heart and expiratory rate; sweating

2. Sexual practices

   a. Healthy sexual activity

      (1) Based on mutual consent

      (2) Physically and psychologically positive

      (3) Not harmful to either participant

   b. Woman's view of herself as female incorporates concepts of gender identity (identification of self as female); the sense of having characteristics customarily defined as feminine, masculine, or both; body image (mental picture of one's body and its relationship to the environment)

   c. Sexual lifestyle provides the pattern and context for a woman's sexuality; options include—marriage with a monogamous partner; serial monogamy; nonmonogamous marriage; heterosexual coupling without marriage; single state; lesbianism; bisexuality; celibacy

3. Sexual dysfunction—impaired or absent expressions of normally recurring sexual desire and responses with associated subjective discomfort

a. May occur during masturbation, or during sexual activity with a partner; may be lifelong or develop after a period of normal responsiveness; may occur only once or recur

b. Traumatic sexual experiences such as incest or rape may precipitate dysfunction; other associated factors include depression, anxiety and life stress

c. Female sexual dysfunctions

   (1) Inhibited sexual desire—lack of desire for sexual activity, lack of sexual dreams or fantasies or frustration if sexual activity does not occur; cause is unknown, but is associated with high levels of stress; treatment is often difficult and usually focuses on sensation enhancement and techniques to improve communication between partners

   (2) Anorgasmia—inability to experience orgasms; defined as disorder only if woman reports receiving sufficient stimulation without orgasm

       (a) Causes include—restrictive home environment, negative cultural conditioning during childhood, unrealistic expectations about performance, relationship problems, lack of knowledge about female anatomy and sexual response

       (b) Most common treatments are behavioral, focusing on increasing the woman's awareness of genital sensations and masturbatory techniques

   (3) Vaginismus—involuntary, spasmodic, sometimes painful contractions of the pubococcygeus and other muscles in lower third of the vagina and introitus

       (a) Causes include—sexual trauma, strong conservative religious values, dyspareunia, and hostile feelings toward sexual partner

       (b) Treatment involves desensitization process including insertion of progressively larger dilators into vagina by the woman and/or her partner and possibly psychotherapy

- Preconception Counseling
    1. Based on principle that the status of a woman's health can influence her ability to conceive, her ability to maintain the pregnancy, and the outcome of pregnancy for the woman and her infant
    2. Key counseling and education
        a. Menstrual cycle charting—to plan pregnancy and to help establish gestational dating
        b. Adequate exercise and nutrition
            (1) Folic acid supplementation (0.4 mg/day for low-risk women) to reduce risk of neural tube defect
            (2) Encourage overweight or underweight women to attain ideal weight prior to conception
            (3) Begin exercise program before pregnancy to help improve cardiovascular status and impart feeling of overall well-being; may help overweight woman attain ideal weight, lessen potential for problems such as diabetes and hypertension during pregnancy
        c. Avoidance of teratogens
        d. Readiness for parenthood
        e. Identification and resolution of substance use/abuse and other unhealthy behaviors
        f. Identification of genetic risk (woman and couple)
        g. Obtain appropriate vaccinations (rubella, tetanus, hepatitis) when indicated
        h. Diabetes control prior to conception

QUESTIONS

Select the best answer

1. The health history includes the history of the present illness, past medical history, and which of the following?

   a. Today's blood pressure, pulse and respirations
   b. Review of systems, family history and psychosocial history
   c. Nutritional assessment, physical exam findings and menstrual history
   d. Review of systems, obstetric history and today's CBC

2. Review of systems documentation includes:

   a. Information from the patient and findings from the physical examination
   b. Information about each body region and organ system, including past and present function and/or problems
   c. A summary of the client's current major health concerns
   d. Identification of potential or actual risk factors

3. The technique of percussion is best defined as:

   a. Dullness, resonance or tympany
   b. Touching the body to feel pulsations and vibrations, to locate structures and to elicit tenderness
   c. Tapping against a body surface to produce distinct sounds and elicit tenderness
   d. Listening to body sounds

4. The screening examination of the ear includes:

   a. Audiogram, otoscopy and irrigation of canals
   b. Assessment of pinna and mastoid; otoscopic exam; gross hearing screen
   c. Palpation of tympanic membrane, if indicated
   d. Otoscopy, audioscopy and Rinne and Weber

5. The general background of the fundus of the eye varies in color depending on a person's:

   a. Eye color
   b. Skin color

    c. Age

    d. Hair color

6. Which of the following statements is true?

    a. Percussion normally elicits resonance over the liver and spleen

    b. Percussion normally elicits dullness over a lower intestine filled with feces and a bladder filled with urine

    c. Percussion normally elicits tympany over the liver and spleen

    d. Percussion is not an appropriate technique when evaluating a client's abdomen

7. Assessing the temperature, shape and consistency of a body region is known as:

    a. Percussion

    b. Palpation

    c. Auscultation

    d. Inspection

8. While palpating a client's thorax, the practitioner assesses respiratory excursion; what does this technique assess?

    a. Chest movement

    b. Breath sounds

    c. Lung vibration

    d. Voice sounds

9. When auscultating the client's heart sounds, the practitioner should hear S_1 best at which site?

    a. Pulmonic area

    b. Aortic area

    c. Erb's point

    d. Mitral area

10. Blood indices are ordered for the following reason:

    a. As a substitute for the white blood cell count with differential

    b. To evaluate and differentiate anemias

    c. As a screening test for iron deficiency anemia

    d. To evaluate inflammatory skin disorders

11. A 57 year-old asymptomatic female is found to have an erythrocyte sedimentation rate (ESR) of 30 mm/hr. The most likely diagnosis in this woman is:

a. Cancer
b. Sickle cell anemia
c. Multiple myeloma
d. Normal

12. Which of the following tests would you expect to be the most helpful in evaluating a patient suspected of having hypothyroidism?

a. T_4
b. TSH
c. T_3
d. T_3 RIA

13. Which of the following is a true statement regarding Leopold's maneuvers?

a. They are techniques used by the practitioner to confirm positive pregnancy test results at or around 12 weeks gestation
b. They give the practitioner information regarding fetal lie, presentation and position after approximately 28 weeks gestation
c. They are a useful clinical tool for evaluation of the fetal heart rate and rhythm
d. They are not useful for evaluating pregnancies after 32 weeks gestation

14. Early uterine enlargement of pregnancy is sometimes difficult to assess. As a general rule in a normal pregnancy, the uterus:

a. Is nonpalpable until 12 weeks gestation
b. Is palpable only as a pelvic organ until about 12 weeks gestation when it becomes palpable right above the symphysis pubis
c. Is palpable as an abdominal organ at 8 weeks gestation
d. Is palpable abdominally at 4-6 weeks gestation if the patient's bladder is full

15. When in pregnancy may the examiner expect that the length in centimeters from the top of the symphysis pubis to the top of the uterine fundus is roughly equal to the weeks of gestation?

a. Between 10 and 20 weeks gestation in primigravidas only
b. Between 20 and 34 weeks gestation
c. After 30 weeks gestation
d. Between 20 and 24 weeks gestation

16. During inspection of the female breasts, which of the following suggests an abnormality?

    a. Bilateral nipple inversion
    b. Nipples that point outward, slightly upward, and lateral
    c. Bilateral nipple eversion
    d. Unilateral nipple inversion

17. Which of the following statements about sexual dysfunction is true?

    a. Sexual dysfunction is defined as impaired or absent expressions of normally recurring sexual desire and responses associated with subjective discomfort
    b. Most sexual dysfunction is caused by psychological trauma
    c. Sexual dysfunction is more common in women with low stress and anxiety levels
    d. Sexual dysfunction is often used interchangeably with dyspareunia (pain with intercourse)

18. Along with increasing fiber and decreasing sodium in the diet, the American Heart Association recommends which of the following?

    a. Total daily caloric intake should include < 60% fat, 25% carbohydrates and 20-30% protein
    b. Total daily caloric intake should include < 30% fat, 50-55% carbohydrates and 15% protein
    c. Total daily caloric intake should include > 75% carbohydrates, 20% protein and 5-10% fat
    d. Total daily caloric intake should include 25% milk and dairy products, 25% meat, fish and poultry, 25% vegetables and fruits and 25% bread, cereals and grains

19. Which of the following history questions would be most helpful in assessing cerebral function?

    a. "How would you describe your eyesight?"
    b. "Have you noticed a change in your ability to remember?"
    c. "Have you noticed a change in your muscle strength?"
    d. "Have you noticed a change in your coordination?"

20. Which documentation statement suggests an abnormal finding?

    a. Tympanic membranes shiny and pink
    b. Bowel sounds auscultated in all four quadrants

   c. Ovaries almond-shaped, firm, mobile and nontender

   d. Conjunctivae clear with multiple small vessels

Answer

1. b	11. d
2. b	12. b
3. c	13. b
4. b	14. b
5. b	15. b
6. b	16. d
7. b	17. a
8. a	18. b
9. d	19. b
10. b	20. a

BIBLIOGRAPHY

Barker, L.R., Burton, J.R., & Zieve, P.D. (Eds.). (1995). *Principles of ambulatory medicine* (4th ed.). Baltimore: Williams and Wilkins.

Bates, B. (1994). *A guide to physical examination and history taking* (6th ed.). Philadelphia: J.B. Lippincott Company.

Bowers, A.C., & Thompson, J.M. (1992). *Clinical manual of health assessment* (4th ed.). St. Louis: C.V. Mosby Company.

Bradley, J., Rubenstein, D., & Wayne, D. (1994). *The clinical manual.* London: Blackwell Scientific Publications.

Graber, M.A., Allen, R.J., & Levy, B.T. (1994). *The family practice handbook* (2nd ed.). St. Louis: C.V. Mosby Company.

Hoole, A.J., Pickard, C.G., Ouimette, R.M., Lohr, J.A., & Greenberg, R.A. (1995). *Patient care guidelines for nurse practitioners* (4th ed.). Philadelphia: J.B. Lippincott Company.

Jarvis, C. (1992). *Physical examination and health assessment.* Philadelphia: W.B. Saunders Company.

Malasanos, L., Barkauskas, V., & Stoltenberg-Allen, K. (1990). *Health assessment* (4th ed.). St. Louis: C.V. Mosby Company.

Pagana, K.D., & Pagana, T.J. (1994). *Diagnostic testing & nursing implications: A case study approach* (4th ed.). St. Louis: C.V. Mosby Company.

Seidel, H.M., Ball, J.W., Dains, J.E., & Benedict, G.W. (1995). *Mosby's guide to physical examination* (3rd ed.). St. Louis: C.V. Mosby Company.

Treseler, K.M. (1995). *Clinical laboratory and diagnostic tests* (3rd ed.). Norwalk, CT: Appleton & Lange.

Wallach, J. (1992). *Interpretation of diagnostic tests: A synopsis of laboratory medicine* (5th ed.). Boston: Little, Brown and Company.

Non-Gynecologic Disorders

Mary C. Knutson

Eyes, Ears, Nose, and Throat

Allergic Rhinitis

- Definition: Inflammation of nasal mucosa in response to inhaled allergens; specific IgE antibodies are present
- Etiology/Incidence
  1. Seasonal
     a. Affects approximately 10% of adults
     b. Typically caused by plants, e.g., ragweed
     c. Occurs at specific times of year when allergens are present ("hayfever")
  2. Perennial
     a. Allergens present throughout the year
     b. Typically dust, mites, feathers, pet dander
- Signs and Symptoms
  1. Nasal obstruction and excessive watery discharge
  2. Sneezing, nasal pruritus
  3. Often accompanied by conjunctivitis and tearing
- Differential Diagnosis
  1. Rhinitis medicamentosus
  2. Vasomotor rhinitis
  3. Upper respiratory infection (URI)
  4. A clear diagnosis cannot always be made
- Physical Findings
  1. Nasal mucosa pale and boggy
  2. Clear, thin rhinorrhea
- Diagnostic Tests/Findings
  1. Usually none indicated

2. Wright stain of nasal secretions (eosinophils present in 65-75% of cases)

3. Positive response to topical corticosteroids

4. Refer for skin tests to determine specific allergens

- Management/Treatment

    1. Avoidance of allergens

    2. Antihistamines

        a. Chlorpheniramine (Chlor-Trimeton)

        b. Terfenadine (Seldane)

        c. Astemizole (Hismanol)—do not use in pregnancy

    3. Corticosteroids (Beconase, Vancenase) by aerosol application

Conjunctivitis

- Definition: Inflammation of the membranous covering of the eye and eyelids

- Etiology/Incidence

    1. Allergy

    2. Infection, e.g., bacterial, viral

    3. Mechanical, e.g., foreign body, chemical

    4. An extremely common eye condition

- Signs and Symptoms

    1. Sensation of grit in eye

    2. Matted eye lashes

    3. Irritation around eye

- Differential Diagnosis

    1. Aimed at determining cause

    2. Rule out acute iritis, acute glaucoma, or herpetic lesions

- Physical Findings

    1. Allergic

    a. Uniformly red

    b. White, elastic mucoid discharge

2. Infection

    a. Bacterial

       (1) Mucopurulent drainage

       (2) Red "cobblestone" conjunctiva

    b. Viral

       (1) Watery discharge

3. Foreign body—exudate, pain

- Diagnostic Tests/Findings—usually none, unless suspect specific pathogens, e.g., chlamydia, gonorrhea (GC)

- Management/Treatment

    1. Allergic

       a. Cold compresses

       b. Antihistamines

          (1) Terfenadine

          (2) Chlorpheniramine

    2. Bacterial

       a. Dramatic clearing within 24 to 48 hours of treatment

       b. Often self-limiting

       c. Topical antibiotics

          (1) Erythromycin ophthalmic solution

          (2) Sulfisoxazole ophthalmic solution

    3. Viral—topical antibiotics (prevent secondary infection)

    4. Foreign body—refer

Sinusitis

- Definition: Acute or chronic inflammation of the frontal or maxillary sinuses

- Etiology/Incidence
    1. Acute sinusitis almost always bacterial; may be complication of URI
    2. Extremely common in ambulatory care
    3. Estimated 25% of people develop sinusitis in their lifetime
- Signs and Symptoms
    1. Aching facial pain, increased with bending over
    2. Headache
    3. Congestion
    4. Foul nasal discharge, yellow or green in color; sometimes unilateral
    5. Malaise
- Differential Diagnosis
    1. Nasal polyps
    2. Tumors
    3. Dental disease
- Physical Findings
    1. Low-grade fever
    2. Mucopurulent secretions in nares
    3. Nasal mucosa swollen, pale, dull red to gray
    4. Pain on firm palpation over sinus area
    5. Decreased transillumination effect in sinuses due to fluid-filled cavities
- Diagnostic Tests/Findings
    1. Cultures marginally useful
    2. White blood cell count possibly elevated
    3. X-ray of sinuses (gold standard) if persistent or recurrent disease; reveals opacity in infected areas
- Management/Treatment
    1. Pharmacologic
        a. Antibiotics

        (1)   Amoxicillin-clavulanate (Augmentin)

        (2)   Trimethoprim-sulfamethoxazole (Bactrim)

   b. Analgesics

        (1)   Aspirin

        (2)   Acetaminophen

   c. Decongestants

        (1)   Sympathomimetics, e.g., Afrin

        (2)   Antihistamines, e.g., Chlorpheniramine

2. Non-pharmacologic

   a. Steam inhalation

   b. Warm compresses

   c. Hydration (2,000-3,000 mL/day)

3. Refer

   a. Patients with no improvement by 2 weeks

   b. Chronic sinusitis

   c. Acute frontal infection on first visit—due to possibility of intracranial extension, abscess, osteomyelitis

Otitis Media

- Definition: An infection of the middle ear; often accompanies or follows URI

- Etiology/Incidence

   1. Causes in adults are viral, bacterial

   2. Highest incidence occurs in children < 10 years-old

- Signs and Symptoms

   1. Initially, feeling of blockage in affected ear

   2. Deep ear pain, throbbing

   3. Hearing diminished in affected ear(s) due to conductive loss

   4. URI symptoms

    5. Foul-smelling, purulent or brown-red waxy discharge if tympanic membrane ruptures

- Differential Diagnosis
  1. Mastoiditis
  2. Cholesteatoma
  3. Otitis externa
  4. Temporomandibular joint (TMJ) syndrome
- Physical Findings
  1. Tympanic membrane red, thickened, bulging
  2. Diminished or absent light reflex
  3. Fever to above 101°F
- Diagnostic Tests/Findings—usually none indicated
- Management/Treatment
  1. Pharmacologic
     - a. Antibiotics
       - (1) Ampicillin, amoxicillin
       - (2) In penicillin allergic—trimethoprim-sulfamethoxazole or cephalosporin
     - b. Decongestants of no proven benefit
     - c. Analgesics
  2. Non-pharmacologic—local heat
  3. Refer suspected extension of infection, mastoiditis, meningitis or perforation of tympanic membrane

Serous Otitis (Secretory Otitis)

- Definition: Collection of serous fluid in the middle ear from obstructed or dysfunctional eustachian tube
- Etiology/Incidence
  1. Allergies

    2. Residual subacute or acute otitis media

    3. Blockage, e.g., enlarged adenoids, edema

    4. Can be sequelae to acute otitis media

- Signs and Symptoms
  1. Initial—crackling sound when yawning or swallowing
  2. Feeling of fullness in affected ear
  3. Pain uncommon, occasionally mild
  4. Discharge uncommon
  5. Diminished hearing
  6. May persist up to 10 weeks
- Differential Diagnosis—rule out acute or chronic otitis media
- Physical Findings
  1. Afebrile or low-grade fever
  2. Tympanic membrane—yellowish, retracted, immobile
  3. Air bubbles may be visible under membrane
  4. Fluid line visible behind membrane
- Diagnostic Tests/Findings—usually none indicated
- Management/Treatment
  1. Controversial; studies inconclusive
  2. Antihistamines and decongestants seem logical; studies inconclusive
  3. Antimicrobial to eliminate residual bacteria
  4. Mechanical effects of chewing, gentle nose blowing may aid clearing eustachian tubes
  5. Refer if persists more than 4 weeks

Respiratory

Asthma

- Definition: A complex disorder with multiple precipitating causes and pathophysiologic abnormalities; clients experience episodic respiratory distress characterized by bronchospasm, secretion and edema of bronchial mucosa
- Etiology/Incidence
  1. Causes
     a. Extrinsic: Provoked by inhaled allergens
     b. Intrinsic: Usually related to infection
  2. Prevalence
     a. About 3% in general population
     b. Can occur at any age
- Signs and Symptoms
  1. Chest tightness
  2. Intermittent wheezing
  3. Breathlessness
  4. Initial nonproductive cough
  5. Chronic productive cough
  6. Anxiety
  7. Occasional nocturnal episodes
  8. Aggravating factors
     a. Viral upper respiratory illness
     b. Cold air and exercise
     c. Exposure to allergens, air pollution, beta blockers
- Differential Diagnosis
  1. Chronic Obstructive Pulmonary Disease (COPD); can overlap with asthma

    2. Bronchogenic carcinoma

    3. Fixed upper airway obstruction

    4. Pulmonary edema, embolism

- Physical findings (not all consistently present)

    1. Wheezing (inspiratory and/or expiratory)

    2. Prolonged expiratory phase

    3. Diminished lung sounds

    4. Hyper-resonance with percussion

    5. Paradoxical pulse or tachycardia

    6. Tachypnea, dyspnea

- Diagnostic Tests/Findings

    1. Pulmonary function test (PFT) demonstrates reversible obstruction

    2. Spirometry and peak flow rates improve with bronchodilator challenge

    3. Absolute eosinophil count elevated

        a. $122/mm^3$ = normal

        b. $85/mm^3$ = corticosteroid treatment

        c. $350/mm^3$ = asthmatics

        d. Eosinophils present in wet mount of sputum (sputum Gram stain marginal)

- Management/Treatment

    1. Goals

        a. Control symptoms

        b. Maintain lung function

    2. Acute

        a. Oxygen therapy

        b. Beta-adrenergics by inhalation, e.g., metaproterenol sulfate (Alupent)

        c. Aminophylline if no response

        d. Hospitalize promptly for signs of severe hypoxia, atelectasis, acute respiratory failure, or inadequate response to medication

   3. Chronic or persistent

        a. Bronchodilators (aerosol and/or oral)

           (1) Metaproterenol sulfate

           (2) Aminophylline/theophylline

           (3) Cromolyn sodium (Intal)

        b. Short course corticosteroids, e.g., beclomethasone, by inhalation

        c. Serial Peak Expiratory Flow Rates (PEFR)—demonstrate degree of obstruction, useful in adjusting medication

   4. Patient teaching

        a. Adequate hydration and humidification

        b. Avoid known allergens

        c. Treat infections promptly

        d. Prophylactic medication, e.g., sustained release theophylline, pre-exercise dosing

Bronchitis

- Definition: Inflammation of the mucous membranes of the bronchial tubes; may be chronic or acute
- Etiology/Incidence
  1. Bacterial
  2. Viral, especially if following viral URI
  3. More prevalent in winter months and among smokers
- Signs and Symptoms
  1. Occasional shallow breathing, tachypnea
  2. Rhinorrhea
  3. Cough—initially unproductive, changing to mucopurulent sputum
  4. Acute—possible chest pain and high fever

     5. Chronic—wider variety of causes and physical manifestations
- Differential Diagnosis
  1. Pneumonia
  2. Asthma
  3. Tuberculosis
- Physical Findings
  1. Low-grade fever
  2. Auscultation
     a. Coarse crackles (rhonchi) that clear or shift
     b. Expiratory wheezes
- Diagnostic Tests/Findings
  1. X-ray clear of areas of consolidation
  2. PPD if tuberculosis risk and/or with chronicity
- Management/Treatment
  1. Often self-limited
  2. Humidification and hydration
  3. Antibiotics in presence of purulent sputum
     a. Ampicillin
     b. Tetracycline
  4. Cough suppressants questionable
  5. Antipyretics

Pneumonia

- Definition: Acute lower respiratory disease with inflammation of the tracheobronchial tree, in which exudates lead to lung consolidation; pneumonia is the most severe of a spectrum of respiratory infections
- Etiology/Incidence
  1. Causes
     a. Most common pathogens: Virus, mycoplasma

      b. Less common: *S. pneumoniae, H. influenzae*

      c. *Pneumocystis carinii*—occurs in AIDS patients

  2. Contributing factors

      a. Preceding viral URI

      b. Compromised tracheobronchial function

  3. More prevalent in males

- Signs and Symptoms

  1. Vary between viral and bacterial infection; severity usually worse in bacterial

  2. May be absent in very young, elderly, immunosuppressed, coexisting chronic disease

      a. Bacterial more frequently characterized by sudden onset of symptoms

      b. Mycoplasma and viral more frequently characterized by a more gradual onset

  3. Ill less than 2 weeks

  4. Symptoms consistent with URI—rhinorrhea, sore throat

  5. Dry, non-productive cough changing to purulent sputum; sometimes blood-tinged ("rusty"); more common in bacterial

  6. Occasionally, cyanosis

  7. Associated symptoms—lethargy, headache, anorexia, nausea, vomiting in bacterial, viral, mycoplasma

- Differential Diagnosis

  1. Bronchitis

  2. Atelectasis

  3. Emphysema

  4. Malignancy

  5. Tuberculosis

- Physical Findings

  1. Physical examination may be normal in early stages; findings may be absent in mycoplasma and viral

   2. Tachycardia (bacterial)

   3. Tachypnea, dyspnea (bacterial)

   4. Percussion—dull over area of consolidation (bacterial, usually)

   5. Auscultation—non-clearing crackles, diminished breath sounds over consolidation

   6. Fever with chills, high spikes (more frequent in bacterial)

- Diagnostic Tests/Findings

   1. X-ray reveals patchy, regional areas of infiltration; may be normal in early stages

   2. Cultures not usually helpful due to contamination from nasopharynx

   3. Gram stain of sputum

      a. No organisms—assume viral or mycoplasma origin

      b. Gram positive—presume *S. pneumoniae*

      c. Gram negative—presume *H. influenzae*

   4. WBC elevation ($10,000/mm^3$ to $25,000/mm^3$) with a shift to left, i.e., increased bands (an immature form of neutrophil); ranges from below normal to a modest elevation in viral and mycoplasma

- Management/Treatment

   1. Pharmacologic

      a. Expectorants

      b. Antipyretics

      c. Analgesics

      d. Antibiotics

         (1) Procaine penicillin

         (2) Erythromycin

         (3) Tetracycline

         (4) Ampicillin

   2. Non-pharmacologic

      a. Bed rest

      b. Hydration, humidity

      c. Improve oxygenation, e.g., stop smoking

  3. Refer

      a. No improvement in 24-36 hours

      b. Fever over 39°C (102°F)

      c. Pallor or cyanosis with tachycardia, tachypnea

      d. Flaring of nares

      e. Mental confusion

Cardiovascular

Hypertension

- Definition
  1. Elevated blood pressure demonstrated on at least 3 separate occasions; can cause morbidity directly (stroke, congestive heart failure), or indirectly by progressive deterioration of organ systems (retinopathy, atherosclerosis, renal failure)
  2. Classifications—usually by etiology or severity
     a. Etiology
        (1) Essential—no known cause
        (2) Secondary—from a disease entity
     b. Severity
        (1) Normal: Systolic < 130/< 85 mm Hg diastolic
        (2) Stage 1 (mild): 140-159/90-99 mm Hg
        (3) Stage 2 (moderate): 160-179/100-109 mm Hg
        (4) Stage 3 (severe): 180-209/110-119 mm Hg
        (5) Stage 4 (very severe): ≥ 210/ ≥ 120 mm Hg
- Etiology/Incidence
  1. Essential hypertension

a. No discernable etiology

b. Comprises 90-95% of diagnosed hypertension

c. Risk factors

    (1) Black race—prevalence doubles

    (2) Advancing age

        (a) Females—peri/postmenopausal

        (a) Males—over age 45

    (3) Positive family history

    (4) Lifestyle—sedentary, stress, obesity, alcohol use

2. Secondary hypertension

a. Due to underlying disease/condition, e.g., diabetes, kidney disease, pheochromocytoma, primary aldosteronism, coarctation of aorta

b. About 5-10% of adult hypertension

- Signs and Symptoms

1. Essential

a. Often none, especially if mild to moderate

b. Occasional lightheadedness, palpitations

2. Secondary hypertension

a. Orthostatic hypotension, severe headaches, palpitations, sweating (pheochromocytoma)

b. Polyuria, polydipsia, muscle weakness, headache (primary aldosteronism)

c. Headaches, epistaxis, coldness of extremities, claudication (coarctation of aorta)

- Differential Diagnosis—focuses on determining if essential or secondary hypertension

- Physical Findings

1. Often none, other than elevated blood pressure

2. Consistently elevated blood pressure over time ($\geq$ 140/90 mm Hg on 3 readings at least a week apart)

3. Possible retinopathy in long-standing hypertension

4. Possible abdominal or carotid bruits

5. Occasional diminished distal pressures and pulses

- Diagnostic Tests/Findings—rule out undiagnosed secondary causes

    1. Renal disease

        a. Urinalysis

        b. Serum creatinine

        c. Blood urea nitrogen (BUN)

    2. Hyperlipidemia—serum lipid levels

    3. Diabetes—blood glucose

    4. Cardiomyopathy, myocardial ischemia, coarctation

        a. Electrocardiogram, echocardiogram

        b. Chest x-ray

    5. Adrenal gland pathology

        a. 24-hour urine for catecholamines, metanephrine

        b. Potassium

- Management/Treatment: Essential hypertension

    1. Refer

        a. When client is under 30 or over 60 years old

        b. Client with diastolic pressure of more than 110 mm Hg

        c. Evaluation and treatment of secondary causes

    2. Patient education

        a. Lifelong condition

        b. Asymptomatic nature

        c. Treatment regimen reduces complications

        d. Follow-up critical

3. Non-pharmacologic

    a. Diet—low sodium, weight reduction if needed

    b. Stop smoking

    c. Reduce alcohol use

    d. Increase moderate exercise

    e. Reduce stress—biofeedback, relaxation techniques

4. Pharmacologic

    a. Thiazide diuretics—initial therapy, e.g., hydrochlorothiazide

    b. Beta blockers—second level therapy, e.g., Propranolol

    c. Vasodilators—third level therapy, e.g., Hydralazine hydrochloride

    d. Calcium channel blockers—e.g., Verapamil

    e. ACE inhibitors—e.g., Enalapril, Captopril

Heart Murmurs

- Definition: Prolonged extra heart sounds heard during either systole or diastole; commonly associated with dynamics of regurgitation or stenosis

- Etiology/Incidence

1. Disruption of blood flow into, through, or out of the heart can result in murmur

2. Characteristics of sound dependent on:

    a. Size of valve opening

    b. Vigor of contraction

    c. Rate of flow

    d. Thickness of chest wall

3. "Innocent" or "functional" murmurs

    a. Transient; pose no direct threat to health

    b. Usually heard in systole

      c.   Often due to high output demands (rapid growth, pregnancy, anemia, fever, thyrotoxicosis)

      d.   Occur in 50-70% of children and 50% of young adults

   4. Pathologic murmurs reflect heart or valvular disease

      a.   Heard almost exclusively in diastole

      b.   Must be investigated, e.g., rheumatic heart disease

- Signs and Symptoms

   1. Functional murmurs—asymptomatic

   2. Pathologic

      a.   Possible chest pain

      b.   Shortness of breath on exertion

      c.   Orthopnea

      d.   Cough or wheeze

      e.   Paroxysmal nocturnal dyspnea

      f.   Growth failure

- Differential Diagnosis—focused on determining whether innocent or pathologic

- Physical Findings

   1. Innocent

      a.   Usually none except audible murmur

      b.   Soft (grade 1 or 2), medium pitch, systolic murmur

      c.   Heard best when patient is supine

   2. Pathologic

      a.   Refer if suspect

      b.   Diastolic murmur or any above grade 3

      c.   Murmur intensifies with exercise or Valsalva maneuver

      d.   Cyanosis

      e.   Jugular vein distention

      f.   Hepatomegaly

g. Pedal edema

h. Diminished femoral pulses or unequal blood pressure in left and right arms

- Diagnostic Tests/Findings—indicated only if suspect pathologic murmur

  1. CBC and hematocrit/hemoglobin—rule out anemia

  2. Chest x-ray—indications of cardiac enlargement

  3. Thyroid function—rule out hypo/hyperthyroid

- Management/Treatment

  1. Asymptomatic systolic murmur with low-risk history can be assumed innocent with follow-up next visit

  2. Refer any suspected cardiomyopathy, diastolic murmurs

Varicosities

- Definition: Form of venous insufficiency characterized by swollen, dilated veins in dependent extremities, diminished blood flow rate and increased intravenous pressure; described as either superficial or deep

- Etiology/Incidence

  1. Causes

     a. Incompetence of vessel wall or venous valves

     b. Obstruction of a more proximal vein

  2. Contributing factors

     a. Genetic predisposition

     b. Hormonal effects, e.g., pregnancy

     c. Phlebitis or trauma

     d. Advancing age

     e. Sedentary lifestyle or job

     f. Stasis or constriction

  3. Prevalence

     a. 2 to 4 times more common in women

b. Commonly encountered in primary care practice

- Signs and Symptoms
    1. Superficial
        a. Usually none
        b. Cosmetic consequence only
    2. Deep—aching pain on prolonged standing
- Differential Diagnosis
    1. Edema of chronic disease
    2. Other obstructions
- Physical Findings
    1. Mild edema in lower extremity
    2. Rarely, ulceration
- Diagnostic Tests/Findings
    1. Trendelenburg test (retarded venous refilling)
    2. Perthes' test (patency of deep veins)
    3. "Stripping" (indicates relative competency of collateral circulation)
- Management/Treatment
    1. Symptomatic relief
        a. Support stockings
        b. Elevate feet and legs
        c. Exercise
    2. Surgical excision or sclerosing therapy

Thrombophlebitis

- Definition: The occlusion or obstruction of venous flow by concomitant inflammation and clotting; classified as superficial or deep
- Etiology/Incidence
    1. Causes
        a. Stasis

  b. Surgery or trauma—stimulates release of tissue thromboplastin leading to increased clotting

  c. Direct injury to vessel wall

  d. Increased coagulability states, e.g., estrogen administration

 2. Frequency in general population unknown

- Signs and Symptoms

 1. "Classic" local signs

  a. Pain

  b. Heat

  c. Swelling

  d. Redness

 2. Occasional low grade fever

- Differential Diagnosis

 1. Lymphangitis

 2. Cellulitis

 3. Ruptured Plantaris tendon

- Physical Findings

 1. Palpable cord along course of saphenous vein

 2. Positive Homan sign (pain with foot dorsiflexion)

 3. Inflammation (local redness, heat, pain)

 4. Swelling, e.g., extremities unequal circumference

- Diagnostic Tests/Findings

 1. Deep venous thrombophlebitis (DVT)

  a. Venography

  b. Doppler ultrasound

 2. Superficial—none indicated

- Management/Treatment

 1. DVT

    a. Bed rest

    b. Elevation of affected area

    c. Local heat application

    d. Anticoagulation therapy

2. Superficial thrombophlebitis

    a. Restricted activity

    b. Local heat application

    c. Anti-inflammatory drugs

Gastrointestinal

Peptic Ulcer Disease

- Definition: Circumscribed, chronic ulcerations in the mucosal lining of the duodenum or stomach, most commonly the duodenum
- Etiology/Incidence
  1. Etiology—exact etiology unexplained
     a. Known aggravating/risk factors
        (1) Hypersecretion of gastric acid
        (2) Hyposecretion of gastric HCO_2
        (3) Increased pepsinogen levels
        (4) Corticosteroid or anti-inflammatory drugs
        (5) Familial predisposition
        (6) *Helicobacter pylori*
     b. Known protective factors
        (1) Bicarbonate production
        (2) Cell repair and regeneration
        (3) Local prostaglandins
        (4) Mucus production

        (5) Blood flow

  2. Incidence

      a. Estimated 5-10% in general population

      b. Affects men 4 times more often than women

      c. Hospitalization and mortality rates have been greatly reduced by improvements in management

- Signs and Symptoms

  1. Pain

      a. Localized, high epigastric; burning or gnawing in nature

      b. Increased with empty stomach, early a.m.

      c. Decreases with food intake

      d. Intermittent, periodic in nature

  2. GI bleeding evidenced in stools or vomitus

  3. Nausea

- Differential Diagnosis

  1. Early appendicitis

  2. Cholecystitis/hepatitis/hepatomegaly

  3. Pancreatitis

  4. Perforated ulcer, obstruction

  5. Angina

- Physical Findings

  1. Uncomplicated duodenal ulcer

      a. Usually entirely normal

      b. Occasional epigastric tenderness

  2. Complications (perforation, penetration)

      a. Abdomen tense, rigid

      b. Vital signs may reflect bleeding, shock (tachycardia, tachypnea, hypotension)

- Diagnostic Tests/Findings

1. Stool for occult blood—positive in 20-70%

2. Hematocrit—evaluate for anemia due to blood loss

3. Fasting serum gastrin normal in uncomplicated duodenal ulcer

4. Endoscopy

5. Upper GI series

6. Abdominal ultrasound

- Management/Treatment

   1. Refer

      a. Acute or severe abdominal pain

      b. Constant pain, vomiting

      c. Over 35 years old with atypical or prolonged symptoms

   2. Treatment

      a. Non-pharmacologic

         (1) Diet—decrease caffeine, acidic foods

         (2) Lifestyle changes—decrease alcohol, smoking

         (3) Stress management

      b. Pharmacologic

         (1) Avoid aspirin and non-steroidal anti-inflammatory agents (NSAIDS)

         (2) Antacids

         (3) Histamine (H_2) Receptor blockers—inhibit gastric acid secretion

            (a) Ranitidine (Zantac)

            (b) Cimetidine (Tagamet)

         (4) Coating agents, e.g., sucralfate

Constipation

- Definition: Infrequent and difficult defecation of hard stools and sensation of incomplete evacuation or straining

- Etiology/Incidence
    1. Causes
        a. Simple
            (1) Low fiber diet
            (2) Laxative overuse
            (3) Inactivity
            (4) Dehydration
            (5) Poor abdominal/pelvic floor musculature
        b. Secondary (acute)
            (1) Obstructive pathology, e.g., cancer
            (2) Neurologic disorder
            (3) Systemic disease or condition, e.g., hypothyroidism, pregnancy
            (4) Medications, e.g., iron, antidepressants
    2. Prevalence
        a. Unknown due to frequent self-treatment, but very commonly reported
        b. More common in women
- Signs and Symptoms
    1. Simple and/or intermittent
        a. Often asymptomatic
        b. Typically fewer than 3 bowel movements per week
        c. Hard feces
    2. Long standing/chronic constipation
        a. Hemorrhoids
        b. Cathartic colon
- Differential Diagnosis
    1. Intestinal pathology

2. Chronic or systemic disease

3. Obstruction

4. Medication/drug use

- Physical Findings

  1. Firm to hard stool present in rectum

  2. Fecal impaction

  3. Abdomen

     a. Normal bowel sounds

     b. Non-tender with simple constipation

- Diagnostic Tests/Findings

  1. Occult blood negative times 3 samples

  2. Rule out suspected underlying disease

     a. Thyroid function

     b. Barium enema

     c. Flexible fiberoptic sigmoidoscopy

- Management/Treatment

  1. Refer any suspected systemic disease or obstructive pathology

  2. Patient education

     a. Prompt response to "urge"

     b. Stress importance of minimal reliance on laxatives

  3. Non-pharmacologic

     a. Increase fluid intake

     b. Exercise

     c. High fiber diet

  4. Pharmacologic

     a. Bulk-forming agents, e.g., Psyllium seed

     b. Stool softeners, e.g., Docusate sodium

Diarrhea

- Definition: Defecation of loose, watery stool; usually frequent evacuation, and increased volume of stool
- Etiology/Incidence
    1. Causes
        a. Viral or bacterial gastroenteritis
        b. Parasites
        c. Medications, e.g., antibiotics
        d. Irritable bowel syndrome
    2. Prevalence
        a. Unknown in general population due to frequent self-treatment
        b. One of most frequent diagnoses in ambulatory care
- Signs and Symptoms
    1. Often abrupt onset
    2. May be accompanied by nausea and vomiting
    3. Crampy abdominal pain
    4. Increased frequency and volume of stools
- Differential Diagnosis
    1. Appendicitis
    2. Acute cholecystitis
    3. Inflammatory bowel disorder, e.g., ulcerative colitis
- Physical Findings
    1. Usually normal
    2. Occasional, low-grade fever, malaise
    3. Hyperactive bowel sounds
    4. Palpation—may have some abdominal tenderness
- Diagnostic Tests/Findings
    1. Usually none indicated for simple diarrhea

2. If persistent or chronic:

    a. Stool evaluation for cause

        (1) Fecal leukocyte exam—leukocytes present if bacterial cause

        (2) Ova and parasites

        (3) Cultures

    b. HIV testing

    c. Liver function and prothrombin time

- Management/Treatment

1. Usually self-limited

2. Non-pharmacologic

    a. Observation

    b. Hydration/electrolyte replacement

3. Pharmacologic

    a. Antidiarrheal drugs, e.g., Bismuth subsalicylate

    b. Absorbents, e.g., Kaopectate

    c. Salicylates—in ulcerative colitis types

    d. Antibiotics

        (1) Indicated when pathogen identifiable

        (2) May exacerbate simple episode

4. Refer—signs of serious disease

    a. Blood or mucus in stools

    b. Clinical dehydration

    c. Irreversible or progressive symptoms

Hemorrhoids

- Definition

1. Varicosities and stretched mucosal/submucosal tissue protruding into anal canal

2. Types

    a. Internal

        (1) Originate above anorectal line

        (2) Covered by rectal mucosa

    b. External

        (1) Originate below anorectal line

        (2) Covered by anal skin

- Etiology/Incidence

    1. Contributing factors

        a. Pressure associated with constipation

        b. Pelvic congestion

        c. Poor pelvic floor musculature

    2. One of most common anorectal conditions

- Signs and Symptoms

    1. Internal—painless, bright red bleeding with defecation

    2. External—itching, pain and bleeding with defecation

    3. Exacerbated by constipation or diarrhea

- Differential Diagnosis

    1. Condyloma acuminata

    2. Rectal prolapse

    3. Rule out other causes for bleeding

        a. Colorectal cancer

        b. Polyps

        c. Anal fissure

        d. Inflammatory bowel disease

        e. Colonic diverticulitis

- Physical Findings

    1. Internal

      a. Usually not visible unless prolapsed

      b. Usually not palpable unless thrombosed

  2. External

      a. Protrude with straining or standing

      b. If thrombosed, blue, shiny masses at anus

      c. Painless, flaccid skin tags (resolved thrombotic hemorrhoids)

- Diagnostic Tests/Findings

  1. Sigmoidoscopy

  2. Anoscopy reveals bright red to purplish bulges

- Management/Treatment

  1. Asymptomatic—no treatment

  2. Symptomatic

      a. Pharmacologic

         (1) Anesthetic, astringent, or steroidal suppositories

         (2) Bulk-forming agents

         (3) Stool softeners

      b. Non-pharmacologic—Sitz baths

      c. Patient education

         (1) Regulation of bowel habits

         (2) Increase bulk/fiber/fluids in diet

      d. Refer

         (1) Acute thrombosis of an external hemorrhoid

         (2) Irreducible prolapse

Functional Bowel Syndrome (Irritable Bowel Syndrome)

- Definition: A physiologic disorder of bowel dysfunction, often occurring intermittently

- Etiology/Incidence

  1. Cause unknown, although commonly associated with stress

    2. Prevalence

        a. As high as 15% in general population

        b. As high as 30% in young adults

- Signs and Symptoms

    1. Diarrhea and constipation, alternately

    2. No weight loss

    3. Flatulence

    4. Intermittent, with exacerbations associated with stress, travel, dietary change

    5. Highly diagnostic

        a. Abdominal distention, discomfort

        b. Frequent loose stools with abdominal pain

        c. Decreased pain following defecation

        d. Mucus in stool

        e. Feeling of incomplete evacuation

- Differential Diagnosis

    1. Lactose intolerance

    2. Intestinal neoplasia

    3. Infectious disease/parasitic infestation

    4. Inflammatory disease (ulcerative colitis, Crohn Disease)

    5. Laxative abuse

- Physical Findings

    1. Diagnosis largely one of exclusion

    2. No findings of organomegaly, rebound tenderness, or abdominal mass

- Diagnostic Tests/Findings

    1. Younger clients with brief episodes—none indicated

    2. Older patients

        a. Fecal occult blood—results should be negative

    b. Sigmoidoscopy and/or barium enema

- Management/Treatment
  1. Refer
     a. Older patients with recent onset of symptoms
     b. Presence of bloody or greasy stools
     c. Pain unrelieved by defecation
     d. Weight loss
     e. Fever
  2. Non-pharmacologic
     a. Reassurance—benign nature of disease
     b. Diet
        (1) Decrease caffeine, gas forming foods
        (2) Increase fiber/bulk/fluids with constipation
        (3) Low-residue diet with diarrhea
     c. Stress management, relaxation techniques, identify "triggers"
     d. Exercise
  3. Pharmacologic
     a. Anticholinergics
     b. Antianxiety agents

Appendicitis

- Definition: Inflammation of the vermiform appendix; may be acute, subacute, or chronic
- Etiology/Incidence
  1. Causes
     a. Fecalith
     b. Stricture
     c. Inflammation
     d. Neoplasm

2. More acute among < 5 year-olds and > 50 year-olds

3. More common among males

- Signs and Symptoms

   1. Acute

      a. Abdominal pain, generalized, periumbilical

      b. Nausea and vomiting follow onset of pain within a few hours

      c. Pain localizes to right lower quadrant (RLQ) with rigidity over right rectus muscle

      d. Tenderness over McBurney's point

   2. Subacute: Symptoms milder and subside after 24-36 hours

   3. Chronic

      a. May follow an acute episode

      b. Gastric indigestion

      c. RLQ tenderness

- Differential Diagnosis

   1. Ovarian etiology, e.g., mittelschmerz, cyst

   2. Ectopic pregnancy

   3. Pelvic inflammatory disease

   4. Pyelonephritis

- Physical Findings

   1. Fever of 99-100°F (> 100°F may indicate peritonitis)

   2. Guarding and rebound tenderness

   3. Absent bowel sounds

   4. Positive iliopsoas sign (pain with pressure applied to upper leg when flexed)

   5. Pelvic and rectal examination—RLQ tenderness

- Diagnostic Tests/Findings

   1. Complete blood count with differential—leukocytosis and shift to left

   2. Negative highly sensitive pregnancy test

3. Abdominal ultrasound and x-ray

- Management/Treatment

  1. Refer if strong suspicion—surgery consult needed within hours

  2. Withhold food, drink, local heat, cathartics, enema

Endocrine Diseases

Diabetes Mellitus

- Definition

  1. A syndrome encompassing a heterogeneous group of chronic diseases characterized by hyperglycemia and associated with vascular complications; insulin deficiency results in faulty metabolism of carbohydrates, fats and proteins

  2. Types

     a. Type I—Insulin-Dependent Diabetes Mellitus (IDDM)

     b. Type II—Non-Insulin-Dependent Diabetes Mellitus (NIDDM)

     c. Other—Gestational; < 10% of cases

  3. Complications

     a. Microvascular lesions (retinopathy, neuropathy, nephropathy)

     b. Macrovascular lesions (accelerated cardiovascular disease)

- Etiology/Incidence

  1. Primary mechanism of disease is abnormal carbohydrate metabolism due to either lack of insulin production or poor insulin utilization

  2. Risks for developing diabetes

     a. Impaired glucose tolerance (normally decreases with age)

     b. Obesity

     c. Specific genetic risk for Type I disease

        (1) Monozygotic twin of individual with Type I (50% concordance)

(2) Sibling of individual with Type I

(3) Offspring of individual with Type I

d. Specific genetic risks for Type II disease

(1) Monozygotic twin of individual with Type II (> 90% concordance)

(2) First degree relative with Type II

(3) Mother of neonate > 9.0 pounds

(4) Racial/ethnic groups

(a) American Indian, especially Pima of Southwestern U.S.

(b) Hispanic

(c) African-American women > 50 years old

3. Between 3-7% of population affected

- Signs and Symptoms

1. "Classic" symptoms

a. Polyuria

b. Polydipsia

c. Polyphagia

2. Weight loss

3. Fatigue and/or weakness

4. Persistent/recurrent candida vaginitis

5. Blurred vision

6. Type II sometimes asymptomatic in early stages

- Differential Diagnosis—Type I vs Type II differentiation usually based on clinical presentation

- Physical Findings

1. Early

a. Over or underweight

Table 1

COMPARISON OF FEATURES OF TYPE I AND TYPE II DIABETES MELLITUS

TYPE I (IDDM)	TYPE II (NIDDM)
No insulin response	Deficient insulin response
Require insulin replacement—ketoacidosis develops w/o it	Relative lack of insulin—no ketoacidosis
Onset more often < 35 years old	Onset > 35 years, ethnic risk
Circulating anti-islet cell antibodies	No increase in antibodies
Fasting insulin levels low—poor response to glucose challenge	Fasting insulin levels high—good response to glucose and glucagon challenge
Thinness common	Obesity common
Orthostatic hypotension	Mild-moderate hypotension

      b. Orthostatic hypotension

      c. Hypertension

      d. Infections

  2. Late

      a. Ulcerations

      b. Absent peripheral hair

      c. Retinopathy, cataracts, glaucoma

      d. Decreased deep tendon reflexes (DTRs)

      e. Foot drop

      f. Decreased circulation, decreased pedal pulses

- Diagnostic Tests/Findings

  1. Random plasma glucose ≥ 200 mg/dL, *OR*

  2. On more than one occasion, fasting plasma glucose ≥ 140 mg/dL, or fasting venous glucose ≥ 120 mg/dL, or fasting capillary glucose ≥ 120 mg/dL, *OR*

  3. Abnormal glucose tolerance test (GTT)

- Management/Treatment

  1. Goals primarily achieved by glucose control

      a. Improve patient well-being

      b. Prevent complications

2. Refer all newly diagnosed cases for complete evaluation

3. Type I and II

    a. Diet

        (1) Regulate carbohydrate (CHO) intake

        (2) Maintain ideal weight

    b. Patient education

        (1) Assure compliance with regimen

        (2) Avoid long-term complications

        (3) Signs of hypo/hyperglycemia

        (4) Foot care

    c. Exercise

        (1) Increases insulin sensitivity

        (2) Improves cellular uptake of glucose

4. Pharmacologic

    a. Type I

        (1) Insulin replacement sufficient to metabolize CHO intake

        (2) Self-monitor blood glucose to adjust dose

    b. Type II—oral hypoglycemic agents (sulfonylureas)

        (1) 1st generation

            (a) Increases insulin release

            (b) Chlorpropamide (Diabinese)

        (2) 2nd generation

            (a) Glyburide (Micronase); glipizide (Glucotrol)

            (b) Increases insulin sensitivity

        (3) Glucagon

Hyperthyroidism

- Definition: A hypermetabolic syndrome affecting all body systems characterized by excess circulating thyroid hormone

- Etiology/Incidence
  1. Causes
     a. Graves' disease (thyrotoxicosis, simple goiter)
        (1) Comprise 90% of hyperthyroid cases
        (2) Disproportionately affects women 30-50 years of age
        (3) Autoimmune mechanism
     b. Thyroiditis
     c. Toxic multinodular goiter
     d. Toxic unilateral goiter (adenoma)
  2. More common among women
- Signs and Symptoms
  1. Nonspecific, affecting all body systems
  2. Generally reflect increased or excess thyroid stimulation
  3. Anxiety, nervousness, distractibility
  4. Fine tremor, hyperreflexia
  5. Skin warm, moist, smooth; heat intolerance
  6. Hair fine, thin
  7. Cardiac palpitations, tachycardia
  8. Dyspnea, hyperventilation at rest
  9. Increased GI motility, diarrhea
  10. Increased appetite with concomitant mild weight loss
  11. Oligo/amenorrhea in women; impotence or decreased libido in men
  12. Fatigue, weakness—especially of proximal muscles
- Differential Diagnosis—focus on differentiating among causes of thyroid enlargement
  1. Graves' disease
     a. Symmetrical and moderate thyroid enlargement
     b. Exophthalmos, lid lag

      c. Pretibial myxedema (non-pitting edema)

      d. Forty to sixty percent become euthyroid after initial one year treatment

  2. Thyroiditis

      a. Slight enlargement of thyroid gland

      b. Slightly tender to painful

  3. Adenoma (toxic multinodular goiter)

      a. Large solitary nodule $\geq$ 3 cm

      b. Gradually enlarging gland, asymmetrical

      c. Insidious symptoms

      d. No myxedema

      e. No exophthalmos

- Physical Findings

  1. Enlarged thyroid gland; possible bruit over gland

  2. Hyperactive deep tendon reflexes (DTR), tremor

  3. Erythema

  4. Arrhythmias—sinus tachycardia, atrial fibrillation

  5. Systolic flow murmur

  6. Exophthalmos, lid lag

  7. Increased bowel sounds

- Diagnostic Tests/Findings

  1. Serum total T_4 elevated

  2. Serum total T_3 elevated

  3. Serum free T_3 elevated, confirms diagnosis

  4. TSH undetectable, unless pituitary disease is present

  5. Radio-iodine uptake usually elevated

- Management/Treatment

  1. Refer new cases for full evaluation and initiation of therapy

2. Graves' Disease

    a. Antithyroid drugs

        (1) Propylthiouracil, methimazole

        (2) Do not give if cardiac disease present

    b. Thyroid ablation with I^{131}

3. Thyroiditis

    a. Often transient, no treatment required

    b. Analgesics, e.g., acetaminophen

    c. Prednisone

4. Toxic multinodular goiter—ablation

5. Adenoma—ablation

6. Education

    a. Diet—increased need for calories

    b. Decrease stimulants

    c. Signs/symptoms of thyroid storm

Hypothyroidism

- Definition: A metabolic syndrome affecting all organ systems characterized by deficient levels of circulating thyroid hormone; may be primary or secondary

- Etiology/Incidence

    1. Primary (thyroidal)—true hypothyroidism

    2. Secondary—pituitary or hypothalamic disease

    3. Eight to ten times more prevalent in females

    4. More often affects those over age 30

- Signs and Symptoms

    1. Often subclinical and nonspecific

    2. Reflect slowed physiologic functioning, affecting all organ systems

    3. Fatigue, lethargy, diminished mental activity

4. Skin cool, dry, pale; cold intolerant

5. Hair dry, brittle

6. Dyspnea on exertion

7. Constipation, abdominal distention

8. Amenorrhea, infertility

9. Arthralgias, muscle cramps

- Differential Diagnosis

    1. Focus on determining possible causes

    2. Primary vs secondary, e.g., pituitary tumor

    3. Transient—history of thyroid blocking drugs, subtotal thyroidectomy

    4. Permanent—history of thyroid destructive process, e.g., irradiation, surgery

- Physical Findings

    1. Thyroid often enlarged

    2. Slow speech, expressionless face

    3. Enlarged tongue and larynx with advanced disease

    4. Galactorrhea

    5. Hearing loss

    6. Edema, especially periorbital ("myxedema")

    7. Paresthesia, neuropathy, carpal tunnel syndrome

    8. Bradycardia

    9. Mild weight gain

    10. Anemia

    11. Diminished bowel sounds

    12. Decreased DTR

- Diagnostic Tests/Findings—see Table 2

    1. Serum free T_4 or T_4 concentration low (specific to hypothyroidism)

    2. TSH high; confirms diagnosis of hypothyroidism

    3. Hypercholesteremia

Table 2

COMPARISON OF LABORATORY VALUES IN THYROID DISEASE

HYPERTHYROIDISM	*HYPOTHYROIDISM*
Serum total T_3 - high	Serum total T_3 - normal
Serum free T_3 - high	Serum free T_3 - normal
Serum total T_4 - high	Serum total T_4 - low
TSH- absent	TSH - high

- Management/Treatment
    1. Primary
        a. Desiccated thyroid hormone
        b. Synthetic thyroid; Sodium liothyronine, Sodium levothyroxine
        c. Monitor T_4 levels and adjust as needed
    2. Refer all secondary causes for evaluation

Thyroid Nodule

- Definition: Solitary or multinodular mass found on examination of thyroid gland in patient with euthyroid status
- Etiology/Incidence
    1. Usually an adenoma, cyst, or nodule that is part of an unrecognized multinodular goiter
    2. Rarely carcinoma
    3. Common; affects about 3% of adults
- Signs and symptoms
    1. Asymptomatic mass
    2. Occasionally pain, dysphagia, hoarseness
- Differential Diagnosis
    1. Cancer
    2. Thyroiditis
- Physical Findings
    1. Asymmetric neck mass
    2. Fixation of nodule to underlying tissue

    3. Hard consistency

    4. Cervical lymphadenopathy

- Diagnostic Tests/Findings

    1. Adenoma

        a. Serum T_4 concentration high

        b. T_3 resin uptake high

    2. Carcinoma

        a. Serum calcitonin elevated

        b. Fine needle aspiration (FNA) biopsy

- Management/Treatment

    1. Monitor for changes

    2. Surgery or suppression with exogenous thyroid

    3. Refer for suspected malignancy

        a. Family history of medullary thyroid cancer

        b. "Hard," fixed nodule

        c. Distant metastasis

        d. Vocal cord paralysis

Infectious Diseases

Acquired Immune Deficiency Syndrome (AIDS)

- Definition

    1. End stage of a spectrum of infection with the Human Immunodeficiency Virus (HIV); complex disease syndrome with variable and unpredictable intervals between infection, onset of symptoms, and death

    2. Several conditions and opportunistic infections occur consistent with immunosuppression

        a. Kaposi sarcoma (KS)

    b. *Pneumocystis carinii* pneumonia (PCP)

    c. Tuberculosis

- Etiology/Incidence

  1. Cause

    a. HIV is transmitted through direct contact with infected blood, blood products and other body fluids.

    b. Risks for acquiring HIV/AIDS

      (1) Exposure to HIV positive individual(s) through unprotected or traumatic sexual activity (multiple or bisexual partners, anal intercourse, sex partner of one who has multiple or bisexual partners)

      (2) Infant of HIV positive mother (20-30% of infants are positive after 18 months)

      (3) Intravenous drug use, sharing needles

      (4) Transfusion of blood or blood products, primarily prior to 1985

  2. Prevalence—diagnosed AIDS cases represent "tip of the iceberg" epidemiologically

    a. Prevalence of HIV infection is unknown in general population due to reluctance to disclose HIV status, reluctance to seek testing, and long asymptomatic interval between infection and clinical manifestations

    b. Diagnosed AIDS rising faster among women than any other group

- Signs and Symptoms

  1. Initial infection and seroconversion

    a. Moderate "flu-like" syndrome 10-30 days after inoculation

    b. Self-limited; patients rarely seek care

    c. Asymptomatic though transmissible period of variable length followsc

    d. Four to six month "window" before blood screening will indicate infection has occurred

2. Progression of HIV positive to AIDS

    a. Two to twelve year asymptomatic interval

    b. Influenced by general physical condition, age, mitigating drug therapy

    c. Appearance of symptoms reflects opportunistic disease

3. Early nonspecific symptoms of progression to AIDS

    a. Fatigue

    b. Rapid weight loss

    c. Night sweats

    d. Arthralgia

    e. Diarrhea

    f. Neurologic manifestations

    g. Gynecologic abnormalities

        (1) Persistent vaginal moniliasis

        (2) Rapidly progressing abnormal Pap

4. *Pneumocystis carinii* pneumonia (PCP)

    a. Dyspnea

    b. Dry cough

5. Kaposi sarcoma (KS)

    a. Patchy, painless skin eruptions; bluish, brown-red, purple

    b. Lesions commonly located on arms, legs, mouth, nose, anus

- Differential Diagnosis

    1. Lymphomas

    2. Pneumonia

    3. Tuberculosis

    4. Chronic fatigue syndrome

    5. Mononucleosis

- Physical Findings

1. Lymphadenopathy
2. Skin lesions
   a. Noninfectious—drug eruptions, malnourishment
   b. Infectious—fungal, viral (herpes), bacterial
   c. Neoplastic—Kaposi sarcoma
3. Oral or vaginal monilia
4. Cervical dysplasia, invasive cancer
5. Fever

- Diagnostic Tests/Findings
  1. Blood testing
     a. Enzyme-Linked Immunosorbent Assay ("ELISA")—positive for antibodies
     b. Western Blot detects HIV presence, confirms ELISA
     c. CD4 lymphocyte count monitors immune function, and stage of disease
        (1) $\geq$ 600 cells/μL normal
        (2) 200-500 cells/μL likely symptomatic
  2. TB skin test—ascertain concomitant opportunistic infection; possible false negative due to severe immunosuppression
  3. Tissue biopsies of suspicious skin lesions
  4. Chest x-ray to evaluate respiratory complaints, positive PPD

- Management/Treatment
  1. Refer all cases for full evaluation
  2. Pharmacologic
     a. Zidovudine
        (1) May retard development and progression of symptoms
        (2) Controversial prophylactic use following known exposure to reduce risk of seroconversion
        (3) Potential use to reduce perinatal transmission

      b. Didanosine

      c. Immunize early in course of infection against

         (1) Hepatitis B

         (2) Pneumococcus

         (3) Influenza (annually)

  3. Non-pharmacologic

      a. Treat diarrhea, fever symptomatically

      b. Frequent Pap smears, colposcopy, as indicated

  4. Client education

      a. Discuss lifelong ability to transmit the virus

      b. Explain modes of transmission

      c. Teach effective ways to reduce fluid exchange

         (1) Breastfeeding contraindicated

         (2) Encourage abstinence, "safer sex"

      d. Emphasize behaviors that protect and enhance immune system

         (1) Stop tobacco, street drug, alcohol use

         (2) Nutritious diet

         (3) Reduce/manage stress

         (4) Exercise as tolerated

Hepatitis

- Definition: Generic term indicating inflammation in the liver, resulting in necrosis and bile stasis; may result from a number of causes, most often viral; consists of four clinical stages

- Etiology/Incidence

  1. Five viral types

      a. Hepatitis A virus (HAV); antiquated term "infectious"

         (1) Spread person-to-person, fecal-oral

         (2) Incubation period 2-6 weeks

   (3) Self-limited, no carrier state or chronic liver disease results

   (4) Accounts for < 10% hepatitis

  b. Hepatitis B virus (HBV); antiquated term "serum"

   (1) Transmitted in blood, blood products, and infected body fluids (saliva, semen) by parenteral, sexual, perinatal exposure

   (2) Incubation period 4-24 weeks

   (3) Up to 10% of infected become chronic carriers; increased risk of cirrhosis, hepatocellular carcinoma

  c. Hepatitis C virus (HCV)

   (1) Transmitted by sexual contact, blood exchange

   (2) Incubation 3-15 weeks

   (3) Majority of post-transfusion cases

  d. Hepatitis D virus (HDV); "Delta"

   (1) Occurs only in those infected with HBV

   (2) Worsens existing HBV

  e. Hepatitis E virus (HEV)

   (1) Waterborne

   (2) Endemic in developing countries

 2. A common liver disease, rising in incidence over the past 20 years

 3. Incidence estimated at 0.25/1,000 population

- Signs and Symptoms

 1. All viral types produce very similar syndromes

  a. Phase 1: Incubation

   (1) Asymptomatic

   (2) May last weeks to months (see above)

  b. Phase 2: Preicteric (Prodromal)

   (1) 3-10 days in length

   (2) Malaise, fatigue

     (3) Anorexia, nausea and vomiting

     (4) "Flu-like" achiness, headache

   c. Phase 3: Icteric

     (1) Two to six weeks in length

     (2) Dark-colored urine

     (3) Clay-colored stools

     (4) Jaundice of skin, sclera, nail beds

     (5) Pruritus, rash

     (6) Upper right quadrant pain

   d. Phase 4: Convalescence

     (1) May last weeks to months

     (2) Possible chronic disease develops

     (3) HBV may be fatal

- Differential Diagnosis
  1. Mononucleosis
  2. Cancer
  3. Obstructive jaundice
  4. Alcoholic hepatitis/cirrhosis
  5. Hepatotoxic drugs
- Physical Findings
  1. Occasional urticaria, erythematous rash
  2. Occasional bradycardia
  3. Occasional liver enlargement and tenderness
  4. Low-grade fever
- Diagnostic Tests/Findings
  1. Viral serologies for typing
  2. Lactic dehydrogenase (LDA) mildly elevated
  3. Urinalysis

     a. Proteinuria

     b. Bilirubinemia

     c. Hematuria

  4. Abnormal liver function tests

     a. Alanine aminotransferase (ALT) *and*

     b. Aspartate aminotransferase (AST) dramatically elevated (20-50 times normal)

     c. Serum bilirubin, LDH, prothrombin time—normal or slightly elevated

- Management/Treatment

  1. Non-pharmacologic

     a. Bedrest

     b. Hydration (3,000-4,000 mL fluid/day)

     c. Bland, high protein/carbohydrate/calorie diet

  2. Pharmacologic

     a. Discontinue all but essential medications

     b. Analgesics, antiemetics if needed

  3. Teaching

     a. Careful disposal of infected wastes

     b. Improved hand-washing, food handling techniques

     c. Inoculation of contacts, household members

Tuberculosis (TB)

- Definition: A destructive, communicable disease transmitted by inhaled infectious droplets, primarily affecting the lungs, but ultimately becoming systemic and causing erosion and destruction in distant sites
- Etiology/Incidence

  1. Cause—inhalation of droplets carrying *Mycobacterium tuberculosis*

  2. Prevalence

      a. Decline in U.S. until 1985; now rising; multidrug resistant TB is a serious public health problem

      b. More than 26,000 active cases reported 1992

      c. Prevalence of asymptomatic infected state many times higher

      d. Highest incidence among immigrants, homeless, incarcerated, intravenous drug users, people with HIV/AIDS or otherwise immunocompromised status

- Signs and Symptoms

  1. Infection with *M. tuberculosis*

     a. Asymptomatic state lasting months to years

     b. 10% of infected go on to develop active TB

  2. Active TB

     a. Generalized symptoms

        (1) Night sweats, fever

        (2) Malaise, weakness

        (3) Anorexia

        (4) Weight loss

        (5) Ill appearance, cachectic

     b. Pulmonary symptoms

        (1) Productive cough

        (2) Chest pain

        (3) Dyspnea

     c. Systemic symptoms (extra-pulmonary sites)

        (1) Pelvic pain, pelvic inflammatory disease (PID)

        (2) Menstrual changes

        (3) Skin eruptions, abscesses

        (4) Flank pain

- Differential Diagnosis

  1. Pulmonary vs extra-pulmonary sites

2. Malignancy

3. Silicosis, histoplasmosis

4. Chronic obstructive pulmonary disease

5. Pneumonia

- Physical Findings

    1. Generally normal appearance in early disease

    2. Chest auscultation—rales, bronchial breath sounds, diminished sounds over affected areas

    3. Unexplained fever

    4. Advanced disease

        a. Purulent green or yellow sputum

        b. Hemoptysis

- Diagnostic Tests/Findings

    1. PPD skin test (antigen response) usually indicates infection, not active disease

    2. PPD positive if diameter of induration (not erythema), measured 48-72 hours after inoculation is:

        a. ≥ 5 mm among

            (1) Immunocompromised/immunosuppressed

            (2) Abnormal chest x-ray consistent with TB

            (3) Recent close contact with infectious TB

        b. ≥ 10 mm among

            (1) Immigrants from areas with high TB prevalence

            (2) Intravenous drug users

            (3) Very low socioeconomic status, homeless

            (4) Aged, nursing home resident or incarcerated

            (5) Individuals with chronic disease

        c. ≥ 15 mm among general population

        d. Conversion to active disease

(1) Change in PPD from < 10 mm to >10 mm, or increase by at least 10 mm

(2) Increase of at least 15 mm in > 35 year-old

3. Chest x-ray—apical lesions, pulmonary infiltrates

4. Sputum smear or culture positive times 3, confirms TB diagnosis

5. Gastric aspiration—culture for acid-fast bacillus

- Management/Treatment

    1. Refer all cases to health department for thorough evaluation and initiation of treatment

    2. Pharmacologic

        a. Preventive treatment

            (1) Prevents progression to active disease

            (2) Isoniazid (INH) or rifampin for 9-12 months

        b. Active disease

            (1) Two or more drugs *must* be used to account for resistant strains

            (2) INH and rifampin most commonly used

    3. Follow-up care

        a. Preventive

            (1) Monitor liver function if on INH

            (2) Stress importance of medication compliance

        b. Active

            (1) Monthly evaluation of sputum and chest

            (2) Chest x-ray every two years for life

        c. Special considerations

            (1) Pregnancy and breastfeeding

                (a) INH and Rifampin safe to use

                (b) Treatment of infant also indicated

            (2) Household contacts need evaluation and treatment as indicated

Miscellaneous Disorders

Headaches

- Definition
    1. Commonly reported experience of pain in cranium and/or neck area; may result from a variety of systemic or local problems; reported symptoms, severity, duration vary widely
    2. Classifications
        a. Primary—no underlying disease
            (1) Common primary headache syndromes
                (a) Tension/stress
                (b) Cluster (sometimes described as sub-type of migraine)
                (c) Migraine
        b. Secondary—identifiable underlying pathophysiology
- Etiology/Incidence
    1. Eighty percent of population report at least one per year
    2. Fifty percent have severe, recurring headaches
    3. Causal mechanism not precisely known
    4. Tension headache—pain from vasoconstriction and muscular spasm
        a. Comprises about 90% of reported headaches
        b. Affects females 3 times more than males
    5. Cluster headache—affects males, especially over 50 years old, more than females
    6. Migraine headache
        a. Results from arterial spasm and dilation
        b. Affects 4-15% of the population; females 3 times more than males
- Signs and Symptoms

1. Tension headache

    a. Onset gradual

    b. Frequency—episodic, daily or frequent, worse in late afternoon

    c. Duration—variable

    d. Pain quality—dull, pressure, constant, variable intensity

    e. Location—diffuse, bilateral, often frontal

    f. Associated symptoms—tension, restlessness, insomnia, neck and shoulder spasms

2. Cluster headache

    a. Onset—nocturnal, awakens with pain

    b. Frequency—occurs in clusters lasting a few weeks with remissions lasting weeks to months

    c. Duration—15 minutes to several hours

    d. Pain quality—abrupt, intense

    e. Location—unilateral, always same side, retro-orbital, sometimes radiating

    f. Associated symptoms—facial pain, ptosis of the affected side, lacrimation

3. Migraine

    a. Onset—sometimes preceded by a prodrome or neurological aura; occasionally associated with "trigger" events, e.g., menses, foods; may awaken with pain

    b. Frequency—recurrent, infrequent to daily

    c. Duration—2 to 12 hours

    d. Pain quality—severe, peaks after first 1-2 hours

    e. Location—unilateral tendency, may alternate sides; frontal, temporal, or orbital

    f. Associated symptoms—photophobia, GI upset, fatigue, chills

- Differential Diagnosis

    1. Rule out brain mass, subarachnoid hemorrhage, meningitis

2. Toxic effects of drugs

3. Hypertension

4. Sinus headache/sinusitis

- Physical Findings

  1. Non-specific, aimed at determining primary vs secondary headaches

  2. General appearance indicates discomfort

  3. Neurological assessment normal in all types of primary headache

- Diagnostic Tests/Findings

  1. None indicated for tension headache

  2. Blood pressure, vital signs

  3. Skull, sinus, cervical x-ray helpful in selected cases of migraine

- Management/Treatment

  1. Refer for neurological studies when:

     a. Neurological exam is abnormal

     b. Specific secondary diagnosis is suspected

     c. Chronic headaches develop new features

     d. Atypical features are described

  2. Non-pharmacologic

     a. Modify trigger factors, food, stress, habits, hormonal or other medication

     b. Relaxation techniques, biofeedback, exercise

     c. Education for danger signs and emergency care

     d. Hypnosis

  3. Pharmacologic

     a. Mild/tension headache

        (1) Acetaminophen

        (2) Aspirin

     b. Mild-moderate migraine and recurring tension

        (1) Non-steroidal anti-inflammatory drugs (NSAIDS)—do not use in pregnancy

        (2) Anaprox

    c. Moderate-severe migraine

        (1) Sumatriptan (Imitrex), IM.

        (2) Ergotamine, sublingual or suppository

        (3) Propranolol

    d. Associated symptoms, e.g., nausea

        (1) Dramamine patch

        (2) Promethazine HCL (Phenergan) suppository

        (3) Prochlorperazine (Compazine) suppository

Trigeminal Neuralgia (Tic Douloureux)

- Definition: A painful condition characterized by paroxysms of stabbing facial pain radiating unilaterally along a branch of Cranial Nerve V (CN V/Trigeminal nerve)

- Etiology/Incidence

    1. Cause: Deterioration or pressure on CN V

    2. More common in patients > 50 years old, females

- Signs and Symptoms

    1. Pain—stabbing, flashing or radiating along CN V

    2. Episodic in nature; may be precipitated by cold, heat, chewing, brushing teeth, touching face

    3. Remissions last from weeks to months

    4. Unilateral; right side more common than left

    5. When active, occurs daily, with bouts lasting up to 5 minutes each

- Differential Diagnosis

    1. Neoplasm (tumor)

    2. Dental disease

3. Multiple sclerosis

4. Vascular lesions/temporal arteritis

- Physical Findings

    1. Facial trigger points may stimulate pain or facial spasms

    2. No other neurologic findings

- Diagnostic Tests/Findings

    1. Skull x-rays (basal, sinus, dental)

    2. CAT scan

- Management/Treatment

    1. Self-limited in about one-half of cases

    2. Refer for pharmacologic or surgical treatment

Lower Back Pain (Muscle Strain)

- Definition: Pain identified by patient as musculoskeletal in nature, felt in spinal column, most often in lumbosacral region, usually episodic

- Etiology/Incidence

    1. Usual cause—ligament or muscle strain, especially if presentation includes risk factors

    2. Risk factors include: Age < 35, sedentary lifestyle, obese, repetitive motion, poor body mechanics

    3. Estimated 65-70% of individuals experience at least one episode

- Signs and Symptoms

    1. Lumbosacral pain

    2. Limited movement due to pain

    3. Sudden onset associated with activity

- Differential Diagnosis

    1. Spinal tumor

    2. Herniated disc

    3. Fracture

  4. Osteoporosis

  5. Arthritis

- Physical Findings

  1. Neurologic examination *must* be normal to safely assume simple muscle strain

  2. Poor posture, some rigidity

  3. Gait possibly affected

  4. Normal pelvic, abdominal, rectal examination

  5. Lateral flexion unrestricted in simple strain; if present, indicative of herniated disc, fracture

- Diagnostic Tests/Findings—generally not indicated

- Management/Treatment

  1. Refer for any signs of disabling disease

  2. Acute

   a. Ice applications for 24 hours, then heat

   b. Massage

   c. Analgesics

   d. NSAIDS

  3. Exercises to improve tone once acute stage has passed—gentle stretching, abdominal "crunches"

  4. Client Education

   a. Medication regimen

   b. Weight reduction, if needed

   c. Moderate activity, proper lifting

Carpal Tunnel Syndrome

- Definition: Neuropathy of the median nerve manifesting as varying degrees of paresthesia of the hand and fingers, usually reversible

- Etiology/Incidence

1. Affects women twice as often as men

2. Caused by local swelling and entrapment of median nerve as it passes beneath the transverse carpal ligament

3. Associated risks

    a. Repetitive hand movement or wrist flexion in two-thirds of cases

    b. Pregnancy

- Signs and Symptoms

    1. Pain in hand and thumb, index, middle and median half of ring finger

    2. Worse at night

    3. Usually dominant hand

    4. Shaking or hanging hand decreases pain

    5. May radiate proximally along forearm

    6. Weakened pincer grip

- Differential Diagnosis

    1. Rule out underlying systemic disease (diabetes, hypothyroidism)

    2. Rule out edema secondary to pregnancy, congestive heart failure, trauma

- Physical Findings—usually none

- Diagnostic Tests/Findings

    1. Tinel sign positive (percussion of median nerve produces proximally radiating paresthesia)

    2. Phalen sign positive (wrist flexion increases paresthesia)

- Management/Treatment

    1. Wrist splint—immobilize hand and forearm

    2. Ergonomic work station and tools

    3. NSAIDS or other anti-inflammatory drugs (do not use in pregnancy)

    4. Diuretics if suspect cause is edema (do not use in pregnancy)

    5. Refer if no improvement for possible corticosteroid injection or surgical correction

Acne

- Definition: Skin condition affecting the upper body, characterized by formation of pustules and/or papules on erythematous base, and comedones (whiteheads)
- Etiology/Incidence
  1. Caused by increased sebaceous gland activity, usually beginning at puberty; increased sebum and skin bacteria produce inflammatory process
  2. Very common in teens (up to 90%)
- Signs and Symptoms
  1. Painful lesions
  2. Aggravated by stress, hot, humid environments
- Differential Diagnosis
  1. Rosacea
  2. Pyoderma
  3. Drug eruptions
  4. Underlying endocrine disease characterized by excess androgen production, e.g., Stein-Leventhal, Cushing syndrome
- Physical Findings
  1. Lesions
     a. Comedones
     b. Pustules, papules
     c. Scarring
     d. Cysts
  2. Distribution
     a. Face, neck
     b. Upper chest and back
- Diagnostic Tests/Findings—none indicated if adolescent or young adult
- Management/Treatment

1. Mild (comedones only)

   a. Meticulous cleansing

   b. Topical benzoyl peroxide, salicylic acid

   c. Topical antibiotics

      (1) Tetracycline solution

      (2) Clindamycin solution

2. Moderate (comedones, pustules, papules)

   a. Oral contraceptives in females

   b. Tetracycline 250 mg q.i.d., then b.i.d.

3. Severe (cystic)

   a. Isotretinoin (retinoic acid)—avoid pregnancy

   b. Intralesional corticosteroids

   c. Ultraviolet (UV) light treatments

Contact Dermatitis

- Definition: An inflammatory reaction evoked when the skin comes in contact with an irritant or allergen
- Etiology/Incidence
  1. Prevalence unknown in general population
  2. Nearly any substance can produce irritation
  3. Variables

     a. Dosage (concentration)

     b. Frequency of exposure

     c. Duration of exposure
- Signs and Symptoms
  1. Report of recent (within 24 hours) exposure to known allergens
  2. Dry skin
  3. Pain, burning sensation
  4. Pruritus

- Differential Diagnosis
  1. Tinea
  2. Bacterial eruptions (associated with stress, asthma, allergies)
  3. Atopic dermatitis eczema
  4. Psoriasis
  5. Scabies/pediculosis
  6. Secondary syphilis
- Physical Findings
  1. Acute—weeping vesicles, urticaria, rash, fissures, erythema
  2. Chronic—lichenification, occasionally hyperpigmentation
- Diagnostic Tests/Findings
  1. Usually none indicated
  2. VDRL—negative
  3. KOH preparation of skin scraping—negative
  4. Lesion—culture negative
- Management/Treatment
  1. Compresses/soaks—Burow solution, Epsom salts
  2. Drying lotions
  3. Topical corticosteroids after acute lesions heal
  4. Pain medication
  5. Antihistamines if pruritus is severe

Herpes Zoster ("Shingles")

- Definition: Inflammation of the dorsal root ganglia characterized by exquisitely painful, unilateral ulcerations; self-limited
- Etiology/Incidence
  1. Caused by reactivation of latent infection by varicella zoster virus in a partially immune host

2. Higher incidence among the elderly and immunocompromised individuals; estimated 10-20% of adults affected at some time in life

- Signs and Symptoms
    1. Malaise
    2. Burning unilateral pain, beginning several days prior to eruption of lesions
    3. Headache

- Differential Diagnosis
    1. Herpes simplex
    2. Eczema, dermatitis
    3. Hodgkin lymphoma
    4. HIV/AIDS

- Physical Findings
    1. Unilateral distribution of vesicular, herpetic lesions along nerve dermatome
    2. Occasional lesions on eyelids and corneas
    3. Adenopathy
    4. Fever

- Diagnostic Tests/Findings
    1. Not usually necessary for diagnosis
    2. Cytologic (Tzanck) smear from lesion for giant cells—not specific for Herpes Zoster

- Management/Treatment
    1. Analgesia
    2. Corticosteroids
    3. Acyclovir may speed resolution if started within 2-3 days of onset
    4. Sleeping medications
    5. Refer any face/eye lesions

Skin Cancer

- Definition
    1. Malignant neoplasms arising in skin cells
    2. Types
        a. Basal cell carcinoma—rarely metastatic, but locally invasive
        b. Squamous cell carcinoma
        c. Malignant melanoma—metastasizing
- Etiology/Incidence
    1. Basal cell carcinoma
        a. Accounts for about 75% of all skin cancers
        b. Associated with UV light exposure and light complexion
        c. Incidence increases with age
        d. Basal cell nevus syndrome (a rarer sub-type)— is congenital
    2. Squamous cell carcinoma
        a. Directly attributable to sun exposure or chronic irritation
        b. Second most common skin cancer
        c. Higher prevalence in oral cavity of smokers and drinkers
        d. Metastasis uncommon
    3. Malignant melanoma
        a. Accounts for 1-2% of all malignancies and is rising
        b. Caused by UV radiation damage to melanocytes—40-50% arise from pigmented moles
        c. Highest skin cancer mortality—two-thirds of skin cancer deaths
        d. Metastasis common
- Signs and Symptoms
    1. Basal cell carcinoma
        a. Painless, slow-growing lesions on exposed skin areas

b. Lesions eventually develop central ulcer with recurrent crusting, bleeding

2. Squamous cell carcinoma

a. Skin lesion that does not heal

b. Occurs on exposed skin, develops nodular or warty appearance

3. Melanoma

a. Usually pigmented lesions that increase in size

b. Pain

c. Pruritus

d. Bleeding

e. Mnemonic for suspicious moles or lesions (see General Assessment Chapter)

- Differential Diagnosis

1. Nevus

2. Sores slow to heal from other causess

- Physical Findings

1. Basal cell

a. Firm, smooth nodules

b. Slight elevation

c. Waxy to translucent

d. May ulcerate in center

2. Squamous cell

a. Ulcerated or healing with crusted appearance

b. Nodular or wart-like appearance over time

3. Melanoma

a. Pigmented lesions (blue, black, gray)

b. Central black papule or nodule with surrounding lentigo

c. Often irregular surface and borders

- Diagnostic Tests/Findings—biopsy confirms malignancy

- Management/Treatment
    1. Physician referral for excision and on-going care (radiation, chemotherapy, immunotherapy)
    2. Prevention
        a. Reduce exposure
            (1) Patient teaching to avoid sun exposure
            (2) PABA sun screen use or sun protective factor (SPF) ≥ 15
            (3) Protective clothing, sunglasses, hats
            (4) Educate about risks of tanning salons
        b. Self-examination—teach ABCD of skin self-examination

Hematologic

Iron Deficiency Anemia (IDA)

- Definition
    1. Low blood hemoglobin concentration due to inadequate intake or absorption of iron
    2. IDA is a microcytic, hypochromic anemia
    3. May be normocytic, normochromic in early stage
- Etiology/Incidence
    1. Causes
        a. Iron loss in excess of intake, e.g., overt or occult bleeding, menorrhagia, poor nutrition
        b. Rapid growth, e.g., adolescence
        c. Metabolic demands in excess of intake, e.g., pregnancy
        d. Impaired absorption of iron, e.g., post-gastrectomy, chronic diarrhea
    2. The most commonly identified nutritional disorder and anemia
        a. Ten to fifteen percent of premenopausal women are affected

      b. Thirty to fifty percent of pregnant women are affected

- Signs and Symptoms
  1. Asymptomatic unless severe, then nonspecific
  2. Fatigue, generalized weakness, dyspnea on exertion
- Differential Diagnosis
  1. Other microcytic anemias—Thalassemia
  2. Macrocytic anemias—B_{12} or folate deficiency
  3. Underlying chronic disease
  4. Lead poisoning
- Physical Findings
  1. Often none
  2. Skin or conjunctival pallor
  3. Glossitis, stomatitis
  4. Tachycardia with/without systolic flow murmur
  5. Tachypnea
  6. Nail changes
     - a. Spoon shaped (koilonychia)
     - b. Brittle, easily split
     - c. Flat, ridged
- Diagnostic Tests/Findings
  1. Routine hematocrit and hemoglobin screening (See General Assessment Chapter)
  2. Baseline CBC with indices, MCV, MCH, MCHC, and reticulocyte count
  3. Diagnostic: Low (< 12 µg/L) serum ferritin concentration (12-150 µg/L normal for women)
  4. Presence of hypochromic, microcytic red blood cells
- Management/Treatment
  1. Diet—increase iron intake

2. Oral replacement—ferrous sulfate 300 mg t.i.d. to q.i.d.

3. Recheck reticulocyte count in 2 weeks, Hct in 4 weeks

4. Refer Hct < 25% or atypical laboratory values

Pernicious Anemia (Vitamin B_{12} Deficiency Anemia)

- Definition: A macrocytic, megaloblastic anemia caused by a lack of intrinsic factor in gastric secretions which results in malabsorption of vitamin B_{12}; insidious and progressive to profound spinal cord involvement

- Etiology/Incidence
  1. Possibly an autoimmune reaction, leading to lack of intrinsic factor production necessary for B_{12} absorption
  2. Prevalence in all races in the U.S. about 0.1%
  3. Risks
     a. Most prevalent around age 60, can occur earlier, familial tendency
     b. Seen in individuals practicing strict vegetarianism
     c. Increased incidence in individuals with immunologic disease

- Signs and Symptoms
  1. None at first, insidious onset
  2. Fatigue, lightheadedness
  3. Weakness, paresthesia of extremities
  4. GI disturbances—anorexia, diarrhea, indigestion
  5. Palpitations
  6. Dyspnea, orthopnea, shortness of breath

- Differential Diagnosis
  1. Anemia of iron or folate deficiency
  2. Anemia of liver disease or other chronic disease

- Physical Findings
  1. Skin pale, occasional jaundice

2. Stomatitis, glossitis

3. Arrhythmias, systolic flow murmur, tachycardia

4. Wheezing rales

5. Organomegaly—hepatomegaly, splenomegaly

6. Neurological—ataxia, hyperactive reflexes

- Diagnostic Tests/Findings

    1. Gastric analysis reveals no acid

    2. Complete blood count (CBC)

        a. Red blood cells (RBCs), hemoglobin, hematocrit low

        b. White blood cells (WBCs) and platelets low

    3. Mean corpuscular volume (MCV) increased >100 μm^3; normal 80-94 μm^3

    4. Serum $B_{12} \leq 100$ pg/mL (normal 150-1,300 pg/mL)

    5. Schilling test (diagnostic)—24-hour urine

- Management/Treatment

    1. Parenteral B_{12} for life

    2. Treat any neurologic symptoms

    3. Watch for hypervolemia due to rapid increase in RBCs after initiation of treatment

Sickle Cell Anemia

- Definition: A hemolytic anemia characterized by distortion of erythrocytes into crescent-shapes as a result of Hgb A being replaced with Hgb S; individuals experience episodic crises resulting in permanent damage from vaso-occlusion

- Etiology/Incidence

    1. Mechanism: Physiologic stressors (decreased O_2, infection) cause Hgb S to destabilize, leading to clumping and "sickling" of cells; resultant vaso-occlusion causes ischemic pain and areas of infarction

    2. An autosomal recessive disorder

3. A homozygous trait in an estimated 0.5% U.S. Blacks

4. A heterozygous trait in an estimated 7.0% of U.S. Blacks, resulting in a "carrier state" (AS)

5. Lesser prevalence among Greeks, Italians, Middle Easterners, Asian Americans

- Signs and Symptoms

    1. Often none during remissions

    2. Retarded growth and sexual maturation

    3. Crises

        a. Pain, especially abdomen, chest and lower legs

        b. Malaise, chills

        c. Headache, epistaxis, vomiting

- Differential Diagnosis

    1. Thalassemia and other hemoglobinopathies

    2. In crises, rule out appendicitis, acute cholecystitis

- Physical Findings

    1. Non-crises, often normal

    2. In crises

        a. Temperature, pulse, respirations elevated; blood pressure low

        b. Pallor, cyanosis due to poor oxygenation

        c. Scleral jaundice

        d. Decreased skin turgor

    3. Chronic findings

        a. Increased susceptibility to infection

        b. Skin ulcers

        c. Degenerative arthritis

        d. Hemorrhagic detached retina

- Diagnostic Tests/Findings

    1. Hgb low (6-9 g/dL)

2. Hgb S detected by sickle cell preparation

3. Hemoglobin electrophoresis determines Hgb types and amounts

- Management/Treatment
    1. In remission
        a. Treat all infections aggressively
        b. Folic acid supplements 1 mg/day
    2. Refer all suspected cases of crises
        a. Hydration
        b. Analgesia
        c. Oxygen
        d. Transfusion

Lifestyle/Family Alterations

Addictive Disorders (Alcoholism and Drug Use)

- Definition
    1. Behavioral patterns in which individuals become progressively dependent, to the point of negative physical, psychological, or social health effects, in pursuit of a particular substance or behavior; a spectrum of use, physical dependence, and tolerance develops insidiously
    2. Commonly encountered addictive disorders
        a. Alcohol use
        b. Drug use
- Etiology/Incidence
    1. Identified predictors of substance abuse among women
        a. Low self-esteem
        b. Childhood sexual abuse/physical abuse
        c. Chronic debilitating physical health problems
        d. Depression, anxiety states

e. Higher incidence among lesbian, separated, divorced, widowed women

2. Alcoholism

a. Familial, possible genetic predisposition

b. Conceptualized on a continuum; described by identifiable stages (see Physical Findings); prevalence controversial and generally ill-defined in the general population

c. Estimated prevalence 5-6% among women aged 18-49 (Vourakis, 1995)

3. Drug abuse

a. Because nature of drug abuse is often illegal and/or stigmatizing, prevalence is uncertain and dependent on type of drug

b. Age and socioeconomic status influence types of drugs used

4. Drug and alcohol use (poly-drug use)

a. Women more likely than men to use several drugs concurrently

b. Women tend to use more prescription psychoactive drugs than men; prevalence is uncertain

- Signs and Symptoms

1. Alcoholism

a. Hallmark: Insidious onset, progressive

b. Periods of remission/abstinence and relapse

c. Reports of alcohol-related problems with relationships, job, school

d. Frequent accidents, legal problems

e. Concurrent use or abuse of other chemicals

f. Denial or defensive reaction to confrontation

g. Physical complaints of fatigue, amenorrhea, gastritis, vomiting, diarrhea

h. Depression, mood disorders, sleep disorders

i. Sexual dysfunction

      j.   Loss of control over alcohol intake

  2. Drug use—generalized signs

      a. Behavior inappropriate to situation

      b. Decline in school or job performance

      c. Anxiety/inattentiveness or lethargy/drowsiness

      d. Change in libido, sleep/wake cycles

      e. Change in appetite, GI function

- Differential Diagnosis

  1. Focus on underlying cause for compulsions

  2. Detect any underlying or associated chronic diseases or depression

- Physical Findings

  1. Alcoholism

      a. Early stage (Level III)

         (1) General appearance usually normal

         (2) Possible tachycardia, B/P elevation

         (3) Possible abdominal tenderness

      b. Mid-Stage/Moderate (Level II)

         (1) General appearance possibly normal; oriented to time, place, person

         (2) Possible tachycardia, arrhythmias, B/P elevation

Table 3

SIGNS AND SYMPTOMS OF DRUG USE SEEN IN CLINICAL PRACTICE

DEPRESSANT/NARCOTIC	*STIMULANT/NARCOTIC*
Nausea, vomiting, constipation	Nausea, vomiting, diarrhea, frequent urination
Apathy, dysphoria, depression, euphoria; mood swings, aggression, combativeness	Unpredictable moods, euphoria to depression or suicidal ideation
Drowsiness, slurred speech, psychomotor retardation	Restlessness, irritability, anxiety, insomnia
Fever, perspiration with withdrawal	Perspiration, chills
Ataxia, lack of coordination	Tremors

        (3) Possible organomegaly, tenderness

        (4) Skin—ecchymosis, unexplained scars

        (5) Hyperreflexia

    c. Late stage (Level I)

        (1) Possibly disoriented to time, place, person

        (2) Tachycardia, arrhythmias, B/P elevation

        (3) Skin—spider nevi, angiomas on face

        (4) Enlarged parotid glands, facial edema

        (5) Possible hepatomegaly, splenomegaly

  2. Drug use

    a. Personal appearance may indicate neglect, poor hygiene; depends on extent of abuse/addiction

    b. Various neurologic, GI, skin findings, based on drug used and route of administration

- Diagnostic Tests/Findings

  1. Alcoholism

    a. CBC and differential—hypochromic, macrocytic anemia

    b. Mean corpuscular volume (MCV) elevated in 50%

    c. Electrocardiogram—tachycardia, arrhythmias, T-wave changes

    d. Serum osmolality increased

    e. Folic acid decreased

    f. Prothrombin time prolonged

    g. Blood alcohol level increased

Table 4

EFFECTS OF DRUGS ON THE CENTRAL NERVOUS SYSTEM (CNS)

CNS TARGET	DEPRESSANT/NARCOTIC	STIMULANT
Vital signs	Depressed	Accelerated
Pupils	Constricted	Dilated
Reflexes (DTR)	Depressed	Exaggerated

2. Drug abuse

    a. CBC generally shows leukocytosis, anemia

    b. Blood or urine screen for specific drugs

- Management/Treatment

  1. Alcoholism

    a. Recovery program that supports abstinence from alcohol

    b. Work site/employee assistance programs

    c. Family centered therapy

    d. Social services referrals

    e. Evaluate for associated conditions—STD, TB, hepatitis, HIV infection

    f. Treat nutritional/vitamin deficit if needed

    g. Treat associated chronic disease

  2. Drug abuse

    a. After acute intoxication phase has passed, group and individual therapy aimed at stopping the compulsive behavior

    b. Change individual's social environment

    c. Supportive or replacement drug therapy occasionally helpful

    d. Evaluate and treat associated conditions—STD, TB, hepatitis, HIV infection

Addictive disorder (Tobacco use)

- Definition: Habitual use of tobacco by inhalation of smoke or chewing tobacco leaf; characterized by active sensation of pleasure, discomfort upon withdrawal, and craving that persists long after obvious withdrawal symptoms are past

- Etiology/Incidence

  1. Associated with significant morbidity, disability from cardiopulmonary damage, and carcinogenicity

  2. Prevalence decreasing among general population; increasing among women, especially adolescent girls

3. Prevalence estimated at 30-40% of adults

- Signs and Symptoms

    1. Cough

    2. Shortness of breath on exertion, dyspnea

    3. Prolonged expiration

    4. Withdrawal

        a. Tension, irritability, anxiety, craving

        b. Nausea, constipation, diarrhea

        c. Slower heart rate

- Differential Diagnosis—rule out associated emphysema, pulmonary carcinoma, chronic obstructive pulmonary disease, bronchitis

- Physical Findings

    1. Tachycardia

    2. Tachypnea

    3. Rhonchi, expiratory wheezes

    4. Later stages—increased anteroposterior diameter of chest

- Diagnostic Tests

    1. None indicated unless suspect cardiopulmonary complications

    2. Later stages

        a. Spirometry—impaired flow volume

        b. Chest x-ray—hyperinflated chest

- Management/Treatment

    1. Nonpharmacologic

        a. Behavior modification

        b. Gradual reduction

        c. Support groups

        d. Relaxation techniques

    2. Pharmacologic

a. Nicorette gum

b. Nicotine adhesive patch

Aging

- Definition: The continuum of physical and mental processes that occur over a lifetime

- Etiology/Incidence

  1. Rate of senescence (biological aging) varies

     a. Intrinsic factors

        (1) Genetic programming

        (2) Cumulative damage, disease

        (3) Hormonal changes

        (4) Perceived effect of consequences of aging

     b. Extrinsic factors

        (1) Exercise, diet

        (2) Smoking

        (3) Parity

        (4) Economic status

  2. Demography

     a. Increasing proportion of population > age 65

     b. Women disproportionately represented due to longer life expectancy

- Signs and Symptoms

  1. Waning fertility, amenorrhea

  2. Gradual loss of flexibility, physical vigor

  3. Changes in cognition—short and long-term memory, learning, motivation

- Differential Diagnosis—onset of new or chronic disease, especially with sudden appearance of new symptoms

- Physical Findings
    1. Diminished lean body mass
    2. Diminished skin turgor
    3. Diminished bone density/osteoporosis
    4. Often dental problems due to periodontal disease, osteoporosis
- Diagnostic Tests/Findings
    1. FSH > 30 diagnostic of menopause
    2. Bone density study benefit controversial
- Management/Treatment
    1. Health maintenance
        a. Encourage adequate nutrition
        b. Calcium
            (1) Dietary recommendation 1,500 total mg/day—not on hormone replacement therapy (HRT)
            (2) Supplementation if dietary intake insufficient, to 1,500 mg/day combined total
            (3) On HRT, 1,000 mg/day
        c. Vitamin D 200 IU/day may reduce incidence of hip fractures in women with osteoporosis
        d. Estrogen replacement therapy often beneficial
        e. Moderate exercise improves mobility, reduces cardiovascular risk and maintains bone density
        f. Reduce alcohol intake, smoking
    2. Social considerations
        a. Family changes—loss of lifetime partner, friends, caregiving responsibilities
        b. Economic status
            (1) Older women more often impoverished
            (2) Health care access may be altered

        (3) Housing, nutrition possibly substandard

    c. Isolation

        (1) More likely to survive spouse

        (2) Retirement from work role

        (3) Possible reduced mobility

Parenting

- Definition
  1. An interactive process of nurturing that begins in the prenatal period and continues until physical and developmental tasks of childhood have been mastered
  2. At its best, represents a developmental process for both parent and child in which each is supported in the mastery of each stage's task

- Stage 1 (Birth to 6 months)
  1. Child learns to communicate appropriate cues
  2. Parent learns to interpret and respond to cues

- Stage 2 (Six to 18 months)
  1. Parent supports early exploration
  2. Safety of environment is crucial
  3. Child mobile, exploring and testing environment, child gains self-confidence

- Stage 3 (Eighteen months to 3 years)
  1. Parent encourages healthy expressive behavior
  2. Child masters emotional expression, verbalization, early social skills and self-control

- Stage 4 (Three to 6 years)
  1. Parent begins to separate
  2. Child begins to connect feelings with thinking

- Stage 5 (Six to 12 years)
  1. Parent assists child with internalization of rules, appropriate structure

2. Child formulates and practices personalized sense of values, sets boundaries, makes own decisions, begins to understand consequences, societal goals

- Stage 6 (Thirteen to 19 years)

  1. Focus is on identity, separation, and sexuality

  2. Child tests independence, may experiment with risk-taking behaviors

- Stage 7 (Age 19 and over)

  1. Letting go, "launching"—letting child run own life

  2. Child successfully transitions to independence, adult living

Domestic Violence and Abuse

- Definition

  1. A pattern of controlling behavior that consists of physical, sexual, and/or psychological assaults; without intervention, becomes more destructive over time

  2. Described as cyclic in nature

     a. Escalating aggression/demeaning behavior

     b. Culminates in abusive or violent event

     c. "Honeymoon" period of remorse follows

     d. Gradually escalating aggressive behavior begins again

     e. Cycles reflect "spiraling" abusive behavior

  3. Three types of violence commonly encountered

     a. Intimate partner abuse (spousal abuse): Victim is the female partner > 90% cases

     b. Child abuse: Physical harm, verbal, sexual abuse or neglect inflicted on child in a way that hinders normal development

     c. Elder abuse: Includes physical harm, sexual abuse, neglect or exploitation of the elderly; usually by caregivers

- Etiology/Incidence

  1. Believed to be primarily a learned behavior

2. Prevalence very difficult to measure due to furtive nature of events comprising abuse

3. Estimated as high as 1.8 million spousal abuse incidents per year; under-reporting acknowledged

- Signs and Symptoms

  1. Psychological manifestations range from anxiety to psychosis

     a. Acute—shock, denial, fear

     b. Late—depression, mental health problems

  2. Dependence on the abuser

     a. Financial support from abuser

     b. Perceived powerlessness, feelings of worthlessness, low self-esteem

  3. Misuse of alcohol or drugs

  4. In children—acting out behaviors, promiscuity

  5. Vague physical complaints—headaches, GI upset

  6. Frequent calls or visits to medical provider, often for minor concerns

- Differential Diagnosis

  1. Underlying acute or chronic disease

  2. Accidental trauma

- Physical Findings

  1. Acute

     a. Cutaneous trauma (burns, bruises, lacerations)

     b. Fractures

     c. Panic response—tachycardia, extreme anxiety

     d. In pregnancy—breasts and abdomen are frequent targets of assault

  2. Chronic

     a. Wasting, malnourishment

     b. Elusive and nagging physical complaints

- Diagnostic Tests/Findings
    1. X-rays may reveal old fractures
    2. Urine—hematuria
    3. Hct—anemia
    4. Colposcopic examination helpful in sexual assault
- Management/Treatment
    1. Reporting of child abuse is mandatory in all states
    2. Acute cases best handled by trained individuals to protect legal rights and proper evidence collection
    3. Documentation
        a. Use body map if possible, photographs
        b. Avoid making conclusive statements
        c. Explicit, descriptive charting
    4. Refer to crisis intervention, case management services, shelter

Sexual Assault

- Definition: A broad continuum of violent acts involving sexual contact of varying intrusiveness; examples include—harassment, indecent liberties, molestation, rape, sodomy
- Etiology/Incidence
    1. Incest
        a. Specific form of sexual abuse in which victim and perpetrator belong to the same family, e.g., child and parent, sibling, etc.
        b. Incidence unknown; often revealed after months to years of abuse; complicated by widely differing definitions
    2. Rape
        a. Legal term for a form of sexual abuse in which intercourse or penetration occurs by use of force or nonconsent; may be marital, acquaintance ("date"), or stranger rape

      b. Incidence unknown due to furtive nature of rape; reported rape and attempted rape is increasing (120/100,000 women > age 12) (Campbell & Landenburger, 1995)

- Signs and Symptoms (Incest or Rape)
  1. Unreported or undetected abuse
     a. Evasive, defensive or inconsistent responses to routine questions
     b. Over-protective, controlling behavior on the part of parent or spouse, e.g., refusing to permit examination of the victim, or to leave victim alone with provider
     c. Vague presenting complaints of pelvic pain, headache, GI discomfort, dyspareunia
     d. Extreme apprehensiveness regarding genital examination, vaginismus
  2. Acute presentation
     a. Expressions of shock, fear, or anger
     b. Appearance of recent physical struggle
- Differential Diagnosis
  1. Dysfunctional relationships and ideation
  2. Trauma from other causes
  3. Bleeding, clotting disorder must be ruled out with bruises
- Physical Findings
  1. Evidence of sexual activity in prepubertal child
  2. Genital and/or anal trauma
  3. Findings consistent with use of physical force
  4. Sexually transmitted diseases, pregnancy
  5. Findings inconsistent with "story"
- Diagnostic Tests/Findings
  1. Fluorescence—presence of semen
  2. STD testing
  3. Colposcopy

- Management/Treatment
  1. Acute presentation
     a. Examination should be conducted by trained sexual abuse team to ensure proper handling of evidence
     b. Surgical or medical intervention for trauma
     c. Emergency contraception, STD evaluation
     d. Reporting to criminal justice system
  2. Long term
     a. STD follow-up including HIV screen
     b. Individual or family counseling
     c. Psychotherapy
     d. Referral to legal or social services
  3. Sexual abuse of a minor is reportable in all states

Depression

- Definition
  1. Mood disorder experienced as a range of feelings from sadness or despondency to psychoses; often described by recognizable pattern, e.g., seasonal, bipolar, dysthymia (chronic)
  2. Most clinical depression is situational, treatable
- Etiology/Incidence
  1. Cause
     a. Primary—reaction to grief, loss, anger
     b. Secondary—metabolic, neurologic, chemical
  2. Prevalence unknown in general population, but commonly reported in clinical practice
     a. Dysthymia most common type encountered
     b. Affects women twice as often as men
- Signs and Symptoms

1. Fatigue, lethargy

2. Anorexia

3. Sleep disturbance—insomnia, hypersomnia

4. Loss of interest in daily activities

5. Feelings of helplessness, pessimism, hopelessness

6. Suicidal ideation

7. Somatic complaints

- Differential Diagnosis

    1. Chronic illness

    2. Hypothyroidism

    3. Medication side effects

    4. Premenstrual syndrome

    5. Substance abuse

- Physical Findings

    1. Mental status—self-deprecating remarks, delusions

    2. Flat affect or agitation

    3. Weight loss or gain

    4. General appearance of neglect, apathy

- Diagnostic Tests/Findings

    1. None specific to depression

    2. CBC, SMA 24, Thyroid panel

- Management/Treatment

    1. Pharmacologic—antidepressants

        a. Tricyclics

            (1) Imipramine hydrochloride (Tofranil)

            (2) Amitriptyline hydrochloride (Elavil)

        b. Serotonin Re-uptake Inhibitors

            (1) Fluoxetine (Prozac)

(2) Sertraline (Zoloft)

  c. Monoamine oxidase inhibitors (MAOI)—Isocarboxazid (Marplan)

  d. Heterocyclic Antidepressants—Bupropion (Wellbutrin)

2. Nonpharmacologic

  a. Psychotherapy

  b. Relaxation techniques

  c. Hypnosis

  d. Exercise

3. Hospitalization if psychotic, suicidal

4. Concern for suicide increased if depressed person suddenly feels better—may have decided on a plan; always ask if person has thought of suicide and whether they have a plan

Stress

- Definition

  1. General term for emotional and physical response to stimuli (stressors) resulting in adjustment and change

  2. External stressors—job, role demands, situational danger

  3. Internal (physiologic)—pregnancy, chronic illness

- Etiology/Incidence

  1. Autonomic response to catecholamine secretion stimulated by physiological or psychological stressors

  2. Physical consequences of prolonged stress—generalized anxiety, diminished immune or protective response to disease

  3. One of most common complaints in practice

- Signs and Symptoms—generalized, nonspecific

  1. Headaches

  2. Lack of appetite, GI complaints

  3. Muscle tension, fatigue

4. Restless, anxious

5. Depressed

- Differential Diagnosis

  1. Rule out underlying problems, e.g., hypertension, asthma

  2. Complete psychosocial assessment to uncover problems

- Physical Findings

  1. Occasionally tachycardia, mildly elevated B/P

  2. Rigidity, muscular tension

- Diagnostic Tests/Findings

  1. Aimed at identifying underlying cause

  2. Investigate headaches if persistent, severe

  3. ECG to evaluate developing cardiac disease

- Management/Treatment

  1. Identify external stresses, separating them into

     a. "Things I can*not* change"

     b. "Things I *can* change"

  2. Alter coping patterns

     a. Biofeedback, relaxation exercises

     b. Improved health maintenance habits

     c. Time management

     d. Assertiveness skills

     e. Counseling to improve coping skills

Anxiety

- Definition

  1. An emotion experienced as feelings of dread, fear, or danger that is situational

  2. May be normal reaction to real, perceived, or anticipated stimuli, or manifestation of underlying disorder

3. Major types

    a. Generalized anxiety

        (1) Unrealistic or excessive worry about 2 or more life circumstances for 2 months or longer

        (2) Most common anxiety disorder

    b. Panic/anxiety state

        (1) Extreme state of fear

        (2) Episodic, minutes to days

    c. Phobic disorder

        (1) Involuntary, morbid fear of specific stimulus

        (2) Leads to avoidance of stimulus; disruptive to life

    d. Post-traumatic stress disorder (PSD)

        (1) Develops after traumatic event

        (2) Usually patient re-experiences the event

        (3) Onset may be many years after traumatic event

- Etiology/Incidence

  1. Causes

    a. Situational stress

    b. Drug use/abuse

    c. Metabolic disturbance

  2. Prevalence

    a. Generalized anxiety—slight predominance among women, usually 20-35 years of age

    b. Panic disorder—twice as prevalent in women; affects 3-5% of population

- Signs and Symptoms

  1. General—hyperventilation, pains, fear, GI symptoms, palpitations, urinary frequency, headache

  2. Panic—sudden sense of fear with accompanying symptoms, urge to scream

3. PSD—sleep disturbances, hyperalertness, restlessness, difficulty concentrating

- Differential Diagnosis—investigate for underlying conditions
    1. Alcohol or substance abuse or withdrawal
    2. Hyperthyroidism, thyroid storm
    3. Hypertension
    4. Hypoglycemia
    5. Paroxysmal tachycardia
    6. Medication side-effects
    7. Physical or sexual abuse—current or past
    8. Organic brain syndrome

- Physical Findings
    1. Vital signs elevated
    2. Restlessness, trembling, screaming
    3. Skin—pallor, sweating/clammy, erythema
    4. Possible loss of bladder or bowel control
    5. Physical examination otherwise normal

- Diagnostic Tests/Findings
    1. None specific to anxiety
    2. Thyroid panel
    3. Electrocardiogram
    4. Blood glucose
    5. Drug/alcohol screens

- Management
    1. Acute
        a. Decrease environmental stimuli
        b. Stay with patient, stay calm
        c. Hospitalization if psychotic or danger to self or others

2. Long-term/Preventive

    a. Pharmacologic—anti-anxiety drugs

        (1) Benzodiazepines

            (a) Alprazolam (Xanax)

            (b) Oxazepam (Serax)

        (2) Beta blockers—Propranolol

    b. Psychotherapy

QUESTIONS

Select the best answer.

1. The "gold standard" diagnostic test for sinusitis is:

    a. Decreased transillumination effect in sinuses
    b. Culture of nasal discharge
    c. Eosinophils on wet prep of nasal discharge
    d. Opaque areas on sinus x-ray

2. Otitis media is suspected when deep ear pain develops concurrent with or following:

    a. An upper respiratory infection
    b. An asthma attack
    c. An allergic reaction
    d. Persistent headache

3. A physical finding consistent with a diagnosis of serous otitis includes:

    a. A bulging, red tympanic membrane
    b. Mucopurulent nasal discharge
    c. A dull, retracted tympanic membrane
    d. High fever

4. An important diagnostic finding in asthma is:

    a. Increased red blood cells
    b. Gram stain of sputum reveals eosinophils
    c. Absolute eosinophil count 3 times normal
    d. Absolute eosinophil count below normal

5. An incidental finding of blood pressure 156/90 during a routine examination of an asymptomatic, 42 year-old African-American woman would indicate:

    a. Essential hypertension
    b. Normal physiologic response to anxiety
    c. Probability of underlying pathology
    d. Necessity for follow-up and further evaluation

6. A systolic heart murmur present in an asymptomatic individual is likely:

    a. Due to valvular disease
    b. A physiologic ("innocent") murmur
    c. Associated with history of rheumatic fever
    d. To intensify with the valsalva maneuver

7. The most common reason for painless rectal bleeding with defecation is:

    a. Internal hemorrhoids
    b. External hemorrhoids
    c. Rectal polyps
    d. Colorectal cancer

8. Linda is a 25 year-old college student with a part-time job. She complains of intermittent, loose stools with pain and flatulence. After defecation, there is a temporary feeling of relief. Symptoms increase during stressful times. You suspect:

    a. Ulcerative colitis
    b. Functional bowel syndrome
    c. Lactose intolerance
    d. Intestinal parasitic infection

9. A recommended dietary change for Linda's episodes of diarrhea includes:

    a. High fiber diet
    b. Low fiber diet
    c. Eliminate dairy products
    d. Vitamin supplements

10. African-American women are at increased risk for hypertension and:

    a. Skin cancer
    b. Pernicious anemia
    c. Hepatitis
    d. Type II diabetes mellitus

11. Monozygotic twins have _____% concordance for developing Type II diabetes:

    a. 20%
    b. > 50%
    c. 70%
    d. > 90%

12. The laboratory finding confirming a diagnosis of hypothyroidism is:

    a. Elevated TSH
    b. Elevated T_3
    c. Elevated T_4
    d. Low T_4

13. A finding of a solitary, asymptomatic mass during examination of the thyroid in a patient whose physical status is otherwise euthyroid, is likely:

    a. Thyroiditis
    b. Thyroid cancer
    c. Grave's disease
    d. Thyroid nodule

14. Karen, a 30 year-old housewife, sees you for an examination and contraceptive prescription. She relates nonspecific symptoms of fatigue, diarrhea, and weight loss. Physical findings include vaginal moniliasis, and her Pap returns with a high grade squamous intraepithelial lesion (SIL). Her husband has been in the military for 14 years and travels all over the world on assignment, sometimes for months at a time.

    Your most serious concern in evaluating Karen's condition is to assess her risk for:

    a. Irritable bowel syndrome
    b. HIV infection/disease
    c. Diabetes mellitus
    d. Progressive/malignant cervical disease

15. The confirmatory test for HIV infection is:

    a. Enzyme-linked immunosorbent assay (ELISA)
    b. Western blot
    c. Culture for HIV
    d. CD4 lymphocyte count

16. An important aspect of care for HIV positive women is:

    a. Mammography every 12 months
    b. Frequent cervical Pap smear evaluation
    c. Recommend therapeutic abortion in the event of pregnancy
    d. Contraceptive sterilization

17. About 10% of those infected with Hepatitis B virus become chronic carriers of the disease, a state putting them at risk for:

    a. Hepatocellular carcinoma
    b. Mononucleosis
    c. Gall bladder disease
    d. Chronic immunocompromised status

18. Aside from transmission due to contact with infected blood/blood products, the most common mechanism of transmission of the Hepatitis B virus is:

    a. Fecal-oral route
    b. Contaminated water source
    c. Perinatal (mother-to-baby)
    d. Air-borne droplets

19. Lan has recently immigrated to the U.S. from S.E. Asia to join her large extended family. They live in a poor section of town in a crowded apartment. She appears to be healthy and has an entirely normal physical examination. She should receive screening for tuberculosis by:

    a. PPD skin test
    b. Sputum culture
    c. Chest x-rays
    d. Gastric aspiration

20. A positive PPD skin test indicates infection with *Mycobacterium tuberculosis.* About what percent of infected individuals will develop active disease?

    a. 100%
    b. 75%
    c. 30%
    d. 10%

21. The most common reason for lumbosacral back pain is:

    a. Herniated disc
    b. Muscle strain
    c. Neoplasm
    d. Arthritis

22. The most important physical finding when making a diagnosis of lower back strain is:

    a. A thorough neurological examination is normal
    b. Normal x-ray of the spinal column
    c. The patient's gait is affected
    d. Typical poor posture and rigidity

23. The usual underlying cause of carpal tunnel syndrome is:

    a. Diabetes mellitus
    b. Pregnancy
    c. Trauma
    d. Repetitive hand movement

24. The most aggressively metastasizing skin cancer in adults is:

    a. Basal cell carcinoma
    b. Basal cell nevus syndrome
    c. Squamous cell syndrome
    d. Malignant melanoma

25. The frequency of sickle cell crises may be reduced by:

    a. Activity restrictions
    b. Oxygen therapy
    c. Aggressive treatment of infections
    d. High protein diet

26. The cardinal feature of alcoholism is:

    a. A positive family history of alcoholism
    b. Concomitant use of other drugs
    c. Alcohol associated with cardiomyopathy
    d. Insidious and progressive compulsion

27. A diagnosis of menopause can be based on:

    a. FSH < 20
    b. FSH 20-30
    c. FSH > 30
    d. Amenorrhea for 11 months

28. Mrs. L. brings her 15 year-old daughter, Patti, to the clinic for evaluation of amenorrhea. From the start, Mrs. L. does all the talking, answers questions directed at Patti, fills out the history forms, and insists on being present while a pregnancy test is being run. She further insists Patti doesn't need an examination, they "just want a pregnancy test." Patti appears ill-at-ease, mutters only monosyllabic answers when addressed, and casts resentful glances at Mrs. L. from time to time. When asked if she has a boyfriend, Patti shakes her head "No," and Mrs. L. says "Yes." Based on the interview, you suspect:

    a. Patti is a rebellious teen with poor rapport with her mother
    b. Mrs. L. is in denial about Patti's sexual activity
    c. Patti is most likely a victim of sexual abuse
    c. Mrs. L. is simply an overbearing, controlling parent

29. The cycle of violence that occurs in domestic violence situations includes periods of:

    a. Emotional withdrawal of the abused partner
    b. Physical retaliation by the abused partner
    c. Evasive responses from the abused partner
    d. Gradually escalating abusive behavior

30. The most commonly encountered form of depression is:

    a. Seasonal
    b. Bipolar
    c. Dysthymia (chronic)
    d. Secondary

ANSWERS

1. d	11. d	21. b
2. a	12. a	22. a
3. c	13. d	23. d
4. c	14. b	24. d
5. d	15. b	25. c
6. b	16. b	26. d
7. a	17. a	27. c
8. b	18. c	28. c
9. b	19. a	29. d
10. d	20. d	30. c

BIBLIOGRAPHY

American Thoracic Society Board of Directors. (1993). Control of tuberculosis in the United States. *American Review of Respiratory Disease*, 146, 1623-1633. Reprinted, 1993. (Publ. #733-260/63561). Washington, DC: U.S. Department of Health & Human Services.

Burkhart, C. (1992). Guidelines for rapid assessment of abdominal pain indicative of acute surgical abdomen. *The Nurse Practitioner*, 17 (6), 39-49.

Bushnell, F. (1992). A guide to primary care of iron-deficiency anemia. *The Nurse Practitioner*, 17 (11), 68-74.

Campbell, J., & Landenburger, K. (1995). Violence against women. In C. Fogel & N. Woods (Eds.), *Women's health care* (pp. 407-426). Thousand Oaks, CA: Sage Publications.

Caulker-Burnett, I. (1994). Primary screening for substance abuse. *The Nurse Practitioner*, 19 (6), 42-48.

Clarke, J., & Dawson, C. (1989). *Growing up again: Parenting ourselves, parenting our children*. San Francisco: Harper & Row.

Costa, A. (1993). Elder abuse. In B. Elliott, K. Halvorson, & M. Hendricks-Matthews (Eds.), *Primary care: Clinics in advanced practice,* 20 (2), 375-378.

Diamond, M. (1995). Older Women's Health. In C. Fogel & N. Woods (Eds.), *Women's health care* (pp. 101-110). Thousand Oaks, CA: Sage Publications.

Fishel, A. (1995). Mental Health. In C. Fogel & N. Woods (Eds.), *Women's health care* (pp. 323-362). Thousand Oaks, CA: Sage Publications.

Garbarino, J. (1993). Psychosocial child maltreatment. In B. Elliott, K. Halvorson, & M. Hendricks-Matthews (Eds.), *Primary care: Clinics in advanced practice,* 20 (2), 307-316.

Hsu, H., Feinstone, S., & Hoofnagle, J. (1995). Acute viral hepatitis. In G. Mandell, J. Bennett, & R. Dolin (Eds.), *Mandell, Douglas, and Bennett's principles and practice of infectious diseases:* Vol. 2 (4th ed.), (pp. 1136-1151). New York: Churchill Livingstone.

Journal of Nurse Midwifery. (March/April, 1995). Primary care for women, 40(2).

Kappas-Larson, P., & Lathrop, L. (1993). Early detection and intervention for hazardous ethanol use. *The Nurse Practitioner*, 18 (7), 50-55.

Kelso, S. (Ed.). (1994). *Public Health Improvement Plan*. Olympia, WA: Washington State Department of Health.

Managing early HIV infection. (1994). Publ. #94-0573. Rockville: U.S. Department of Health and Human Services.

Manderine, M., & Brown, M. (1992). A practical, step-by-step approach to stress management for women. *The Nurse Practitioner, 17* (7), 18-28.

Millonig, V. (Ed.). (1994). *Adult nurse practitioner certification review guide* (2nd ed.). Potomac, MD: Health Leadership Associates.

Onion, D. (1993). *The little black book of primary care: Pearls and references.* New York: Norton Medical Books.

Perry, M., & Anderson, G. (1992). Assessment and treatment strategies for depressive disorders commonly encountered in primary care settings. *The Nurse Practitioner, 17* (6), 25-36.

Sassetti, M. (1993). Domestic violence. In B. Elliott, K. Halvorson, M. Hendricks-Matthews (Eds.), *Primary care: Clinics in advanced practice, 20* (2), 289-303.

Schnare, S. (1994). *Protocols of the Harbor-UCLA women's health care nurse practitioner program.* Torrance, CA.

Schwartz, R. (1994). The diagnosis and management of sinusitis. *The Nurse Practitioner, 19* (12), 58-63.

Seidel, H., Ball, J., Dains, J., & Benedict, G.W. (1991). *Mosby's guide to physical examination* (2nd ed.). St. Louis: Mosby-Year Book.

Vourakis, C. (1995). Drug abuse problems among women. In C.Fogel & N. Woods (Eds.), *Women's health care* (pp. 497-516). Thousand Oaks, CA: Sage Publications.

Youngkin, E., & Davis, M. (1994). *Women's health: A primary care clinical guide.* Norwalk, CT: Appleton & Lange.

Normal Women's Health Care

Carolyn M. Sutton

Life Cycle Changes of the Adolescent - Adult Woman

- Overview of Reproductive Physiology
    1. Functional reproductive physiology requires intact hypothalamus, anterior pituitary, ovaries, and feedback systems; interfaces with other systems and is affected by the stress response
        a. Hypothalamus—a region of the brain that contains specialized cells which secrete releasing and inhibiting hormones into portal blood system to act on anterior pituitary
            (1) Hormones classified as releasing factors include
                (a) Gonadotropin releasing hormone (GnRH), regulates gonadotropins
                (b) Corticotropin releasing hormone (CRH), regulates ACTH secretion, and activates sympathetic nervous system
                (c) Growth hormone-releasing hormone (GHRH)
                (d) Thyrotropin releasing hormone (TRH), regulates thyroid hormones, T_3 and T_4
            (2) Dopamine, a prolactin inhibiting factor (PIF) is also released from hypothalamus
        b. Hormones released from anterior pituitary regulate gonadal, thyroid and adrenal function, lactation, bodily growth and somatic development; hormones include
            (1) Follicle-stimulating hormone (FSH)
            (2) Luteinizing hormone (LH)
            (3) Thyroid-stimulating hormone (TSH)
            (4) Adrenocorticotropic-stimulating hormone (ACTH)
            (5) Prolactin (PRL)
            (6) Growth hormone (GH)
        c. Oxytocin released from posterior pituitary—stimulates milk ejection by contracting cells around the alveoli and ducts in mammary gland; release controlled by stimulation of touch receptors in nipple

    d. Ovaries are responsible for

        (1) Sex steroid formation and secretion (estradiol and progesterone)

        (2) Gamete production

    e. Positive and negative feedback systems act directly on hypothalamus and anterior pituitary to control pattern of hormone secretion throughout menstrual cycle

- Preadolescence

    1. Period of maximal hypothalamic suppression

    2. Little response of pituitary to GnRH

    3. Low levels of gonadotropins

    4. GnRH, thyroid, insulin, glucocorticoid, FSH and LH play primary roles in timing and progression of growth and development

- Puberty

    1. Time when endocrine and gametogenic functions activate and reproduction becomes possible

        a. Major influence on timing of puberty is genetics

        b. Other factors include

            (1) Geographic location

            (2) Exposure to light

            (3) General health and nutrition

        c. Onset of menarche dependent upon

            (1) Attainment of critical body weight (47.8 kg)

            (2) Percent body fat in range of 16.0-23.5%

    2. *Usual sequence* of pubertal development

        a. Acceleration of growth

        b. Thelarche—breast budding (median age 9.8 years)

        c. Adrenarche—increased secretion of adrenal androgens (median age 10.5 years) causing growth of axillary and pubic hair

    d. Peak height velocity—year in which height in centimeters (cm) increases on average 6-11 cm (requires growth hormone and estrogen); occurs 1 year prior to menarche

    e. Menarche

        (1) First menstrual period (average age 12.8 years)

        (2) Menses for first 12-18 months usually anovulatory, irregular and occasionally heavy

        (3) Growth in height much slower after menarche

    f. Tanner staging often used as guideline to assess adolescent pubertal development

        (1) Stage 1 (prepubertal)—elevation of papilla only; no pubic hair

        (2) Stage 2—elevation of breast and papilla, appear as small mound; enlargement of areola diameter; sparse, long pigmented hair along labia majora (median age 9.8)

        (3) Stage 3—further breast enlargement without separation of breast and areola; dark, coarse, curled pubic hair sparsely distributed over mons (median age 11.2 years)

        (4) Stage 4—secondary mound of areola and papilla above the breast; adult type hair abundant but limited to the mons (median age 12.1 years)

        (5) Stage 5—recession of areola to contour of breast; adult-type hair in distribution and quantity (median age 13.7 years)

3. Developmental changes in female reproductive system

    a. Breasts

        (1) Major hormonal influence estrogen

        (2) Full glandular development also requires progesterone, thyroxine, cortisol, insulin and prolactin

        (3) Oxytocin released from the posterior pituitary; required with prolactin for lactation

        (4) Full breast development reached on average by 14.6 years

    b. Growth of pubic and axillary hair requires adrenal androgen

c. Vulvar changes (estrogen influence)

   (1) Fat deposits increase mons and labial size

   (2) Labia majora fuller; assume wrinkled appearance

   (3) Labia minora smaller, pink, moist

   (4) Clitoris and urethral mound enlarge

   (5) Hymenal opening increases

d. Vaginal changes (estrogen influence)

   (1) Lengthens to approximately 10-11 cm; more elastic

   (2) Epithelial transition to stratified squamous cells

   (3) Vaginal pH decreased (normal range 3.2-4.5)

   (4) Milky white discharge

      (a) Presence of discharge considered normal physiologic occurrence

      (b) Some variation in amount throughout lifespan (most abundant in reproductive years and pregnancy)

      (c) Imbalance in vaginal ecology and pH can result in vaginal infections such as monilia vaginitis and bacterial vaginosis

      (d) Factors which may alter vaginal pH include menses, inoculum with infectious agent, excessive douching, ejaculate, vaginal lubricant, and large amount of cervical eversion (ectropion)

e. Uterus (estrogen and progesterone influence)

   (1) Corpus to cervix ratio reaches 1:1 at menarche (estrogen influence); mature corpus to cervix ratio $2/3$ to $1/3$

   (2) Proliferation of endometrium (estrogen influence)

   (3) Cervical glands secrete mucus (estrogen influence)

   (4) After ovulation, secretory endometrium (progesterone influence)

     f. Ovaries

        (1) Enlarge (to 3-4 cm) and assume adult almond shape; ovaries atrophy after menopause (1-1.5 cm) and become non-palpable

        (2) Estradiol secretion greatly increased

        (3) Approximately 300,000 follicles present at onset of puberty, number decreases steadily throughout reproductive life

- Normal Menstrual Cycle

   1. Ovarian cycle

     (1) Follicular phase—estrogen dominant

        (2) Usually 14 days, but highly variable with range of 7-22 days, ending with ovulation; FSH predominates

        (3) FSH stimulates maturation of ovarian follicles, end result is one dominant follicle

        (4) LH stimulates theca cells of ovary to produce androgens which are converted to estrogen in granulosa cells

        (5) FSH levels decline in mid-late follicular phase as result of rising estradiol levels

     b. Ovulation

        (1) FSH and LH surge triggered by rise in estradiol at mid-cycle

        (2) Ovulation occurs about 10-16 hours after LH surge

        (3) Mature follicle releases oocyte, and follicle then becomes functioning corpus luteum with a lifespan of 14 days

     c. Luteal phase—progesterone dominant

        (1) Begins with ovulation, ends with onset of menses

        (2) Corpus luteum produces progesterone and estrogen; rising levels inhibit secretion of pituitary gonadotropins (FSH, LH) and suppress new follicular growth

        (3) Unless fertilization occurs, corpus luteum regresses, causing onset of menses

   2. Endometrial cycle

a. Proliferative phase (approximately 10 days)

  (1) Estrogen dominant phase—major effects

    (a) Stimulates growth of uterine smooth muscle (myometrium) and glandular epithelium (endometrium)

    (b) Induces synthesis of receptor sites for progesterone

  (2) Other estrogen effects

    (a) Liver—increased Thyroxine-binding globulin (TBG)

    (b) Breast—increased mammary duct cells

    (c) Vagina—thickens vaginal mucosa

    (d) Endocervix—causes watery, clear and stretchy cervical mucus (*spinnbarkeit*)

b. Secretory phase—lasts about 14 days

  (1) Progesterone dominant

    (a) Endometrial growth arrested

    (b) Number of estrogen and progesterone receptors decreased

    (c) Secretory endometrium prepared for implantation

    (d) Without fertilization, corpus luteum regresses, progesterone falls and the endometrium sloughs

  (2) Other progesterone effects

    (a) Breast—increased glandular growth

    (b) Vagina—thinning of mucosa

    (c) Endocervix—thick, sticky mucus

    (d) Promotes renal excretion of salt

c. Menstrual phase

  (1) Fall of estrogen and progesterone

    (a) Deprives endometrium of hormonal support

    (b) Endometrial sloughing occurs marking first days of menses

        (2) Prostaglandins released just prior to menses

            (a) Cause smooth muscle to contract

            (b) Can result in headache, dysmenorrhea and nausea

        (3) Ovulatory bleeding pattern—cyclic, predictable in onset, amount and duration

            (a) Cycle length: 28-30 days

            (b) Duration: 4-6 ± 2 days

            (c) Blood loss: 30-40 mL

3. Cultural factors related to menstrual cycle

    a. Cultural assessment

        (1) Woman's attitudes and beliefs about health

        (2) Communication styles

        (3) Role socialization (role within a group population)

    b. Factors which influence cultural attitudes about the menstrual cycle

        (1) Taboos and symbolism about menstruation

        (2) Myths and traditions held by social groups about women and their bodies

        (3) Personal beliefs about being a woman

    c. Strategies should be designed that promote health and allow women to operate within their own cultural framework

- Climacteric

  1. Definition

    a. Transitional period from reproductive capability to cessation of menses marked by waning ovarian function

        (1) May span 10-15 years

        (2) Term perimenopause may be used interchangeably

    b. Menopause

(1) Single point in time that marks the last episode of menstruation signaling the termination of reproductive capability

(2) Mean age in U.S. is 51 years

c. Postmenopause—period following menopause characterized by complete termination of ovarian activity and signs of estrogen deficiency

2. Hormonal changes

a. Number of follicles responsive to gonadotropins decrease and those remaining are not as responsive

b. Fewer available follicles to produce estradiol (most potent estrogen)

c. Hormones

(1) Lower estradiol levels

(2) Increased FSH levels

(3) LH usually remains normal

d. After menopause

(1) Primary estrogen becomes estrone which is derived from the conversion of androstenedione to estrone in extraglandular sites

(2) FSH is elevated 10-20 fold (or > 30 mIU/mL)

(3) LH is elevated 3-fold (20-100 mIU/mL)

3. Physical changes

a. Several alterations in menstrual pattern may occur

(1) Anovulation

(2) Decreased menstrual flow

(3) Hypermenorrhea

(4) Eventually amenorrhea

b. Vasomotor instability (hot flushes and night sweats) often begins in perimenopause

c. Atrophy of estrogen-dependent urogenital sites

           (1)   Vaginal epithelium and canal

           (2)   Urethra

           (3)   Cervix

           (4)   Vulva/introitus

  d. Skin changes including

           (1)   Hyperpigmentation (senile lentigo)

           (2)   Hypopigmentation (vitiligo)

           (3)   Decreased sweat and sebaceous gland activity

           (4)   Atrophy and thinning of epidermal and dermal skin layers

           (5)   General decrease in scalp, pubic and axillary hair

  e. Musculoskeletal changes

           (1)   Accelerated bone loss

           (2)   Osteoporosis

  f. Psychological symptoms reported include

           (1)   Anxiety, depression, irritability

           (2)   Libido changes

           (3)   Insomnia

4. Signs and symptoms

  a. Irregular menses—wide variation in cycle length characterized by shortened follicular phase and anovulatory cycles

  b. Hot flashes/flushes occurring during day or at night

  c. Urogenital

           (1)   Vaginal dryness, decreased rugae, increased vaginal pH

           (2)   Dyspareunia and pruritus

           (3)   Urinary difficulties—urethritis; urgency, dysuria, frequency, nocturia; incontinence; recurrent urinary tract infections (UTI)

           (4)   Symptoms of atrophic vaginitis—itching, burning, dyspareunia, and sometimes vaginal bleeding

5. Psychosocial changes

   a. Important to emphasize health-promoting behaviors—adequate nutrition, exercise, stress reduction, disease prevention, smoking cessation

   b. Specific mental health problems for older women—alcohol and drug abuse, loneliness, depression, stress-induced illness, cigarette smoking, violence victimization, poverty

6. Sexuality

   a. Decreased estrogen may cause dryness, tightness, irritation and burning with coitus; postcoital spotting and soreness

   b. Sexually active women experience less atrophy

   c. Decline in sexual activity may be influenced by culture and attitude as well as physiology

   d. Most important reason for decreased sexual activity is unavailability of partner

   e. Strength of relationship and health status of each partner strongly influence sexual intimacy in older couples

7. Health considerations

   a. Available contraceptive options

      (1) Barrier methods

      (2) Progestin-only methods

      (3) IUD

      (4) Healthy non-smoker without cardiovascular risks may use low-dose oral contraceptives (OC) until menopause (to determine onset of menopause while on OCs, draw FSH on 7th day of placebo week)

      (5) Assure availability of emergency postcoital contraception

   b. Encourage annual screening for breast, cervical, colorectal, ovarian and endometrial cancer

   c. Explore nutrition issues

      (1) Caloric requirements decrease with aging

      (2) Adjust diet to maintain optimal weight

        (3) Decrease intake of saturated fats, nitrates, sodium, caffeine, sugar, alcohol and fat (all may aggravate menopausal symptoms)

  d. Calcium supplementation reduces bone loss and decreases fractures

        (1) Average woman ingests 500 mg of dietary calcium daily

        (2) If on estrogen therapy, minimal daily supplement of 500 mg required (total 1000 mg)

        (3) If not on estrogen, minimal daily supplement of 1000 mg required (total 1500 mg)

  e. Hormone replacement therapy (HRT)

        (1) Indications

            (a) To relieve menopausal symptoms related to estrogen deficiency

            (b) For prevention and treatment of osteoporosis

            (c) To protect against cardiovascular disease (estrogen causes decreased LDL, increased HDL, decreased total cholesterol)

        (2) Progestin should be added to estrogen regimen to decrease risk of endometrial cancer if uterus present

        (3) Regimen options for HRT

            (a) Sequential regimen—0.625 mg conjugated estrogens *or* 1.0 mg micronized estradiol either daily or from day 1-25 of each month; daily dose of 10 mg medroxyprogesterone acetate (Provera) added for the first 14 days of the month or for last 10 days of estrogen administration, respectively

            (b) Continuous/Combined regimen—daily administration of 0.625 mg conjugated estrogens, or 0.625 mg estrone sulfate, or 1.0 mg micronized estradiol with daily progestin administration of 2.5 mg medroxyprogesterone acetate, or 0.35 mg norethindrone

        (c)   Transdermal delivery of estradiol is a popular option; add medroxyprogesterone acetate 10 mg for 12 days of month or 2.5 mg continuously

        (d)   When estrogen contraindicated, medroxyprogesterone acetate may occasionally be used to relieve vasomotor symptoms

(4)   Risks of HRT

        (a)   May increase risk of gallbladder disease

        (b)   Relationship between HRT and breast cancer inconclusive; research is ongoing

(5)   Benefits of HRT

        (a)   Relieves/improves hot flashes, urinary symptoms, vaginal dryness

        (b)   Effective in prevention and treatment of osteoporosis

        (c)   Does not negatively alter lipid profile

        (d)   Reduces incidence of mortality from stroke

        (e)   Reduces risk of coronary heart disease and related mortality when estrogen used

        (f)   May improve overall feeling of well-being

        (g)   May protect against rheumatoid arthritis

        (h)   Does not impair glucose tolerance

        (i)   Does not negatively impact blood pressure

(6)   Contraindications to HRT

        (a)   Past or present history of deep vein thrombosis

        (b)   Known or suspected breast cancer

        (c)   Estrogen-dependent cancer

        (d)   Liver dysfunction or disease

        (e)   Undiagnosed abnormal vaginal bleeding

        (f)   Thrombophlebitis

(7)   Guidelines for HRT

(a) Decision about using HRT should rest primarily with the woman after she has received thorough counseling and education

(b) Use lowest dose of estrogen that relieves symptoms

(c) Refer if contraindications for estrogen exist

(d) Must have negative clinical breast examination and mammogram; endometrial biopsy indicated before initiating HRT in presence of abnormal vaginal bleeding

(e) Forty to sixty percent experience breakthrough bleeding during first 6 months of continuous therapy; if bleeding persists after first 6 months, further evaluation is needed

(f) Periodic follow-up required after HRT initiation

f. Non-hormonal therapy

(1) Diet low in saturated fats, nitrates, sodium, caffeine, sugar and alcohol

(2) Vitamin and mineral supplementation—vitamin E, B-complex vitamins, vitamin C, zinc

(3) Calcium supplementation to prevent osteoporosis (controversial)

(4) Studying preventative effects of vitamin D, sodium fluoride, phosphorus and calcitonin

(5) Regular aerobic exercise 3-5 times per week (weight-bearing exercise best for osteoporosis prevention)

(6) Kegel exercises to improve vaginal tone and prevent urinary stress incontinence

(7) Eliminate smoking and alcohol use

Fertility Control

- Combination Oral Contraceptives (OCs)
  1. Description

   a. Pill used for contraception that contains an estrogenic and a progestational agent

      (1) Only two estrogens available in U.S., mestranol and ethinyl estradiol; most OCs contain ethinyl estradiol

      (2) First generation progestins currently available

         (a) Norgestrel and levonorgestrel (two most potent)

         (b) Norethynodrel

         (c) Norethindrone

         (d) Norethindrone acetate

         (e) Ethynodiol diacetate

      (3) New generation progestins derived from levonorgestrel—gestodene, norgestimate, desogestrel

      (4) Types of combination OCs

         (a) Monophasic—deliver constant dose of hormones throughout cycle

         (b) Multiphasic—deliver varying amounts of hormones throughout cycle

      (5) Goal is to prescribe OC with 35 μg or less of estrogen when possible

2. Mechanism of action—combined effects of estrogen and progestin

   a. Suppression of FSH and LH inhibits ovulation

   b. Ovum transport accelerated

   c. Cervical mucus thickens, inhibiting sperm mobility

   d. Uterine secretions and endometrium altered, interfering with implantation

3. First year failure rates

   a. Perfect use: 1%

   b. Typical use: 3%

4. Advantages—noncontraceptive health benefits

   a. Affords protection against

   (1) Ovarian and endometrial cancer

   (2) Pelvic inflammatory disease (PID)

   (3) Ectopic pregnancy

   (4) Functional ovarian cysts

   (5) Iron deficiency anemia

   (6) Benign breast disease

   (7) Osteoporosis

   (8) Endometriosis

  b. May improve acne and premenstrual syndrome (PMS) symptoms

  c. May decrease menstrual cramps and blood loss

 5. Disadvantages—potential side effects are caused by estrogenic, progestational and androgenic properties of OCs

  a. Potential estrogenic effects—nausea, breast tenderness, increased breast size, fluid retention and cyclic weight gain, spider angiomas

  b. Potential progestational effects—breast tenderness, headaches, breakthrough bleeding

  c. Potential androgenic effects—increased appetite and weight gain, depression and fatigue, decreased libido, acne, increased breast size

  d. Provides no protection from HIV or sexually transmitted disease (STD)

 6. Precautions/Risks

  a. OCs should not be provided to women with current or past

   (1) Thrombophlebitis or thromboembolic disorder

   (2) Cerebrovascular accident

   (3) Coronary artery or ischemic heart disease

   (4) Undiagnosed breast mass or breast cancer

   (5) Known or strongly suspected estrogen-dependent neoplasia

      (6)   Benign hepatic adenoma or liver cancer

      (7)   Markedly impaired liver function (current)

  b. Carefully screen and monitor closely for development of adverse effects

      (1)   Over 35 years old and smokes $\geq$ 15 cigarettes per day

      (2)   Migraines that begin after initiating OCs

      (3)   Hypertension with resting diastolic of $\geq$ 90 mm Hg, or a resting systolic of $\geq$ 140 mm Hg on three separate visits, or a diastolic of $\geq$ 110 mm Hg on a single visit

      (4)   Diabetes mellitus

      (5)   Impending major surgery

      (6)   Undiagnosed abnormal vaginal bleeding

      (7)   Sickle cell disease or sickle C disease

      (8)   Lactation

      (9)   Gestational diabetes

     (10)   Active gallbladder disease

     (11)   Congenital hyperbilirubinemia

     (12)   Age over 50

     (13)   Completion of term pregnancy within 10-14 days

     (14)   Cardiac or renal disease

     (15)   Family history of hyperlipidemia

     (16)   Family history of death of a parent or sibling due to heart attack before the age of 50

  c. Risks associated with OC use

      (1)   Serious cardiovascular system disease (CVD) is rare with low dose OCs

        (a)   Hypertension—is dose-related effect of estrogen and progestin; rare with low-dose pills; return to normotensive state when OCs discontinued; no impact on blood pressure with new progestins

(b) Coagulation—heavy smoking is risk factor for thrombosis in OC users; changes in coagulation factors are due to estrogen content of OCs; OCs with ≤ 35 µg estrogen have minimal impact on blood clotting mechanisms

(c) Lipid metabolism—estrogen increases HDL and decreases LDL; synthetic progestins decrease HDLs and increase LDLs; new progestins have lipid neutral or lipid positive effect

(2) OCs and cancer

(a) Current data suggest that OC use does not increase a woman's risk for breast cancer; *may* have breast cancer promoting effect on specific subgroup of women; research ongoing

(b) Protective effect for ovarian and endometrial cancer which continues for at least 10 years after OCs discontinued

(c) Association between OC use and cervical cancer unclear

(d) Hepatocellular adenoma and cancer—benign liver tumors have been associated with use of combination OCs; risk increased with long-term use and women over 30 using higher dose OCs; very low risk with current formulations; uncertain link with hepatocellular carcinoma (very rare condition)

(3) Glucose intolerance—current low dose OCs do not adversely affect carbohydrate metabolism; higher dose OCs may affect, but following OC discontinuation, glucose tolerance returns to normal

(4) Gallbladder disease—recent studies suggest OCs do not increase the risk for development of gallbladder disease or cancer; may accelerate gallbladder disease in susceptible women

d. OCs and drug interaction

(1) Efficacy of low dose OCs may be lowered when used concurrently with

      (a) Anticonvulsants—phenytoin (Dilantin), carbamazepine (Tegretol), primidone (Mysoline)

      (b) Antibiotics, especially ampicillin and tetracycline

      (c) Barbiturates (such as phenobarbital)

      (d) Griseofulvin

      (e) Rifampin

      (f) Antacids

   (2) OCs may decrease clearance of certain tranquilizers; lower doses of these medications may be indicated while on OCs

   (3) OCs may decrease clearance and increase the half-life of anti-inflammatory corticosteroids; lower doses may be indicated when on OCs

   (4) Clearance of bronchodilating drugs and caffeine may be reduced by 30-40% in OC users

   (5) One gram of vitamin C increases serum ethinyl estradiol levels by 50%, changing OC into a high dose pill; alteration may cause spotting; to counteract effect, take Vitamin C 4 hours apart from OC

- Progestin-Only Pills (Mini-pills)

   1. Description—contraceptive pills consisting of a fixed dose progestational agent (norethindrone or norgestrel)

   2. Mechanism of action

      a. Creation of thin, atrophic endometrium

      b. Thickened cervical mucus affects sperm permeability

      c. May affect tubal physiology, decreasing ovum transport

      d. Inhibits sperm capacitation

      e. Does not consistently suppress gonadotropins; 40% will ovulate normally

   3. First year failure rates

      a. Perfect use: 3%

      b Typical use: 5%

    c. Almost 100% effective in lactating women

    d. Higher failure rate in younger women (3.1 per 100 woman years), compared to women over 40 (0.3 per 100 woman years)

4. Advantages

    a. No adverse effect on lactation; may be initiated immediately after delivery

    b. Fewer side effects than combined OCs

    c. May be an alternative for women who cannot use estrogen

    d. Immediate return to fertility upon discontinuation

5. Disadvantages

    a. Must take daily at the same time; vulnerable efficacy

    b. If pregnancy occurs, ectopic must be suspected

    c. Increased incidence of functional ovarian cysts

    d. Irregular menstrual bleeding; major reason for discontinuation

6. Precautions/Risks—FDA labeling in package insert includes same contraindications as for combined OCs

    a. No data to support increased risk of cardiovascular complications, malignant disease, or metabolic changes

    b. Precaution should be exercised when prescribing OCs for any woman with unexplained abnormal vaginal bleeding during the last 3 months, symptomatic functional cysts, or who uses medications such as rifampin or anticonvulsants

- Intrauterine Devices (IUDs)

  1. Description

    a. Two types available in United States

        (1) Progesterone T (Progestasert System)

            (a) Releases 65 mcg progesterone per day

            (b) Must be replaced annually

            (c) Has a blue-black double string

        (2) Copper T 380A (Paragard)

       (a)   T-shaped device bound in fine copper wire

       (b)   Has clear or whitish knotted double string

       (c)   Lowest failure rate of IUDs; approved for 10 years

       (d)   Most widely used IUD in U.S.

2. Mechanism of action (postulated)

   a. Immobilizes sperm

   b. Interferes with migration of sperm from vagina to fallopian tubes

   c. Speeds transport of ovum through fallopian tube

   d. Possible inflammation of endometrium

3. First year failure rates

   a. CuT 380A—typical use: 0.8%; perfect use: 0.6%

   b. Progesterone T—typical use: 2%; perfect use: 1.5%

4. Advantages

   a. Progesterone-releasing IUD decreases menstrual blood loss and dysmenorrhea

   b. Can be used during lactation

   c. Good option in women who have medical contraindications to OCs

   d. Less expensive per year than other methods

5. Disadvantages

   a. Increased risk of PID occurring at time of insertion

   b. Provides no HIV or STD protection

   c. May experience increased dysmenorrhea and/or menstrual spotting

   d. Spontaneous expulsion may occur

6. Precautions/Risks

   a. IUDs should not be provided to women with

       (1)   Active, recent, or recurrent pelvic infection

       (2)   Known or suspected pregnancy

b. Women with following conditions who want IUDs should be carefully screened, counseled thoroughly on risk factors, and monitored closely for development of adverse affects

   (1) Risk factors for PID—purulent cervicitis, recent positive test for gonorrhea or chlamydia, recurrent history of gonorrhea or chlamydia

   (2) High risk for STD—multiple sexual partners or partner with multiple partners

   (3) Impaired immune response—diabetes, steroid treatment, HIV disease

   (4) Risk factors for HIV infection

   (5) Undiagnosed, irregular, heavy or abnormal vaginal bleeding

   (6) Known or suspected cervical or uterine cancer

   (7) Unresolved abnormal Pap smear (can still have IUD, but need Pap follow-up)

   (8) History of ectopic pregnancy

   (9) Previous complication with IUD use

   (10) History of severe vasovagal response

   (11) Valvular heart disease (aortic stenosis, mitral valve prolapse)—can use prophylactic antibiotics

   (12) Uterine abnormalities—fibroids, endometrial polyps, cervical stenosis, bicornuate or small uterus

   (13) Nulliparity

   (14) History of anemia

   (15) Lack of access to medical care if IUD-related complication should arise

c. Side effects and complications

   (1) Spotting, bleeding, hemorrhage

      (a) May be sign of pregnancy or infection

      (b) Common in first 3 months after insertion

      (c)   Perform Hgb or Hct

      (d)   If associated with pain, rule out PID and pregnancy

      (e)   If thought to be associated with endometritis, remove IUD, culture for chlamydia and gonorrhea, treat presumptively with antibiotics, provide alternative contraception

      (f)   If over 40 and bleeding is prolonged, remove IUD; refer if bleeding persists

  (2) Anemia

      (a)   If Hgb < 11.5 g at insertion, prescribe $FeSO_4$ 300 mg once daily for 1-2 months, then repeat Hgb at 3 month follow-up; if IUD desired, consider Progestasert

      (b)   For Hgb < 9 g, remove IUD, provide alternative contraceptive method, provide iron supplement for 2 months, repeat Hgb in one month

      (c)   If Hgb falls ≥ 2 g, remove IUD, treat as in (2)(a)

      (d)   Check Hgb in presence of abnormal bleeding

  (3) Cramping/Pain

      (a)   Common at time of insertion; could indicate perforation; analgesic helpful with menses

      (b)   If perforation is suspected and strings are present, remove IUD and treat as infection

      (c)   If perforation is suspected and strings are not visible, refer to physician

  (4) Expulsion

      (a)   Symptoms may include—unusual vaginal discharge, cramping or pain, intermenstrual spotting, postcoital spotting, dyspareunia, absence or lengthening of string, and palpation of device at os or in vagina

      (b)   If partial expulsion—remove IUD, evaluate for pregnancy or infection; if neither are present, reinsert another IUD, give 5-7 days of doxycycline 100 mg every 12 hours

(5) Pregnancy

    (a) One-third or fewer of IUD-related pregnancies are caused by undetected or partial expulsion

    (b) Increased risk of spontaneous abortion (50%) and sepsis if IUD left in place

    (c) Five percent of pregnancies will be ectopic; at highest risk if previous history of ectopic; Progestasert users have 6-10 fold higher ectopic rate than copper IUD users

(6) Uterine perforation, embedding, and cervical perforation

    (a) Range of incidence 1 in 1,000 to 1 in 2,500

    (b) Rate 2.0-2.8 per 100 users at 24 months with immediate postpartum insertion

    (c) Most common perforation sites—uterine fundus, body of uterus, cervical wall

(7) Pelvic inflammatory disease (PID)

    (a) Can be serious, life-threatening condition; requires aggressive treatment and follow-up

    (b) Initial 2-3 months following insertion is time of highest risk

    (c) Remove IUD with any degree of PID

    (d) If patient is pregnant, pregnancy is desired, and IUD strings visible, remove IUD

    (e) If pregnancy is desired and IUD strings are *not* visible, may leave in place with strong warning signs regarding infection and ectopic

- Diaphragm

  1. Description—thin, dome-shaped rubber cup stretched over flexible ring that is inserted into the vagina prior to intercourse with the posterior rim resting in the posterior fornix, and the anterior rim positioned snugly behind the pubic bone

  2. Available in range of sizes (50 to 100 mm in diameter) and in several spring types

    a. Arcing spring—folds into arc shape which facilitates correct insertion; indicated for women with fair to relaxed vaginal muscle tone; firm spring strength

    b. Coil spring—intermediate spring strength; suited for women with average vaginal muscle tone

    c. Flat spring—folds flat; thin rim; good choice for women with very firm vaginal tone or shallow pubic notch

3. Mechanism of action—provides barrier plus spermicide

4. First year failure rates

    a. Perfect use: 6%

    b. Typical use: 18%

5. Advantages

    a. Safe

    b. Few side effects

    c. Provides some protection against STDs, including gonorrhea and chlamydia, and against cervical neoplasia

    d. Protection for HIV risk uncertain

6. Disadvantages

    a. Device is prescriptive; must be fit by a clinician

    b. Dyspareunia if fit is too large

    c. Interference with spontaneity of lovemaking

    d. Increases risk for bacterial vaginosis, candidiasis and urinary tract infection

7. Precautions for use

    a. History of toxic shock syndrome (TSS)

    b. Allergy to latex or spermicide

    c. Chronic UTI despite refit efforts

    d. Inability to achieve satisfactory fit due to anatomic abnormality

        (1) Uterine prolapse

        (2) Severe cystocele

(3) Rectocele or extreme uterine retroversion

- Cervical Cap (Prentiff Cavity-Rim)

    1. Description—deep, soft rubber cup with a firm, round rim creating suction over cervix; available in four sizes (22, 25, 28, 31 mm); should cover cervix completely with rim resting at the base of the cervix

    2. Mechanism of action—provides barrier plus spermicide

    3. First year failure rates

        a. Perfect use

            (1) Parous: 26%

            (2) Nulliparous: 9%

        b. Typical use

            (1) Parous: 36%

            (2) Nulliparous: 18%

    4. Advantages—continuous contraception for 48 hours

    5. Disadvantages—requires examination for fitting

    6. Precautions

        a. History of TSS

        b. Allergy to latex or spermicide

        c. Acute PID, cervicitis, or undiagnosed vaginitis

        d. Cervical biopsy or cryosurgery during past 6-12 weeks

        e. Full-term delivery during past 6-12 weeks

        f. Anatomic abnormalities—cervix flush with vaginal vault or asymmetry of cervix

        g. History of abnormal Pap smear

        h. Known or suspected cervical or uterine malignancy

        i. FDA specifies 48-hour maximum wearing time, 3-month follow-up Pap smear, and annual cap replacement

- Vaginal Sponge—no longer produced after March 1994 due to problems with manufacturer standards

- Spermicides (Nonoxynol-9 or Octoxynol-9)
    1. Description
        a. Inert base plus spermicidal chemical
        b. Spermicidal products—foams, creams, jellies, suppositories, tablets and contraceptive film
    2. Mechanism of action—destroys sperm cell membrane, killing sperm
    3. First year failure rate
        a. Perfect use: 6%
        b. Typical use: 21%
    4. Advantages
        a. Inexpensive and available
        b. Some protection against STDs and PID
        c. Risk for STD is greatly reduced with condom use
    5. Disadvantages
        a. Allergic reactions
        b. Increased risk of symptomatic candidiasis
        c. Relationship between spermicide use and HIV risk is not established
    6. Precautions
        a. Severe allergic reaction
        b. Inability to learn correct insertion technique
        c. Abnormalities in vaginal anatomy (vaginal septum, prolapse, double cervix)
- Condoms
    1. Male condoms
        a. Description
            (1) One of most popular contraceptive methods in U.S.
            (2) Three types
                (a) Latex (rubber)

        (b) Polyurethane (plastic)

        (c) Lambskin (intestine membrane)—not recommended for STD protection

  b. Mechanism of action

     (1) Mechanical barrier; prevents semen from entering vagina

     (2) Added protection with brands coated with spermicide (nonoxynol-9)

  c. First year failure rates—perfect use 3%; typical use 12%

  d. Advantages

     (1) Effective component of safer sex practice to prevent transmission of STDs, including HIV (latex)

     (2) Accessible, inexpensive

     (3) In women who produce sperm antibodies, condom use for 3-6 months can decrease antigen release into vagina

     (4) *May* prevent development of or promote regression of cervical intraepithelial neoplasia (CIN) by preventing contact with semen

     (5) By decreasing STD risk, may decrease infertility risk

     (6) May help prolong erection and prevent premature ejaculation

  e. Disadvantages—allergy to latex; male involvement essential; cultural attitudes about use; sensitivity may be reduced; possibility of breakage; interference with erection

  f. Precautions

     (1) Must be placed on erect penis prior to any genital contact

     (2) Petroleum based lubricants (Vaseline) and some vaginal medications break down latex

     (3) Penis must be removed from vagina while still erect to prevent spillage

2. Female condom

  a. Description—polyurethane sheath with flexible polyurethane rings at each end

    b. Mechanism of action

        (1) Physical barrier that lines the vagina and partially covers the perineum (*no* spermicidal action)

        (2) Open ring at longer outer end covers the labia

        (3) Closed diaphragm-like ring at inner end covers the cervix and serves as an internal anchor

    c. First year failure rate—perfect use 5%; typical use 21%

    d. Advantages

        (1) Theoretically provides protection against STD exposure comparable to latex male condom

        (2) Does not require prescription

        (3) May be inserted up to 8 hours before intercourse

        (4) Less breakage with impermeable polyurethane material than with latex

    e. Disadvantages

        (1) For single use only; expensive

        (2) May be displaced

        (3) Petroleum-based products can deteriorate polyurethane

        (4) May be noisy during use; unattractive

    f. Precautions

        (1) Latex allergy may occur

        (2) Difficult to use if anatomic abnormalities exist

        (3) Insertion may be difficult

- Voluntary Sterilization—most prevalent contraceptive method among married women in U.S.

    1. Female Sterilization—bilateral tubal ligation (BTL)

        a. Description—surgical ligation of fallopian tubes; may be performed during cesarean section, after vaginal delivery or abortion, or as interval procedure

(1) Surgical approaches used—laparotomy; minilaparotomy; laparoscopy; colpotomy/culdoscopy

(2) Methods include—surgical ligation; excision; electrocoagulation; use of mechanical devices

b. Mechanism of action—operative procedure that interrupts fallopian tube and prevents union of ovum and sperm

c. Failure rate 1:400

d. Advantages

(1) Permanent; highly effective

(2) Can be performed during immediate postpartum period

(3) No significant long-term effects

e. Disadvantages/Cautions

(1) General risk of surgery (mortality: 3.6/100,000 women)

(2) Pain associated with procedure

(3) Infection/hemorrhage

(4) Anesthesia related complications

(5) Ectopic pregnancy (absolute risk is lowered after BTL, but if subsequent pregnancy occurs, increased risk of ectopic)

f. Reversal

(1) Requires major surgery; very expensive

(2) Chance for success depends on how sterilization was performed; success rate highest for occlusion techniques

(3) Success cannot be guaranteed

(4) Success possible with minimal tubal damage and 3.5 cm of tube available

(5) High risk for ectopic following reversal

2. Male sterilization—vasectomy

a. Description—male sterilization operation that blocks the vas deferens, preventing passage of sperm

b. Mechanism of action—as above

    c. Failure rate 1:600

    d. Advantages

       (1) Extremely low mortality rate

       (2) Inexpensive and simple procedure (new non-scalpel technique may help reduce anxiety and complications)

       (3) Increasing popularity; estimated 7.5 million men have had vasectomy; significant factor in male acceptance is personal contact with another male who has had vasectomy and is satisfied with method

    e. Disadvantages

       (1) Vasectomy reversal difficult, costly and not widely available; success rates vary based on individual circumstances (16-85% reported) and length of time lapsed between procedure and reversal attempt

       (2) Minor postoperative side effects—bruising, swelling, hematoma, epididymitis, and infection at operative site

    f. Precautions

       (1) Contraindications

          (a) Local skin infections (scabies, genital tract infections)

          (b) Varicocele, large hydrocele, inguinal hernia, and scar tissue from previous surgery

          (c) Special precautions required for clotting disorders, diabetes, and recent coronary heart disease

          (d) Surgery should be discouraged if procedure is performed as cure for sexual dysfunction

          (e) Some consider history of marital, psychosocial or sexual instability a contraindication

       (2) Vasectomy failures are usually due to

          (a) Having unprotected coitus before reproductive tract is cleared of sperm

          (b) Spontaneous recanalization of the vas deferens

   (c) Surgical error

   (d) Missed congenital duplication of the vas deferens

  (3) Barriers to vasectomy option

   (a) Religious ambivalence

   (b) Cultural attitudes or fear regarding sexual performance (impotence, decreased fertility, decreased virility)

- Fertility Awareness Methods

 1. Description—methods used to identify fertile days of menstrual cycle include calendar rhythm method, basal body temperature method, ovulation or Billings method, and sympto-thermal method

 2. Mechanism of action—calculation of fertile period rests on 4 assumptions

  a. Ovulation occurs on day 14 (± 2 days) before the onset of next menses

  b. Sperm remain viable for 2-7 days (average 3 days)

  c. Ovum survive approximately 24 hours

  d. Span of fertility may be from 7 days before ovulation to 3 days after

 3. First year failure rate—typical use 20%; perfect use 1-9%

 4. Advantages

  a. Low cost; no side effects

  b. Can be used to plan conception, detect pregnancy, detect impaired fertility, and to prevent pregnancy

 5. Precautions and disadvantages

  a. No protection against STDs or HIV

  b. Not recommended for women

   (1) With irregular menstrual pattern

   (2) Approaching menopause

   (3) Not able to keep careful records

(4) Postpartum prior to resumption of normal menses

c. Women must abstain when libido is at peak

6. Specific fertility awareness methods

a. Calendar charting—charts cycle over time

(1) Fertile days are predicted based on past menstrual cycle records

(2) The earliest day of fertility is computed by subtracting 18 days from length of shortest cycle

(3) The latest day of fertility is computed by subtracting 11 days from length of longest cycle

(4) If using method to achieve pregnancy, determine first and last fertile days in any given month, have intercourse beginning 2-3 days prior to predicted fertile days and continue throughout fertile cycle

(5) If using method to prevent pregnancy, avoid intercourse, or use back-up method during fertile period

b. Basal body temperature (BBT) charting

(1) BBT defined as lowest temperature of healthy person upon awakening

(2) Time of ovulation can be determined by recording BBT for 3-4 successive months

(3) Determination possible because drop in BBT often precedes ovulation by about 12-24 hours, followed by sustained BBT increase for several days

(4) Progesterone increases BBT 0.4-0.8°F

(5) To prevent pregnancy, abstain until temperature has remained elevated for 3 consecutive days

c. Cervical mucus method (Billings or Ovulation Method)

(1) Mucus changes

(a) Before and during ovulation—mucus clear, thin, wet, elastic and abundant

(b) After ovulation, under influence of progesterone—mucus thick, viscid, white and scant

(2) In addition to cervical mucus, use cyclic changes in position and texture of cervix and presence of mittelschmerz to identify fertile days

(3) To prevent pregnancy, couples should abstain during days of wet cervical mucus; intercourse permitted beginning 4th day after last days of wet mucus or when no mucus present

(4) Douching, vaginal infection, semen, foam, diaphragm jelly, lubricants, medications, and normal lubrication during sexual arousal can interfere with ability to identify mucus changes

d. Sympto-thermal method

(1) Usually combines awareness of ovulation symptoms (mucus and cervical changes) and BBT changes

(2) Abstain or use back-up contraception until 4 days after appearance of fertile mucus and 3 days after temperature rise

- Postcoital Options for Emergency Contraception

1. No product approved specifically for emergency or post-coital use in the U.S.

2. Mechanism of action

   a. Hormonal methods—temporarily disrupt ovarian hormone production causing dysfunctional luteal phase and unsuitable endometrium for implantation, interference with fertilization and tubal transport

   b. IUD—makes endometrium unsuitable for implantation; interferes with fertilization and transport

3. Efficacy: Approximately 75%

4. Indications for emergency postcoital hormonal contraception

   a. Unprotected intercourse within 72 hours

b. Potential for contraceptive failure (missed OCs, condom slippage, incorrect insertion of diaphragm, partial expulsion of IUD, etc.)

c. Sexual assault

d. Exposure to possible teratogen

5. Current options used by providers

a. Combination OCs that contain ethinyl estradiol (EE) and norgestrel—emergency contraceptive pills (ECPs)

(1) Two doses, 12 hours apart, totaling 200 mg EE and 2.0 mg norgestrel or 1.0 mg levonorgestrel ("Yuzpe" regimen)

(2) Most effective when initiated within first 12-24 hours after unprotected intercourse; not likely to be effective after 72 hours

(3) Most commonly used regimen

(4) Should not be used in women for whom OCs are contraindicated

b. Danazol treatment

(1) Synthetic androgen; not widely used

(2) Regimens of two 400 mg doses, 12 hours apart, totaling 800 mg, and three 400 doses, 12 hours apart, totaling 1,200 mg have been studied

(3) Contraindicated in presence of breastfeeding, abnormal vaginal bleeding, impaired liver, kidney, or heart function

c. Postcoital IUD insertion

(1) Must be good candidate for IUD use

(2) Copper IUD inserted 5-7 days after ovulation if unprotected intercourse has occurred during cycle

(3) Should not be used in women at risk for STDs, women who have been raped, or women who have history of ectopic pregnancy

d. DES no longer approved by the Food and Drug Administration (FDA) for postcoital contraception

      e. Side effects

          (1) Nausea and vomiting with ECPs; may provide non-prescription anti-nausea medication (dimenhydrinate)

          (2) Timing of next menstrual period may be altered

  6. Other considerations

      a. Follow-up care within 3-4 weeks after treatment

      b. If vomiting occurs, may require extra OC dose

      c. Offer interim contraception

      d. Possible treatment failure

- **Long-Acting Hormonal Methods (Progestin-Only)**

  1. Norplant

      a. Description

          (1) Six silastic rods 2.4 mm X 34 mm, each containing 36 mg of levonorgestrel

          (2) Rods are implanted beneath skin of upper arm; effective for 5 years

      b. Mechanism of action

          (1) Ovulation inhibited by suppression of LH

          (2) Tubal changes—altered tubal transport, contractility, and histology

          (3) Thickened, decreased cervical mucus inhibits sperm penetration

          (4) Creates thin, atrophic endometrium

      c. Effectiveness

          (1) Failure rate less than 1 per 100 woman-years of use

          (2) Failure rate increases slightly with succeeding years

          (3) Effectiveness of current implants unaffected by woman's weight

    (4) Insert within 7 days of onset of menses, or while using another effective method of contraception to decrease chance of inserting while pregnant

  d. Advantages

    (1) Long-lasting and effective

    (2) Unrelated to sexual intercourse

    (3) Easily reversible

    (4) Contains no estrogen

    (5) Avoids hormonal surges

    (6) Noncontraceptive benefits

        (a) Scanty or no menses

        (b) Decreased anemia, dysmenorrhea, pain with ovulation, risk for endometrial and ovarian cancer, PID, and pain caused by endometriosis

        (c) Lower risk of ectopic pregnancy compared with women using no contraceptive method; if pregnancy occurs, need to rule out ectopic

  e. Disadvantages

    (1) Implants may be slightly visible

    (2) Initial expense high

    (3) Removal requires minor surgery and is sometimes difficult, especially if inserted too deeply or incorrectly

    (4) Alterations in bleeding patterns (most common reason for removal in first 2 years of use)

    (5) Special training required for insertion and removal

    (6) Side effects—weight gain/bloating; breast tenderness; acne/hair loss

    (7) Decreased efficacy with use of anticonvulsants and rifampin

    (8) Ovarian cysts may occur

    (9) Local inflammation or infection at implantation site

     f. Precautions/Risks

        (1) Contraindications

            (a) Unexplained abnormal vaginal bleeding

            (b) Active thrombophlebitis or pulmonary emboli

            (c) Known or suspected pregnancy

            (d) Use of anticonvulsants (except valproic acid) and rifampin

            (e) Known or suspected breast cancer or history of breast cancer

        (2) Precautions—exercise caution and monitor carefully for adverse effects

            (a) Intolerant of irregular bleeding due to personal or cultural reasons

            (b) Migraine or other headaches

            (c) Heart lesions that predispose to acute bacterial endocarditis

            (d) History of heart attack or stroke; chest pain due to diagnosed heart disease; thrombophlebitis; pulmonary embolism; diabetics with predisposition to cardiovascular disease

            (e) History of allergic reaction on OC containing levonorgestrel

            (f) History of increased acne on OCs

2. Depo-Provera (DMPA)

     a. Description—injectable progestin (Depo-medroxyprogesterone acetate)

     b. Mechanism of action

        (1) Microcrystallized hormone distributed in aqueous solution to storage sites in adipose tissue and slowly released into circulation over a 4 month period

        (2) Increased level of circulating progestin blocks LH surge and suppresses ovulation

        (3) Thickened cervical mucus inhibits sperm penetration

        (4) Endometrium is thinned, creating poor environment for ovum implantation

  c. Effectiveness—first year failure rate of 0.3% with 150 mg per 1 cc of medication

  d. Advantages

        (1) Studies reveal no serious short or long-term effects of use

        (2) Lack of interference with intercourse

        (3) Long acting

        (4) Freedom from compliance concerns

        (5) No estrogen-related side effects

        (6) Amenorrhea

        (7) Non-contraceptive benefits

            (a) May increase quantity and quality of breastmilk

            (b) Decreased risk of endometrial and ovarian cancer, PID, endometriosis, and ectopic pregnancy

            (c) No drug interactions

            (d) Decreases frequency of seizures

  e. Disadvantages

        (1) Necessity to return every 3 months for injection

        (2) Intramuscular injections may be uncomfortable

        (3) Changes in bleeding pattern (amenorrhea more likely with DMPA than Norplant; the longer DMPA used, the more likely woman is to experience amenorrhea)

        (4) Delayed return to fertility

        (5) Decrease in bone density (currently under study); reversible when DMPA discontinued

        (6) Decrease in HDL cholesterol levels

  f. Precautions/risks

        (1) Contraindications to use

      (a)   Known or suspected pregnancy

      (b)   Unexplained abnormal vaginal bleeding in past 3 months

   (2)   Exercise caution and monitor carefully for adverse effects

      (a)   Woman with desire for pregnancy in near future

      (b)   Concern about weight gain

      (c)   Severe, acute liver disease or liver tumors and/or severe gallbladder disease

   (3)   Side effects—weight gain; headaches; breast tenderness; menstrual changes (major reason for discontinuing method); anaphylactic reactions possible following injections

  g. Dosage and administration

   (1)   Dosage—150 mg distributed in single dose 1 cc vial

   (2)   Shake vial vigorously before use

   (3)   Administer deep IM. into gluteal or deltoid muscle with 21 or 23 gauge needle

   (4)   Do not massage injection site; may lower effectiveness

   (5)   Administer

      (a)   During first 5 days after onset of normal menses

      (b)   Within 5 days postpartum if not breastfeeding

      (c)   At 6 weeks postpartum, if breastfeeding

      (d)   Pregnancy test required before administration if more than 13 weeks since last injection

- Other Contraceptive Practices

  1. Abstinence—refraining from vaginal or anal intercourse

    a. Completely effective in preventing pregnancy and STDs

    b. Until age 17, abstainers outnumber those who have had intercourse

  2. Withdrawal (coitus interruptus)

a. Description—interrupts intercourse by withdrawing penis from vagina before ejaculation; used by 2% sexually active women

b. Mechanism of action—prevents fertilization by preventing contact between spermatozoa and ovum

c. First year failure rate—perfect use 4%; typical use 19%; depends on male's ability to withdraw prior to ejaculation

d. Advantages

   (1) Requires no devices or chemicals

   (2) Available in any situation

   (3) No medical side effects

e. Disadvantages

   (1) Requires high degree of self control by male partner

   (2) Interruption of excitement or plateau phase of sexual response can diminish pleasure for couple

   (3) No HIV or STD protection

3. Lactation amenorrhea method (LAM)

a. Mechanism of action

   (1) Contraceptive effect due to hyperprolactinemic state which suppresses the release of LH; although FSH returns to normal by 3 weeks, ovary does not promote follicular development

   (2) Most authorities believe infant diet needs to be supplemented by 6 months to promote normal growth and development; breastfeeding mothers should be advised to use another contraceptive method before the 6th month after delivery

b. Effectiveness—depends on mother's level of nutrition, intensity of suckling, and amount of supplementation infant receives

c. During first 6 months after delivery, provides contraceptive effectiveness equal to OCs for women who are amenorrheic and exclusively breastfeed at regular intervals including throughout night

    4. Douching

        a. Considered ineffective and unreliable as a contraceptive method

        b. Practice is associated with increased risk of pelvic infection and ectopic pregnancy

        c. If woman chooses to douche after intercourse, should wait 6-8 hours if vaginal spermicide used as contraceptive

- Experimental Methods

    1. Vaginal Rings

        a. Most current research on ring that contains levonorgestrel released at a rate of 20 µg/day

        b. Also testing ring that contains estrogen and progestin

        c. Problems with vaginal irritation have slowed commercialization

    2. Lea's Shield—one-size fits all diaphragm-like device with one-way valve to allow air to escape during placement; creates better retention against cervix; valve allows escape of uterine and cervical fluids but prevents entrance to sperm; approval anticipated for 1998

    3. Femcap—cervical cap-like method; 3 sizes; size selection based on user's parity

    4. Disposable diaphragm—clinical studies yet to begin; releases nonoxynol-9

    5. Norplant II—improved version Norplant containing 2 rods; similar drug levels and duration of action; may be available 1995

Diagnostic Studies and Laboratory Tests

- Papanicolaou (Pap) Smear

    1. Screening test to detect cancerous and precancerous lesions of the cervix, vulva and vagina

    2. American Cancer Society & ACOG Guidelines

        a. Annual cervical smear and pelvic exam in women who are or have been sexually active or by age 18

        b. After 3 or more annual, consecutive negative tests, may perform less frequently unless client has risk factors

    c. High risk categories

        (1) Coitus before 18-20 years of age

        (2) More than 3 partners in lifetime

        (3) Male partner with history of multiple partners or history of STDs

        (4) History of STD (especially human papillomavirus subtypes)

        (5) Previous abnormal Pap smear

        (6) Cigarette use

        (7) Infection with HIV

        (8) DES-exposure in utero

3. Technique of cytologic screening

    a. High false negative rate (10-30%); sampling errors a major factor

    b. Must collect cellular sample from endocervical canal and a scraping from the entire transformation zone (TZ)

    c. Cytobrush recommended for best yield; use in pregnancy controversial

    d. Steps for obtaining adequate sample

        (1) Collect prior to bimanual exam

        (2) No lubricant on speculum

        (3) Take Pap before STD tests

        (4) If large amount discharge present, carefully remove

        (5) Sample ectocervix, then endocervix

        (6) Apply evenly to slide and fix within 5 seconds

        (7) If DES-exposed, may also take smears from upper two-thirds of the vagina or perform 4-quadrant vaginal smear

    e. Endocervical cells needed for accurate diagnosis

4. The Bethesda System—most current classification system used to interpret cytologic findings; format of report

  a. Statement of specimen adequacy

    (1) Satisfactory for evaluation

    (2) Satisfactory but limited

    (3) Unsatisfactory

  b. General categorization

    (1) Within normal limits

    (2) Benign cellular changes

    (3) Infection

    (4) Reactive changes (repair, atrophy, inflammation, IUD)

    (5) Epithelial cell abnormality

      (a) Squamous abnormalities

      (b) Glandular cell abnormalities

    (6) Other malignant neoplasms

  c. Descriptive diagnosis

    (1) Squamous cell abnormalities

      (a) Atypical cells of undetermined significance (ASCUS)—indicates some abnormality but cause is unclear (infection common)

      (b) Low-grade squamous intraepithelial lesion (LSIL)—HPV, mild dysplasia/CIN I

      (c) High-grade squamous intraepithelial lesions (HSIL)—moderate and severe dysplasia, CIS/CIN II and CIN III

      (d) Squamous cell carcinoma

    (2) Glandular cell abnormalities

      (a) Endometrial cells—menstruating or postmenopausal women

      (b) Glandular atypia—atypical glandular cells of undetermined significance (AGCUS)

(c) Adenocarcinoma—endocervical, endometrial or extrauterine adenocarcinoma

- Wet Mounts

    1. Description—inexpensive and simple test that allows direct microscopic examination of specimens (cervical, breast, urine)

    2. Types

        a. Saline wet prep

            (1) Provides diagnosis of bacterial vaginosis (BV), trichomoniasis and monilia, and assists in presumptive diagnosis of other cervical infections such as gonorrhea and chlamydia

            (2) Can identify normal epithelial cells, clue cells, white blood cells, red blood cells, mobiluncus, motile trichomonads, mycelia, spores, lactobacilli, lepothrix, round parabasal cells and sperm

        b. Potassium hydroxide (KOH) prep used to establish

            (1) Positive amine test or "whiff test"—distinctive fishy odor released when vaginal discharge is alkalinized by adding 1-2 drops of 10% KOH to sample; may assist with diagnosis of bacterial vaginosis

            (2) Diagnosis of candida vaginitis

                (a) One or 2 drops of 10% KOH mixed with vaginal specimen

                (b) KOH lyses epithelial cells and white blood cells, candida cell walls resistant—easier to visualize

- Colposcopy

    1. Primarily used to evaluate abnormal cervical, vaginal and vulvar cytologic findings, and to direct biopsies for definitive diagnosis

    2. Instrument is a stereoscopic binocular microscope of low magnification used with a strong light

    3. Indications for use

        a. Evaluation of abnormal Pap smear reports

        b. Evaluation of visible cervical lesions

     c. Baseline examination in DES-exposed women

     d. Follow-up screening for cervical, vaginal or vulvar cancer

     e. Evaluation of suspicious vulvar or vaginal lesions

     f. Direct tissue biopsies

4. Technique

     a. Procedure takes about 30 minutes

     b. Examine the external genitalia (tissue may be moistened with normal saline)

     c. A non-lubricated speculum is inserted to visualize the cervix; colposcopic exam of cervix is directed toward the transformation zone (TZ)

     d. Application of 3-5% acetic acid solution dissolves mucus, shrinks blood vessels and causes certain cells to shrink, enhancing structures

     e. Colposcopically directed biopsy performed on most atypical lesions for definitive diagnosis

     f. Endocervical curettage provides definitive histologic diagnosis

     g. Evaluation unsatisfactory if entire TZ not visualized

5. Should be performed by a trained and experienced colposcopist

- Pregnancy Tests

1. Detect human chorionic gonadotropin (hCG) in blood or urine

2. Indications

     a. Rule out or confirm pregnancy

     b. Aid in the differential diagnosis of intrauterine or ectopic pregnancy, threatened or missed abortion, or hydatidiform mole

3. Interpretation errors

     a. False negative (rare)

         (1) About 1% false negative rate with urine sensitivity of 50 mIU/mL

         (2) Lab error; elevated lipids; severe kidney disease; high immunoglobulins

b. False positive

    (1) Uncommon

    (2) Lab error; LH or FSH cross-reaction; protein or blood in urine; tumors of pancreas, ovaries or breast

4. Pregnancy test options

  a. Immunometric tests

    (1) Based on enzyme-linked immunosorbent assay (ELISA)

    (2) Specific for beta sub-unit of hCG (no cross-reactions)

    (3) Reported as positive or negative

    (4) Specificity—accurate qualitative results with hCG levels as low as 5-50 mIU/mL

    (5) Test results are positive for 98% of women within 7 days of implantation

    (6) Indications

      (a) Confirm or rule out pregnancy

      (b) Suspected ectopic

  b. Quantitative beta hCG radioimmunoassay (blood test)

    (1) As a qualitative test, no specific advantage over immuno-metric urine tests

    (2) Provides accurate quantitative results with hCG levels as low as 5 mIU/mL reliably detecting pregnancy within 7 days after fertilization

    (3) Indicated when quantitative results needed—ectopic pregnancy, impending spontaneous abortion, retained placental fragments, molar pregnancy

  c. Agglutination inhibition slide tests

    (1) Results depend on binding between hCG (from urine or serum) and an anti-hCG antibody in test solution

    (2) Low sensitivity; not specific for beta subunit; cross-reaction possible with FSH and LH

(3) Good for confirming pregnancy at 6-16 weeks of gestation; may miss early or late pregnancy, ectopic pregnancy or impending abortion

d. Home pregnancy kits

(1) Popular because of convenience and privacy; use immunochromatology tests (color change occurs with antibody reaction to hCG)

(2) Excellent theoretical accuracy, but user skill lowers actual accuracy rates; can detect hCG levels in urine as low as 25-50 mIU/mL as early as 1 week postconception

- Ultrasonography

1. Pelvic ultrasound

a. Examines area from umbilicus to pubic bone

b. Two approaches

(1) Transvaginal—uses vaginal probes; often provides diagnosis at time of procedure; does not require full bladder

(2) Abdominal—not invasive; requires full bladder; satisfactory visualization often difficult in obese women

c. Indications for transvaginal versus abdominal scanning

(1) Better visualization of ovaries and fallopian tubes to monitor growth and development of ovarian follicles (infertility patients); assist in diagnosis of polycystic ovary syndrome, ovarian pathology, ovarian cancer screening

(2) Used more frequently to determine if mass solid or cystic

(3) Aid in tumor radiation therapy

(4) Evaluate for endometriosis, fibroids, ectopic and congenital anomalies (uterine or vaginal agenesis, streak ovaries, double or bicornuate uterus)

(5) Postpartum investigation of retained products of conception, uterine or adnexal hematoma, thromboembolism, or abscess

(6) Assist in evaluation of abnormal uterine bleeding and endometrial thickness in post-menopausal women

(7)   Detect decidual reaction in uterus; highly suggestive of pregnancy in very early stages

(8)   Earlier detection of intrauterine pregnancy

2. Breast ultrasound

a. Primary role is to determine if lesion is cystic or solid; also used to direct needle into mass for aspiration

b. Can be done in an office setting; not sensitive enough to be used for routine screening for breast cancer in asymptomatic women

c. Misses approximately 50% of lesions less than 2 centimeters in diameter; cannot replace mammography

- Mammography

1. Imaging technique used to screen women for breast cancer and/or to aid in diagnosis of a suspicious breast mass

2. Only reliable test to detect breast cancer before a mass can be palpated; 40% of early breast cancers can be detected with mammography

3. Three techniques used

a. Plain-film mammography (lowest dose of radiation)

b. Xeromammography (detects microcalcifications)

c. Electron radiography

4. False negative rate of 5-10%

5. Accuracy depends on equipment, skill, and experience of radiologist

6. An excisional biopsy indicated even though

a. Mammogram is negative in the presence of a suspicious lesion

b. Mammogram is suspicious and no lesion is palpated

7. May be used to localize small lesion prior to surgery

8. American Cancer Society (ACS) recommendations for breast cancer screening

a. All women should be taught self breast examination by age 20

b. Baseline mammogram by age 40 or earlier if high risk factors present

    c. From age 40-49, mammography every 1-2 years for low risk women, annual if risk factors present

    d. Annual mammogram for women age 50 and over

  9. Some advocate baseline at age 30 for women with strong risk factors for breast cancer

- Biopsy

  1. Endometrial biopsy

    a. Simple, inexpensive office procedure sampling the uterine lining

    b. Indications

      (1) Aids in diagnosis of ovarian dysfunction

      (2) Useful in infertility evaluation to assess ovulation and luteal phase

      (3) Rule out endometrial hyperplasia or carcinoma

      (4) Monitor women on HRT

  2. Cervical biopsy

    a. Colposcopic directed biopsy to diagnose cervical lesions

    b. Multiple biopsies are often performed

    c. Bleeding from biopsy site may occur and procedure may be uncomfortable

  3. Breast biopsy

    a. Used as definitive diagnosis of breast cancer

    b. Types

      (1) Fine needle—used when mass is likely fluid-filled; after aspiration, send aspirate for pathology evaluation; if negative and mass disappears, follow closely for recurrence; refer if

        (a) Lesion persists or recurs after aspiration

        (b) No fluid is aspirated

        (c) Aspirated fluid is bloody

(2) Wide-needle—used to a withdraw small amount of tissue; may require local anesthesia (negative finding does not rule out cancer)

(3) Surgical—used most for solid masses

    (a) Excisional—removes entire mass ("lumpectomy")

    (b) Performed with local anesthesia for mass less than 3 cm in diameter

    (c) For mass larger than 3 cm—may require general anesthesia

    (d) If pathology report is positive, a hormonal receptor assay needed to determine tumor's response to estrogen and progesterone; assists with prognosis and therapy decisions

  4. Vulvar biopsy

    a. Used to diagnose suspicious vulvar lesions

    b. Use aqueous solution (1-2%) of local anesthetic; sample obtained with scalpel or skin punch

    c. Minimal bleeding may occur; rarely is suture required

- Hysterosalpingogram (HSG)

  1. Used in infertility evaluations to determine tubal patency with indirect visualization of the reproductive tract

  2. Under fluoroscopic visualization, radiopaque iodine-based dye is injected through the cervix; dye follows normal anatomic pathway into uterus, tubes and abdomen

  3. Reveals degree of tubal patency and any abnormalities of uterine cavity or congenital abnormalities

  4. Performed 2-5 days after cessation of menstrual flow; may be uncomfortable; usual pre-operative preparation includes NSAID and antibiotic prophylaxis

  5. Forcing dye through the tubes may have a beneficial effect; if tubal patency results from procedure, possibility of pregnancy is increased

- Hysteroscopy
    1. Use of lighted hysteroscope provides endoscopic view of interior uterus; technique compliments HSG
    2. Indications
        a. Differentiating between endometrial polyps and submucosal fibroids
        b. Definitive diagnosis and treatment of uterine adhesions
        c. Diagnosis and treatment of intrauterine congenital anomalies
- Postcoital Testing (PCT, Sims-Huhner Test)
    1. Provides information on receptivity of cervical mucus and viability of sperm within the mucus
    2. Couples advised to abstain from intercourse for 48 hours prior to test
    3. Performed around time of LH surge as predicted by previous BBT chart, 2-8 hours after coitus
    4. Endocervical mucus examined for viscosity, spinnbarkeit, clarity, water, cell, and sperm count
    5. Results interpreted as favorable for chance of pregnancy if
        a. Mucus is clear and abundant
        b. Good spinnbarkeit (stretches 8-10 cm)
        c. Ferning pattern present
        d. Sperm are found in mucus (indicates adequate coital technique)
        e. Motile sperm are found (indicates pH is not hostile)
        f. Sperm count is adequate (5-10 motile sperm/HPF)
- Screening Test for Sexually Transmitted Diseases (STDs)
    1. Syphilis testing
        a. Indication—serologic testing of populations at risk for syphilis or when lesion suspicious for syphilis present
        b. Nontreponemal tests
            (1) Not specific to the treponeme; good for screening and follow-up treatment

(2) Types

    (a) Rapid Plasma Reagin (RPR)

    (b) Venereal Disease Research Laboratory (VDRL)

(3) Reported as either reactive (positive) or nonreactive (negative)

(4) All reactive results require confirmation with a treponemal test

(5) Reactive results are quantitated with a titer; fourfold titer increase or greater indicates infection, reinfection or treatment failure

c. Causes for false positive nontreponemal test—acute fever; immunization; pregnancy; acute bacterial or viral infections; aging; drug addiction; autoimmune disease such as systemic lupus erythematosus, arthritis; idiopathic or unknown causes

d. Treponemal tests detect specific antibodies to *T. pallidum;* results reported as reactive or nonreactive; 1% false positive rate

(1) Fluorescent Treponemal Antibody Absorption (FTA-ABS)

(2) Microhemagglutination Assay (MHA-TP)

e. Once treponemal test is reactive, will remain reactive for life, even with adequate treatment

f. Darkfield microscopy

(1) Indications—test of choice when moist lesions present and/or presence of papules or condyloma lata suggestive of secondary syphilis

(2) Results—positive when treponemes present; shaped like corkscrews; shine luminously against dark background

(3) Implications

    (a) Expertise necessary to recognize treponemes

    (b) Lesions on or near mucous membranes need thorough cleaning; non-pathogenic spirochetes colonize oral and genital mucosa

2. Human Immunodeficiency Virus (HIV) Tests—see General Assessment Chapter

3. Gonorrhea (GC)

   a. Culture—modified Thayer-Martin medium most sensitive and specific diagnostic method

      (1) Indications

          (a) Screening in high risk populations

          (b) History of contact

          (c) Signs and symptoms of infection

      (2) Specimen for culture may be collected from the urethra, endocervix, rectum, pharynx, or conjunctivae

      (3) Culture results

          (a) Presumptive positive—treat (see Gynecologic Disorders Chapter)

          (b) Consider sensitivity studies for strains resistant to usual antibiotics, e.g., spectinomycin, penicillin, erythromycin

          (c) Overgrown or unsatisfactory—repeat

      (4) Implications

          (a) Culture for *N. gonorrhoeae* cervical infections 80-90% accurate

          (b) Follow-up culture for test of cure not recommended by CDC if recommended drugs are used

   b. Gram stain

      (1) Positive for GC when typical gram negative intracellular diplococci are identified within polymorphonuclear leukocytes (PMN)

      (2) Gram negative—red; gram positive—purple

      (3) False positive results possible with gram stain

      (4) In women, gram stain sensitivity only 40-70%

4. Herpes simplex virus (HSV-2)

a. Tissue culture—"Gold standard"

    (1) Indication—tender genital lesion(s)

    (2) Culture results

        (a) Positive by 4 days (80%)

        (b) Positive by 7 days (95%)

        (c) May require 10-14 days for positive growth

    (3) Implications

        (a) HSV isolated from greater than 90% vesicular or pustular lesions; culture yield less from ulcerated and early maculopapular or late crusted lesions

        (b) Negative culture does not rule out HSV

        (c) Greatest number HSV particles in vesicles and at first episode

b. Tzanck preparation

    (1) Indication—confirmation of suspected HSV lesion by scraping edge of "unroofed" lesion with sterile swab and fixing the prepared slide in solution

    (2) Findings—multinucleated giant cells positive for HSV

    (3) Implications—if in doubt, confirm with culture; cannot differentiate HSV-1 from HSV-2 infection

c. Herpes titer

    (1) Indications

        (a) History of lesion suggestive of HSV but no active lesion

        (b) History indicating possibility of asymptomatic carrier

    (2) Technique—venipuncture

    (3) Implications

        (a) Not indicated if lesion suitable for culture present

        (b) Serologic testing available that discriminates between HSV-1 and HSV-2, but interpretation sometimes confusing because of some cross-reactivity between them

     (c)   Cost effective way to identify asymptomatic carrier

5. Chlamydia

    a. Growth is restricted to the intracellular environment of host cells

    b. Indications for testing

        (1) Inflammatory cervicitis with mucopurulent discharge

        (2) Known or suspected exposure

        (3) Areas of high prevalence

        (4) Symptoms of PID, gonorrhea

    c. Culture is "gold standard" for diagnosis; requires special media and specific collection technique

        (1) Technique—collect specimen with as many epithelial cells as possible; prevent bacterial overgrowth during transport by adding antibiotic to medium

        (2) Findings—positive if mature "inclusion bodies" found in cells

    d. Nonculture tests

        (1) Types available

            (a) Enzyme immunoassays (EIA)

            (b) Direct fluorescent antibody (DFA)

            (c) ELISA

            (d) Nucleic acid hybridization tests (DNA probe)

            (e) Pap smear—not specific, but findings of inflammatory cells may indicate need for specific chlamydia test

        (2) Findings reported as positive or negative; positive interpreted as presumptive infection

• Serum Hormonal Tests

    1. Prolactin assay

a. Indications

    (1) Amenorrhea with galactorrhea

    (2) Persistent galactorrhea 12 months after last pregnancy

    (3) Overt symptoms of pituitary adenoma (amenorrhea, galactorrhea, visual disturbances, headaches)

b. Normal range: 0-25 ng/mL—draw fasting without breast stimulation

c. Hypothyroidism may cause elevation

2. Follicle-stimulating hormone (FSH) and luteinizing hormone (LH)

a. Indications

    (1) Suspected hormonal dysfunction

    (2) Confirm primary ovarian failure

    (3) Amenorrhea evaluation

b. Normal range—FSH: 5-20 mIU/mL; LH: 2.0-20 mIU/mL (normal range of both varies with menstrual cycle)

- Laparoscopy

1. Surgical procedure that involves use of a laparoscope to directly visualize internal organs under local or general anesthesia

2. Requires a one or two puncture technique

a. Small incision so that abdomen can be inflated with gas

b. After insufflation, laparoscope passed through small incision made close to the umbilicus

3. Common indications

a. Pelvic pain and dysmenorrhea

b. Acute lower abdominal pain

c. Identify pelvic mass

d. Known or suspected endometriosis

e. Staging and second-look with cancer

f. Assessment of tubal pathology

4. Contraindications

     a. Obesity

     b. Current peritoneal infection

     c. Serious cardiac or lung disease

  5. Post-procedure—abdominal pain from remaining insufflation gas

Male Issues Affecting Women's Health

- Sexual Disorders/Dysfunction

  1. Premature ejaculation

     a. Ejaculation which occurs prior to or early in foreplay or intromission, and which is problematic to the couple

     b. Approximately 33% of men under 25 and 10% of men over 40 are affected

     c. Initial onset may be from earliest sexual experience

     d. High success rate with behavioral training—"stop-start" or "squeeze" techniques

  2. Impotence (erectile difficulty)

     a. Inability to sustain erection sufficient to complete desired sexual act; accompanied by high anxiety regarding sexual performance

     b. Cause may be primary or secondary due to psychological, medical, or pharmacological factors

     c. Organic disease can cause impotence and requires careful medical evaluation and consultation

       (1) Endocrine disease—diabetes, low serum testosterone, hyperprolactinemia

       (2) Vascular disease—penile small vessel disease, aortic aneurysm, arterial disease

       (3) Neurologic disease—spinal cord lesion

       (4) Debilitating disease—carcinoma, malnutrition

     d. Pharmacologic induced impotence

       (1) Antihypertensives

       (2) Antidepressants and antipsychotics

      (3) Antiulcer agents (except simple antacids)

      (4) Alcohol

      (5) Muscle relaxants

   e. Psychogenic impotence

      (1) Not uncommon for most men to experience at some time

      (2) May resolve if performance anxiety issues are treated

- Male Contraception (refer to Fertility Control section)
- Infertility
  1. Semen analysis
     a. Performed in infertility evaluation to assess process of normal spermatogenesis
     b. Procedure
        (1) Requires abstinence for 2-3 days prior to semen collection
        (2) Specimen collection by masturbation
        (3) Specimen must be protected from cold and delivered in a clean container to laboratory within an hour of collection
        (4) Specimen is analyzed for
            (a) Sperm count ($\geq$ 20 million/ml)
            (b) Volume (2.6 mL)
            (c) Motility ($\geq$ 50%)
            (d) Morphology ($\geq$ 60%)
            (e) Liquefaction (within 20-30 minutes of ejaculation)
     c. Variability common in semen specimens obtained from same individual; if laboratory report on initial semen analysis abnormal, repeat test
     d. Causes for abnormal sperm quality and quantity
        (1) History of testicular injury, surgery, or mumps
        (2) Increase in scrotal temperature
        (3) Severe allergic reactions

       (4) Exposure to radiation, industrial or environmental toxins

       (5) Heavy marijuana use, smoking and certain drugs

       (6) Frequent coitus

       (7) DES exposure postulated, but not proven

2. Varicocele

   a. Abnormal twisting of the veins within the spermatic cord

   b. Approximately 25-30% of infertile males have varicocele, usually on left side

   c. Presence of varicocele raises testicular temperature

   d. No treatment necessary if normal semen characteristics

   e. Ligation of varicoceles results in 30-35% pregnancy rate

3. DES exposure

   a. No well controlled studies on male offspring

   b. Possible sequelae for male DES-exposed offspring

       (1) Epididymal cysts

       (2) Hypotrophic testes

       (3) Decreased ejaculate volume

       (4) Urethral meatus stenosis

       (5) Varicocele

QUESTIONS

Select the best answer.

1. Ovulation generally occurs:

   a. 14 days, ± 2 days before onset of next menses
   b. 24 hours after the LH surge
   c. As a result of rupture of the corpus luteum

2. A women presents for diaphragm fitting. Her exam reveals a shallow pubic notch and firm vaginal muscle tone. The best diaphragm choice would be:

   a. Arching spring
   b. Flat spring
   c. Coil spring

3. To calculate fertile days for a woman using the calendar rhythm method for contraception, you would:

   a. Subtract 15 days from longest cycle, and 12 days from shortest cycle
   b. Subtract 11 days from longest cycle, and 18 days from shortest cycle
   c. Subtract 11 days from longest cycle, and add 7 days to shortest cycle

4. Use of Danazol as a postcoital contraceptive is contraindicated in the presence of:

   a. Breastfeeding, abnormal vaginal bleeding, or impaired liver, kidney, or heart function
   b. Acne, obesity, and hirsutism
   c. Crohn's disease, gastric ulcer, or diverticulitis

5. The action of Mifepristone (RU 486) is to:

   a. Suppress estrogen effect on endometrial proliferation
   b. Prevent maturation of a dominant follicle
   c. Block action of progesterone on the endometrium

6. Effectiveness of lactation as a contraceptive method in the first 6 months postpartum is equal to that of oral contraceptives under the following circumstances:

   a. Amenorrhea and breastfeeding exclusively

    b. Infrequent intercourse

    c. Maternal weight not greater than 154 lbs.

7. The action of the hormones in combined oral contraceptives provides protection against:

    a. Breast cancer

    b. Pituitary adenoma

    c. Ovarian and endometrial cancer

8. Functional reproductive physiology requires:

    a. Intact hypothalamus, anterior pituitary, ovaries, and feedback systems

    b. Integrity of lymphatic system

    c. Intact cortical function

9. The following statement is true about serum radioimmunoassay pregnancy tests:

    a. May cross react with FSH and LH

    b. Reliable within 7 days after fertilization

    c. Not indicated if ectopic suspected

10. Accuracy of a routine, screening Pap smear requires the presence of:

    a. Endometrial cells

    b. Cervical mucus

    c. Endocervical cells

11. Estrogen stimulates the production of:

    a. Cloudy, tenacious cervical mucus

    b. Liver hormone binding globulins

    c. Endometrial prostaglandins

12. The source of progesterone in the menstrual cycle is the:

    a. Corpus luteum

    b. Primordial follicle

    c. Theca cells

13. A woman presents with the following menstrual history:

Menarche: Age 11
Frequency of bleeding: every 30-31 days
Duration of bleeding: 5 days

Amount: light to moderate
Preceded by breast tenderness and mild lower abdominal discomfort
This history is consistent with:

   a. Ovulation
   b. Oligomenorrhea
   c. Anovulation

14. In a woman with a history of adequately treated syphilis, reinfection is best determined by:

   a. MHA-TP
   b. Tzanck prep
   c. VDRL

15. To be effective, postcoital contraceptives must be administered within:

   a. 24 hours
   b. 48 hours
   c. 72 hours

16. A client with an IUD in place for 7 weeks is complaining of mild pelvic cramping and lengthening of her string. She should be examined for:

   a. Cervicitis
   b. Uterine perforation
   c. IUD expulsion

17. Calculation of the fertile period depends on which of the following physiologic assumptions:

   a. Ovulation is occurring
   b. Ovum lifespan is 24-28 hours
   c. Sperm viability is 12-24 hours

18. A client on oral contraceptives reports nausea and a very bad headache localized over her right eye. She reports other episodes of sudden onset severe right temporal headaches accompanied by double vision. The first step in managing this patient is to:

   a. Change to a less estrogenic pill

b. Discontinue the oral contraceptive today

c. Schedule for headache evaluation

19. A client who is 6 weeks pregnant with a ParaGard IUD in situ wishes to continue the pregnancy. The patient should be told that:

a. The IUD should be left in place to reduce the risk of spontaneous abortion

b. There is an increased risk of fetal congenital anomalies from the copper in the IUD

c. The IUD should be removed today and there is a risk of spontaneous abortion

20. Endometrial biopsy is indicated:

a. Yearly beginning age 45

b. To evaluate endometrial hyperplasia

c. As part of colposcopic evaluation

21. The "gold standard" used to diagnose HSV-2 is:

a. Tzanck smear

b. Gram stain

c. Tissue culture

22. A disadvantage of the progestin-only pill is:

a. Incidence of functional cysts is increased

b. Its adverse effect on lactation

c. Delayed return to fertility after discontinuation

23. The most common contraceptive method used among married women in the U.S. is:

a. Condoms

b. Oral contraceptives

c. Voluntary sterilization

24. Which of the following is an indication for hormone replacement therapy?

a. Irregular vaginal bleeding

b. Vasomotor instability

c. Uterine prolapse

25. A 55 year-old woman presents with complaints of hot flashes and night sweats.

Her last menstrual period was 3 years ago. Her medical history reveals a history of migraine headaches and a lumpectomy for breast cancer last year. An appropriate treatment for the hot flashes is:

   a. Estrogen vaginal cream
   b. Medroxyprogesterone Acetate
   c. Low dose oral contraceptives

ANSWERS

1. a		14. c
2. b		15. c
3. b		16. c
4. a		17. a
5. c		18. b
6. a		19. c
7. c		20. b
8. a		21. c
9. b		22. a
10. c		23. c
11. b		24. b
12. a		25. b
13. a		

BIBLIOGRAPHY

Centers for Disease Control. (1993). 1993 Sexually transmitted diseases treatment guidelines. *Morbidity and Mortality Weekly Report,* 42 (No. RR-14).

Hatcher, R.A., Guest, F., Stewart, F., Stewart, G.K., Trussell, J., Kowal, D., & Cates, W. (1994). *Contraceptive technology* (16th ed.). New York: Irvington Press.

Garner, C. (1991). Midlife women's health. In C. Garner (Ed.), NAACOG's *clinical issues in perinatal and women's health nursing: Midlife women's health* (pp. 473-481). Philadelphia: J.B. Lippincott Co.

Herbst, A.L., Mishell, D.R., Stenchever, M.A., & Droegemueller, W. (1992). *Comprehensive gynecology* (2nd ed.). St. Louis: Mosby Year Book.

Lehne, R. (1994). *Pharmacology for nursing care* (2nd ed.). Philadelphia: W.B. Saunders Co.

Mishell, D., & Brenner, P. (Eds.). (1994). *Management of common problems in obstetrics and gynecology* (3rd ed.). Boston: Blackwell Scientific Publications.

Professional handbook of diagnostic tests. (1995). Springhouse, PA: Springhouse Corporation.

Rubin, M., & Lauver, D. (1990). Assessment and management of cervical intraepithelial neoplasia. *Nurse Practitioner,* 15, 23-30.

Segal-Gidan, F., & White, G. (1991). Treatment of infertility. *Clinician reviews,* 1 (1), 44-64.

Speroff, L., Glass, R., & Kase, N. (1994). *Clinical gynecologic endocrinology and infertility* (5th ed.). Baltimore, MD: Williams & Wilkins.

Stenchever, M.A. (Ed.). (1992). *Office gynecology.* St. Louis: Mosby-Year Book.

Wilson, J.R., & Carrington, E.R. (Eds.). (1992). *Obstetrics and gynecology* (9th ed.). St. Louis: Mosby-Year Book.

Youngkin, E., & Davis, M. (1994). *Women's health: A primary care clinical guide.* Norwalk, CT: Appleton & Lange.

Gynecologic Disorders

Carolyn M. Sutton

Menstrual and Endocrine Disorders

Premenstrual Syndrome (PMS)

- Definition: The cyclic recurrence of symptoms which occur in the luteal phase of the menstrual cycle and cease shortly after the onset of menstruation

- Etiology/Incidence
  1. Etiology unknown; hypotheses include fluid imbalance, changes in gonadotropin levels (low progesterone, excess estrogen, change in estrogen and progesterone ratios), increased prolactin secretion, altered response to prostaglandins, vitamin deficiencies, endogenous endorphin withdrawal, and alteration in glucose metabolism
  2. Estimate of incidence ranges 20-95% of all women

- Signs and Symptoms
  1. Related to menstrual cycle, begin 7-10 days before menses
  2. Wide variety, ranging from mild to severe; may include
     a. Mood alterations, e.g., anxiety, crying spells, depression, lethargy, sleep disorders, decreased libido and loss of concentration
     b. Breast tenderness, swelling
     c. Fluid retention, abdominal bloating, edema of extremities, weight gain
     d. Headache/migraine
     e. Thirst and appetite changes (food cravings)

- Differential Diagnosis
  1. Anxiety or depressive disorder
  2. Endocrine abnormalities, e.g., diabetes, thyroid disorder, hyperprolactinemia
  3. Alcohol/substance abuse
  4. Perimenopause

- Physical Findings

    1. No characteristic physical findings

    2. No specific laboratory tests

- Diagnostic Tests/Findings

    1. Diagnosis based on data obtained from menstrual, sexual, reproductive, family, medical, surgical, nutritional, and psychiatric histories

    2. Basal body temperature recording will document occurrence of symptoms in luteal phase

    3. Laboratory tests individualized based on symptoms; may consider complete blood count (CBC), fasting blood sugar, thyroid studies, FSH/LH, serum prolactin and progesterone level to rule out underlying disorders; laboratory studies to be conducted 1-7 days prior to menses or when symptoms most severe

    4. Complete gynecologic exam to rule out underlying disorders

- Management/Treatment

    1. No universally accepted treatment; goal of therapy to isolate and treat specific symptoms

    2. Treatment options may include

        a. Self-help measures

            (1) Stress reduction techniques

            (2) Participation in support groups

            (3) Exercise (20-30 minute aerobic workout at least four times/week)

            (4) Dietary revisions to include restriction of refined sugar (< 5 tsp/day), salt (< 3 g/day) red meat (up to 3 oz/day), fat intake, and caffeine intake helpful for some women

            (5) Effectiveness of nutritional supplements in relieving symptoms not well documented. Those commonly prescribed include Vitamin B_6, 50-100 mg/daily throughout cycle, daily allowance of Vitamin A, and Vitamin E, 150-600 units/day for breast symptoms

        b. Pharmacologic intervention

            (1) Spironolactone, 25 mg 4 times daily during luteal phase for severe bloating or fluid retention

(2) Prostaglandin inhibitors, specifically naproxen sodium, 500 mg twice daily for 10 days prior to menses

(3) Natural progesterone used, although controversial; give IM., vaginally, or rectally during luteal phase

(4) Combination oral contraceptives (OCs) to eliminate cyclic hormonal fluctuation (may increase symptoms for some)

(5) Depo Provera, 150 mg every 3 months or Provera 10-30 mg daily

(6) Bromocriptine for breast tenderness or Danazol for severe breast discomfort

(7) Use of antidepressants help some; best results with fluoxetine (Prozac) 20-60 mg daily or alprazolam, 0.25 mg 2-3 times daily during luteal phase

(8) Gonadotropin-releasing hormone (GnRH) agonist combined with estrogen/progestin "addback" for severe cases; long-term use carries heart disease and osteoporosis risk

(9) Oophorectomy used as last resort

Dysmenorrhea

- Definition
  1. Primary: Severe painful cramping sensation just before or during menses without organic cause
  2. Secondary: Pelvic pain associated with menses caused by organic conditions
- Etiology/Incidence
  1. Primary—action of prostaglandins on smooth muscle; affects over 50% of all menstruating women; 10% incapacitated
  2. Secondary—underlying pelvic pathology; most often in women over 20
- Signs and Symptoms
  1. Primary

a. Initial onset approximately one year after menarche; associated with ovulatory cycles

b. Pain begins with onset of menses or several hours before; described as crampy or spasmodic; may radiate to lower back and upper thighs

c. Associated symptoms—nausea, vomiting, diarrhea, dizziness, headaches

2. Secondary

a. Pain may occur at any point in cycle; less likely to be relieved with over-the-counter analgesics

b. May be accompanied by change in duration and amount of menstrual flow

- Differential Diagnosis

1. Primary—underlying pelvic pathology

2. Secondary—conditions such as endometriosis, adenomyosis, cervical stenosis, pelvic congestion, leiomyomas, endometrial polyps, pelvic inflammatory disease (PID), chronic pelvic pain, sexually transmitted diseases (STDs), IUD use, and urinary tract infection (UTI)

- Physical Findings

1. Primary—normal gynecologic exam

2. Secondary—pelvic pathology consistent with one of conditions listed in Differential Diagnosis section

- Diagnostic Tests/Findings

1. Primary

a. Detailed symptom analysis of pain and complete gynecologic exam reveals no pelvic pathology

b. No specific laboratory tests available

2. Secondary

a. Detailed symptom analysis of pain to narrow range of diagnoses

b. Diagnostic evaluation may include one or all of following

(1) Vaginal ultrasound to identify pelvic abnormalities

(2) Hysterosalpingogram or hysteroscopy to evaluate endometrial cavity

(3) Diagnostic laparoscopy to evaluate pelvic structures

(4) Appropriate tests/cultures if pelvic infection suspected

(5) Urinalysis to rule out bladder problem

(6) Barium enema to rule out bowel etiology

- Management/Treatment

    1. Primary

        a. If contraception not needed, prostaglandin synthetase inhibitors (PGSI) drug of choice; most effective: mefenamic acid, ibuprofen, naproxen; administer prior to onset of bleeding; side benefitreduces amount of blood loss

        b. When contraception needed, oral contraceptives (OCs) drug of choice; reduces prostaglandin production and amount of blood loss

        c. Combined low-dose contraceptives and PGSI treatment needed for some women

        d. Laparoscopy considered if no response to above therapies

        e. Self-help measures include—increase exercise, promote natural diuresis (limit salt, increase fiber and water intake), heat application, use of relaxation techniques

        f. For severe cases, presacral neurectomy

    2. Secondary—treatment depends on underlying cause

Amenorrhea

- Definition

    1. Clinical expression of a variety of disorders which cause absence or cessation of menstrual flow

    2. Traditionally classified as primary (no previous menstruation) or secondary (cessation of menses after a period of menstruation)

    3. Speroff, Glass, & Kase (1994) suggest that any of the following criteria meet the definition for amenorrhea

      a. No period by age 14 in the absence of growth or development of secondary sexual characteristics (primary)

      b. No period by age 16, regardless of normal growth or development of secondary sexual characteristics (primary)

      c. No menses for 3 cycle lengths or 6 months in a woman with previously established menses (secondary)

- Etiology/Incidence

  1. Etiologies unrelated to pregnancy include—anatomic deviations, genetic factors, endocrine abnormalities or imbalances, autoimmune disease, weight abnormalities, excessive exercise, certain medications, and chronic diseases

  2. Incidence estimated at 5% of reproductive age women who are not pregnant, lactating or menopausal

- Signs and Symptoms

  1. Absence of menarche

  2. No menses and abnormal growth or development of secondary sexual characteristics

  3. No menses for 3 cycle lengths or 6 months in a woman with previously established menses (secondary)

- Differential Diagnosis

  1. Pregnancy

  2. Defects or interruption of hypothalamic-pituitary-ovarian axis—gonadotropin deficiency, extreme exercise or stress, pituitary tumors, Sheehan's syndrome, amenorrhea-galactorrhea syndrome, Chiari-Frommel syndrome, Stein-Leventhal syndrome, premature ovarian failure, severe pelvic inflammatory disease, primary gonadal disorder, thyroid disorders

  3. Anatomical disorders—congenital absence of ovaries, absent or hypoplastic uterus, imperforate hymen, transverse vaginal septum, absence of vagina

  4. Chronic diseases—tuberculosis, alcohol abuse, Type I diabetes mellitus, adrenal disorders, obesity

  5. Use of certain medications—combination OCs; progestin-only contraceptives; phenothiazines; dilantin; reserpine

- Physical Findings
  1. Assess weight, height and vital signs
  2. Evaluate visual fields, thyroid gland for underlying endocrine disorder
  3. Nipple discharge, obstructive disorders of genitalia may indicate endocrine problem
  4. Enlarged uterus, soft, bluish cervix may indicate pregnancy
  5. Hirsutism, clitoromegaly, acne are signs of androgen excess
  6. Pink, moist vagina with rugae and clear cervical mucus indicate adequate estrogen

- Diagnostic Tests/Findings
  1. Serum beta-hCG to rule out pregnancy
  2. Measure TSH and T_4 to rule out thyroid disorder; refer if abnormal
  3. Perform prolactin serum assay; refer if greater than 20 ng/mL
  4. If beta-hCG, thyroid function and prolactin assay tests are normal, evaluate estrogen status with administration of medroxyprogesterone acetate, 5-10 mg twice daily for 5 days
     a. Withdrawal bleeding within 7 days demonstrates adequate estrogen and normal outflow tract, which indicates anovulation
     b. If withdrawal bleeding does not occur, give estrogen to stimulate endometrial proliferation and withdrawal
        (1) If bleeding still does not occur, refer
        (2) If bleeding occurs, measure gonadotropins to determine if problem is with ovaries or CNS pituitary axis; high gonadotropins indicate ovarian failure; low or normal requires further medical studies

- Management/Treatment
  1. Primary—refer to endocrinologist
  2. Secondary
     a. Pregnancy—discuss options and refer appropriately
     b. Elevated TSH—treat hypothyroidism
     c. Anovulation—medical consult

    d. Pituitary adenoma—refer to endocrinologist

    e. Ovarian failure—evaluate for hormone replacement therapy

Oligomenorrhea

- Definition: Infrequent menstrual bleeding characterized by intervals of 35 days or greater
- Etiology/Incidence
    1. Multiple etiologies
        a. Abnormalities of ovaries, pituitary, or hypothalamus
        b. Thyroid, adrenal, or other endocrine disease
        c. Chronic illness
        d. Drug use/abuse
    2. Occurs frequently in perimenopause
- Signs and Symptoms
    1. May present as normal menstrual pattern for first year after menarche, or for several years prior to menopause
    2. May alternate with periods of heavy vaginal bleeding or amenorrhea
- Differential Diagnosis
    1. Endocrine causes—pregnancy, pituitary-hypothalamic problems, or menopause
    2. Systemic cause—excessive weight loss or gain
- Physical Findings—include evidence consistent with pathology in Differential Diagnosis section
- Diagnostic Tests/Findings
    1. Serum beta hCG to rule out pregnancy
    2. Careful menstrual and medical history
    3. Appropriate tests to rule out dysfunction of ovaries, pituitary, or hypothalamus
- Management/Treatment
    1. Rule out pregnancy

2. Goal of therapy—diagnose and treat underlying cause

3. Progestin therapy to control withdrawal bleeding; give medroxyprogesterone acetate, 10 mg daily for 10 days each month

Polycystic Ovarian Syndrome (PCO), Stein-Leventhal

- Definition: Syndrome resulting from combination of anovulation and excess androgen

- Etiology/Incidence—unclear

  1. Primary hormonal abnormality is increased LH with normal or low FSH (LH:FSH ratio, > 3:1); increased production rates of testosterone and androstenedione causing androgenic effects

  2. Affects women 15-30 years old

  3. Present in 1-4% of reproductive age women

- Signs and Symptoms

  1. History of irregular menses (oligomenorrhea or amenorrhea) with gradual onset of hirsutism, beginning at puberty or in early 20s

  2. May have acanthosis nigricans and symmetrically enlarged ovaries (unilateral enlargement less common)

  3. Signs of androgen excess—hirsutism, acne, male pattern baldness, deepening of voice

  4. Obesity may be present

  5. Infertility

- Differential Diagnosis

  1. Obesity

  2. Dysfunctional uterine bleeding

  3. Hyperprolactinemia

  4. Congenital adrenal hyperplasia

  5. Cushing's disease

  6. Thyroid dysfunction

  7. Adrenal/ovarian tumors

- Physical Findings

    1. Physical exam usually normal

    2. Fifty percent will have enlarged ovaries

    3. Hirsutism, frontal balding, increased muscle mass, clitoral enlargement and decreased breast size indicate increased androgen

- Diagnostic Tests/Findings

    1. Serum beta hCG

    2. Progestin challenge to endometrium; bleeding establishes diagnosis of anovulation

    3. LH level elevated, FSH low or normal (3:1 ratio)

    4. Serum testosterone and free testosterone—mild to moderate elevation reflects ovarian androgen excess

    5. Dehydroepiandrosterone sulfate (DHEAS)—normal or elevated

    6. Prolactin—normal or mildly elevated

    7. Thyroid function tests—high or low TSH

    8. Basal Body Temperature—for indication of ovulation and scheduling endometrial biopsy

    9. Endometrial biopsy—to diagnose hyperplasia

    10. Laparoscopy—to determine and treat infertility

    11. Vaginal ultrasound—to assess ovaries

- Management/Treatment

    1. Based on symptoms and desire for pregnancy

    2. If pregnancy desired, refer for ovulation induction

    3. For chronic ovulation with resulting endometrial hyperplasia, medroxyprogesterone acetate, 10 mg daily for first 10 days of month to induce withdrawal bleeding

    4. Low dose combination OCs used to provide cyclic bleeding and effective contraception; select OC with low androgenic activity

    5. The overweight, hyperandrogenic, anovulatory patient may be at risk for diabetes mellitus, breast cancer, and endometrial cancer

Dysfunctional Uterine Bleeding (DUB)

- Definition: Uterine bleeding secondary to chronic anovulation
- Etiology/Incidence
    1. Dysfunction of hypothalamic-pituitary-ovarian axis, resulting in continued estrogen stimulation of endometrium
    2. Organic causes for anovulation—thyroid disorder or adrenal abnormalities
    3. Others—hormone replacement, OC and IUD use, use of corticosteroids, androgens, hypothalamic depressants, digitalis, and anticoagulants
    4. Blood dyscrasias—idiopathic thrombocytopenia purpura, von Willebrand disease, anemia and leukemia
    5. Trauma—sexual assault or foreign body
    6. Early pregnancy disorder (spontaneous abortion/ectopic)
- Signs and Symptoms
    1. Report of irregular bleeding most commonly at extremes of reproductive age (during adolescence and perimenopause)
    2. Evidence of anemia
    3. May have signs and symptoms of hypo- or hyperthyroidism
- Differential Diagnosis
    1. Intrauterine or ectopic pregnancy
    2. Organic gynecologic disease—endometrial and cervical cancer, leiomyomata, adenomyosis, uterine polyps, PCO, vaginitis, cervicitis
    3. Blood dyscrasia
    4. Perimenopausal status
    5. Severe stress
    6. Liver disease
- Physical Findings—include evidence consistent with Etiology/Incidence section
- Diagnostic Tests/Findings

1. Diagnosis made by exclusion of other causes of abnormal uterine bleeding

2. The following tests may be used to rule out other causes

    a. Quantitative beta pregnancy test

    b. Complete blood count

    c. Papanicolaou smear

    d. Thyroid function tests, prolactin assay, liver function tests, FSH and LH levels

    e. Appropriate tests/cultures, if STDs suspected

    f. Coagulation studies, if heavy bleeding

    g. Complete endometrial sampling by curettage for older women to rule out endocervical and endometrial cancer

- Management/Treatment

    1. Low-dose combination OC first choice of therapy, if contraception needed; prescribe one pill 4 times/day for 5-7 days, then normal OC regimen for 6 months; if bleeding continues, refer

    2. If no contraception needed, single dose options include

        a. IM. injection of progesterone in oil, 25-50 mg; bleeding should cease within few days of injection; may experience heavy bleeding within 1-2 weeks, then resume normal menses

        b. Medroxyprogesterone acetate, 10 mg q.d. for 10-14 days (medical D&C); expect heavy bleeding with first menses after therapy

    3. Estrogen used if bleeding is heavy and endometrial support needed (IV. or oral conjugated estrogen)

    4. Cyclic estrogen-progesterone therapy for 3-4 cycles helpful

    5. PGSI for non-hormonal treatment of menorrhagia

    6. When bleeding persists after above treatments, hysterectomy may be indicated; alternative is endometrial ablation

    7. Dilatation and curettage is diagnostic and therapeutic

Hyperprolactinemia, Galactorrhea and Pituitary Adenoma

- Definition
    1. Hyperprolactinemia: Elevated circulating concentration of prolactin (PRL)
    2. Galactorrhea: Spontaneous milky nipple discharge unrelated to pregnancy
    3. Pituitary adenoma: A benign tumor of anterior pituitary gland that secretes prolactin

- Etiology/Incidence
    1. Etiology of pituitary adenoma is unknown; considered the most common type of pituitary neoplasm; greatest incidence in 60s, but can occur at any age
    2. Most common cause of hyperprolactinemia and galactorrhea is pituitary tumor or other lesions of the hypothalamus; additional causes are
        a. Use of tranquilizers, narcotics, antihypertensives, and OCs
        b. Excessive stimulation of nipples of breast
        c. Hypothalamic-pituitary dysfunction
        d. Hypothyroidism, chest lesions, chronic renal disease, nonpituitary prolactin-producing tumors of the lungs or kidneys, and excessive stress
    3. Elevated PRL interferes with release of gonadotropin-releasing hormone (GnRH), which causes lowered levels of follicle-stimulating hormone (FSH) and luteinizing hormone (LH); directly impact ovarian function
    4. Approximately $1/3$ of women with hyperprolactinemia have galactorrhea; $1/3$ of women with galactorrhea will have normal menses; $1/3$ of women with secondary amenorrhea will have a pituitary adenoma

- Signs and Symptoms
    1. Hyperprolactinemia—may complain of infertility, normal or irregular menses, milky breast discharge, headache/visual field disturbances
    2. Galactorrhea—may include bilateral milky breast discharge, amenorrhea or irregular menses; if pituitary adenoma is the cause, may report headache, blurred vision, loss of peripheral vision

3. Pituitary adenoma—may include milky breast discharge and amenor-rhea, visual field disturbances, headaches and blurred vision

- Differential Diagnosis
  1. Hyperprolactinemia
     a. Galactorrhea
     b. Oligomenorrhea/amenorrhea
     c. Ovarian dysfunction
     d. Hypothalamic/pituitary lesion; pituitary adenoma
     e. Hypothyroidism
     f. Pregnancy
     g. Excessive stress/breast stimulation
     h. Certain categories of medications (See Etiology/Incidence 2.a..)
  2. Galactorrhea—includes all of above
  3. Pituitary adenoma—benign and malignant neoplasms of the brain
- Physical Findings
  1. Hyperprolactinemia and galactorrhea
     a. Bilateral milky breast discharge
     b. Fundoscopic exam is normal
     c. Normal gynecologic exam
  2. Pituitary adenoma
     a. Bilateral milky breast discharge
     b. Fundoscopic may reveal papilledema
     c. Abnormal visual fields examination
- Diagnostic Tests/Findings
  1. Hyperprolactinemia/Galactorrhea
     a. Serum prolactin assay (refer if > 20 ng/mL)
     b. Pregnancy test
     c. Wet prep of breast discharge (fat globules indicate milk)

d. Measurement of TSH level (normal value: < 10 µU/mL)

e. CT scan of sella turcica to rule out pituitary adenoma

2. Pituitary adenoma

a. Serum prolactin assay (abnormally high range, 100-300 ng/mL highly suspicious)

b. CT scan of sella turcica (to identify tumor)

c. Visual fields measurement (if visual complaints voiced or if CT scan abnormal)

- Management/Treatment

1. Nulliparous woman with galactorrhea and amenorrhea must be evaluated for pituitary adenoma

2. Management of above disorders requires evaluation and management by endocrinologist

3. Medical management options include

a. Bromocriptine to inhibit production of PRL; 80% of women with hyperprolactinemia and/or galactorrhea will respond to treatment, ovulate, and conceive

b. Surgery may be necessary for adenoma that does not respond to bromocriptine therapy; if tumor is small and slow-growing, endocrinologist may observe for change

c. If TSH is elevated, treat hypothyroidism

Benign and Malignant Neoplasms

Abnormal Papanicolaou (Pap) Smear

- Definition

1. Cervical dysplasia = cervical intraepithelial neoplasia (CIN) = squamous intraepithelial lesion (SIL)

a. Synonymous terms that encompass all epithelial abnormalities that are precursors to invasive squamous cell carcinoma

    b. Degree of severity determined by proportion of epithelial thickness showing deranged maturation

       (1) CIN I = mild dysplasia

       (2) CIN II = moderate dysplasia

       (3) CIN III = severe dysplasia, carcinoma-in-situ

    c. The greater the degree of dysplasia, the more likely and quickly is progression to invasive squamous cell carcinoma

- Etiology/Incidence

    1. Peak in late 20s, early 30s

    2. Most likely multifactorial; risk factors support sexual transmission

    3. Accepted risk factors are covered in Normal Women's Health Chapter

    4. Cervical cancer rate decreased in last 45 years, but CIN has increased dramatically

    5. Human papillomavirus (HPV) is the biggest risk factor for lower genital tract neoplasia; suspected as a co-factor with smoking

- Recommended Screening for CIN—Pap smear cytology is the recommended screening test

    1. Women who are or have been sexually active or have reached age 18

    2. After 3 or more consecutive, satisfactory, normal Paps, may perform less frequently (every 2-3 years) depending on risk factors

- Diagnostic Tests/Findings

    1. Diagnosis of CIN is histologic and requires biopsy

    2. Colposcopic evaluation of cervical transformation zone (TZ) to evaluate epithelial thickness, contour, degree of acetowhiteness, presence of vascular changes, and lesion borders

    3. Colposcopy directed punch biopsy of abnormal appearing areas provides histologic data

    4. Endocervical curettage (ECC) performed under direct colposcopic visualization

- Management/Treatment of Abnormal Pap Findings

    1. Management

a. Within normal limits—repeat Pap smear annually, or as indicated by risk factors

b. Unsatisfactory—specimen is inadequate for diagnosis, or no endocervical cells are found; repeat Pap in 2-3 months

c. Atypical squamous cells of undetermined significance (ASCUS)

   (1) Unqualified or favors reactive process—repeat Pap every 4-6 months for 2 years until 3 consecutive, negative and satisfactory smears; if second ASCUS Pap occurs in 2-year follow-up, consider colposcopy

   (2) Unqualified with inflammation—treat specific cause, repeat Pap in 2-3 months

   (3) Postmenopausal, not on hormone replacement therapy—course of topical estrogen, then repeat Pap; if ASCUS reported, consider colposcopy

   (4) If favors neoplastic process—advise colposcopy, biopsy and endocervical curettage (ECC)

   (5) High risk women—consider colposcopy

d. Low-Grade Squamous Intraepithelial Lesion (LSIL)— advise colposcopy with directed biopsy and endocervical curettage (ECC)

e. High-Grade Squamous Intraepithelial Lesion (HSIL)—colposcopic evaluation of TZ with directed biopsies

f. Glandular cell abnormalities—refer for further evaluation immediately

2. Treatment

a. After invasive cancer ruled out, one of the following ablative procedures is appropriate

   (1) Local excision by excision or punch biopsy

   (2) Cryosurgery—destruction of TZ by freezing lesion which does not extend into canal

   (3) Laser vaporization—destruction of TZ with high-power focused beam for lesions that are too large for cautery probe, extend into the endocervical canal or have deep gland involvement

(4) Diagnostic conization—use of knife, laser beam or loop electrosurgical excision procedure (LEEP) to surgically remove entire TZ

b. Colposcopic evaluations should be performed by trained and experienced colposcopist

Cervical Polyps

- Definition
    1. Small pedunculated, often sessile neoplasms; usually benign
    2. Most originate from endocervix, few from endometrium
- Etiology/Incidence
    1. Possible etiologies include hyperestrogen states, chronic inflammation, abnormal local response to hormonal stimulation, or localized vascular congestion of cervical vessels
    2. Cervical polyps relatively common, especially in multiparas older than 20; rare before menarche, occasionally after menopause
    3. Endometrial polyps common at all ages, highest incidence after age 50
- Signs and Symptoms
    1. Endocervical
        a. Abnormal vaginal bleeding, including but not limited to, intermenstrual or postcoital bleeding
        b. Leukorrhea and hypermenorrhea
    2. Endometrial
        a. History of regularly recurring menorrhagia
        b. May appear as sudden occurrence of bleeding in a postmenopausal woman
- Differential Diagnosis (both types)
    1. Adenocarcinoma of endometrium
    2. Small pedunculated myomas
- Physical Findings
    1. Endocervical

      a. Visible at os as red or pink growth

      b. Usually attached to endocervical mucosa; very soft

      c. Variable in size, few millimeters to 2-3 centimeters

      d. Otherwise normal pelvic exam

  2. Endometrial

      a. May be single or multiple

      b. Range in size, 1-2 millimeters to size large enough to fill uterine cavity

      c. May project through cervical os or even introitus

- Diagnostic Tests/Findings

      a. Pap may reveal atypia

      b. Removal required for pathology evaluation

- Management/Treatment

  1. Polypectomy is usually curative, but recurrence frequent

  2. If abnormal pathology report, refer

Leiomyomata uteri (Fibroids, Myomas)

- Definition

  1. Most common benign gynecologic pelvic neoplasm; arise from uterine smooth muscle

  2. Types include

      a. Interstitial—stays within uterine wall, most common

      b. Submucosal—protrude into uterine cavity; comprise only 5%, but highly associated with symptomatology

      c. Subserosal—bulges through outer uterine wall

      d. Intraligamentous—within broad ligament

      e. Pedunculated—on thin pedicle, attached to uterine base

- Etiology/Incidence

  1. Exact cause unknown; estrogen thought to be important growth factor

2. Incidence—20-25% of all reproductive age women; 1% of pregnant women; higher incidence among African American women

- Signs and Symptoms

    1. Present in 35-50% of women with leiomyomas

    2. Abnormal bleeding (hypermenorrhea or metrorrhagia)

    3. Pressure symptoms when enlarge and encroach on other organs

        a. Bladder—suprapubic discomfort, urinary retention, or overflow incontinence

        b. Colon—constipation, painful defecation

    4. Pain if twisted or infarcted

    5. Abdominal enlargement

    6. Potential complications

        a. Premature labor

        b. Spontaneous abortion

        c. Infertility (2-10%)

        d. Anemia

        e. Barrier to thorough pelvic assessment

- Differential Diagnosis

    1. Pregnancy

    2. Benign and malignant ovarian tumors

    3. Tubo-ovarian abscess

    4. Endometriosis

    5. Adenomyosis

    6. Diverticulitis

- Physical Findings

    1. Wide variance in size; 3-4 mm up to weight of 1-15 pounds

    2. Enlarged, irregularly shaped, firm uterus

    3. Uterus may be displaced if tumor large

    4. Tumors usually movable and painless

5. Abdominal enlargement if growth exceeds true pelvis (12-14 weeks size or greater)

- Diagnostic Tests/Findings

    1. Presumptive diagnosis made by careful abdominal, pelvic and rectal exam

    2. Pelvic ultrasound to identify and confirm location

    3. Hysteroscopy assists in identification and removal

    4. If abnormal bleeding present, fractional curettage to rule out endometrial cancer

    5. Laboratory

        a. CBC may reveal anemia when heavy bleeding present

        b. Urinalysis to rule out UTI

        c. Pregnancy test

        d. Stool guaiac to rule out gastrointestinal problem when abdominal mass palpated

- Management/Treatment

    1. No treatment required if asymptomatic, discovered on pelvic exam, and not of excessive size; monitor closely for changes

    2. If symptomatic, pregnancy desired, or large enough to obscure other pelvic structures, options include

        a. Medroxyprogesterone acetate to suppress menorrhagia and inhibit growth

        b. Gonadotropin-releasing hormone (GnRh) agonists—reduce size by decreasing estrogen; often given prior to surgery

    3. Daily iron supplementation, if anemic

    4. Surgery indicated with rapid growth, excessive size, hypermenorrhea causing anemia, encroachment on other organs, and when differentiation from pelvic mass is inconclusive

        a. Myomectomy—for younger women desiring fertility

        b. Total hysterectomy is curative; indicated when symptoms are severe

Cysts

- Definition

  1. Functional ovarian cysts—physiologic and related to menstrual cycle; 2 types

     a. Follicular—formed during follicular phase when process of fluid resorption does not occur

     b. Corpus luteum—forms after ovulation when mature corpus luteum does not degenerate

  2. Benign cystic teratoma (dermoid)—most common ovarian germ cell neoplasm in reproductive age group

- Etiology/Incidence

  1. Follicular—caused by failure of fluid in an incompletely developed follicle to resorb; may occur at any age before menopause

  2. Corpus luteum—forms when mature corpus luteum becomes cystic or hemorrhagic and fails to degenerate after 14 days

  3. Dermoid—derived from germ cell and contains elements from all 3 embryonic cell types; accounts for 1-25% of all ovarian neoplasms, excluding functional cysts; only 1% contain malignant component

- Signs and Symptoms

  1. Follicular

     a. Usually asymptomatic; occasionally cause irregular menses

     b. Large cysts may cause feeling of heaviness, fullness and aching on affected side

     c. Pain, if torsion occurs

  2. Corpus luteum

     a. Menstrual irregularities (delay in onset, irregular flow)

     b. Dull crampy feeling on affected side

  3. Dermoid

     a. Usually asymptomatic

     b. Local pressure and vague abdominal discomfort if large

    c. Abnormal uterine bleeding (rare)

  4. Signs of rupture include—sudden, severe abdominal pain; mimics ectopic

- Differential Diagnosis

  1. Endometriosis

  2. Pregnancy (intrauterine/ectopic)

  3. Other ovarian neoplasms/cancer

  4. Salpingitis

- Physical Findings

  1. Functional—bimanual may reveal 4-8 cm, mobile, slightly soft, sometimes tender adnexal mass, occurring unilaterally

  2. Dermoid—bimanual reveals 6-15 cm round, smooth, non-tender, moveable ovarian mass; 12% bilateral

- Diagnostic Tests/Findings

  1. Careful menstrual and contraceptive history

  2. Pregnancy test to rule out ectopic

  3. Diagnostic ultrasound to distinguish between solid or cystic mass; calcifications and teeth may be seen with dermoid

- Management/Treatment

  1. Presence of adnexal mass in premenarchal or postmenopausal patient—refer immediately

  2. Follicular—re-examine in 1-2 months; if present, may require laparotomy

  3. Corpus luteum—most will regress; observation and expectant management appropriate

  4. Dermoid—surgical removal

Malignant Disease of the Cervix

- Definition

  1. A progressive, slow growing disease with histologically definable stages; may be in-situ or invasive

2. Spectrum of stages called cervical intraepithelial neoplasia (CIN); highly curable if detected early

- Etiology/Incidence

   1. Risk factors include—first intercourse ≤ age 18, multiple sexual partners, partner with multiple sex partners, cigarette smoking, HPV types 16, 18, 31 (leading cause), DES exposure, history of sexually transmitted diseases

   2. Peak incidence 40-45 age group, although rates of abnormal cytology in adolescents increasing

   3. Squamous cell carcinoma most common (85%)

- Signs and Symptoms (may be asymptomatic)

   1. Abnormal vaginal bleeding/discharge (most common symptom)

   2. Postcoital spotting/bleeding

   3. Anemia, if acute blood loss

   4. Pelvic or epigastric pain (late sign)

   5. Urinary or rectal symptoms

- Differential Diagnosis

   1. Cervical ectopy or polyps

   2. Ulceration secondary to syphilis, chancroid, lymphogranuloma venereum

   3. Acute or chronic cervicitis

   4. Condyloma acuminata

   5. Cervical tuberculosis (rare)

- Physical Findings

   1. Cervix may appear normal

   2. Sanguineous or purulent, odorous discharge

   3. Cervical lesion/ulcer

   4. Very firm cervix

- Diagnostic Tests/Findings

   1. Screening

    a. Pap smear is standard screening test

    b. Schiller test—malignant cells do not contain glycogen and do not stain when Lugol's or Schiller's iodine applied

    c. Colposcopic evaluation of vulva, vagina and cervix

  2. Diagnostic

    a. Colposcopy and directed biopsy

    b. Endocervical curettage

- Management/Treatment

  1. Options for CIN, microinvasive and invasive cancer

    a. Excisional biopsy

    b. Conization

    c. Hot cautery

    d. Radiation laser surgery

    e. Chemotherapy

  2. Radiation and radical hysterectomy for advanced disease

  3. Follow-up with cytologic evaluation imperative

Malignant Disease of the Uterus (Endometrial Cancer)

- Definition—malignancy of the uterine endometrium
- Etiology/Incidence

  1. Exact etiology unknown, but estrogen implicated

  2. Risk factors include

    a. Nulliparity

    b. Unopposed estrogen stimulation

    c. Feminizing ovarian tumors

    d. Family history endometrial cancer or diabetes

    e. Hypertension

    f. Polycystic ovaries

  3. Peak age group 50-70 years; 2-5% before age 40

    4. Most common cancer of reproductive organs

- Signs and Symptoms
    1. Painless abnormal uterine bleeding (80%)
    2. Mucosanguineous discharge
    3. Lower abdominal cramping pain (10%)
- Differential Diagnosis
    1. Endometrial hyperplasia
    2. Cervical and endometrial polyps
    3. Leiomyomas
    4. Other genital cancers
    5. Dysfunctional uterine bleeding
- Physical Findings
    1. May see blood in vaginal vault
    2. If advanced, uterus may be enlarged and soft
    3. Routine laboratory findings are normal; anemia may be present with prolonged bleeding
- Diagnostic Tests/Findings
    1. Routine Pap test will miss 40% of symptomatic women (not a screening test for endometrial cancer)
    2. Presence of benign endometrial cells on Pap of menopausal women may be associated with occult endometrial cancer
    3. Endometrial sampling may be performed in office setting
    4. Hysteroscopy if polyps suspected
    5. Fractional curettage of endocervix and endometrium is diagnostic
- Management/Treatment
    1. Hysterectomy, bilateral salpingo-oophorectomy
    2. For extensive disease—radiotherapy, steroid hormones (progesterone) and chemotherapy

Malignant Disease of the Ovary (Ovarian Cancer)

- Definition: A malignant neoplasm of the ovary
- Etiology/Incidence
  1. Majority of ovarian cancer is epithelial in origin
  2. Risk factors
     a. Nulliparity, low parity, late onset of childbearing
     b. Family history of ovarian cancer
     c. Personal history of breast, endometrial, colorectal cancer, or ovarian dysfunction
     d. Early menopause (before age 45) or late menarche (after 14)
     e. Increases with age until 70, then decreases
     f. Talc contaminated with asbestos (suggested)
     g. Combination OC use decreases risk of epithelial ovarian cancer; protection persists for 10 years after discontinuation of OC
     h. High dietary fat intake (inconclusive)
  3. Peak age group 65-84; infrequent under age 35
  4. Malignant tumors of ovary occur at all ages, including infancy and childhood
  5. Leading cause of death from genital cancers in U.S.; accounts for 5% of all cancers among women
- Signs and Symptoms
  1. Early symptoms—often "silent," vague lower abdominal discomfort and mild digestive complaints
  2. Late symptoms—increasing abdominal girth, abdominal pain, abnormal vaginal bleeding, cachexia, anemia and ascites
- Differential Diagnosis
  1. Leiomyomas
  2. Benign ovarian tumors
- Physical Findings—bimanual exam detects 1 in 10,000 asymptomatic women, but still most practical method for early detection

1. Palpation of irregular, non-tender, fixed adnexal mass usually first diagnostic finding (70% of ovarian cancer is bilateral)

2. Risk of ovarian cancer significantly higher in premenarchal and post-menopausal women with adnexal mass than in women of reproductive age

- Diagnostic Tests/Findings

    1. Pelvic sonogram/CT Scan

    2. CA-125—elevated CA-125 levels (35 is upper limits of normal) not diagnostic for ovarian cancer; elevated levels can occur with endometriosis, leiomyomata, PID, hepatitis and other malignancies; helpful to assess response of ovarian cancer to chemotherapy and in follow-up

    3. Laparotomy required for definitive diagnosis

- Management/Treatment

    1. Surgery

        a. Total abdominal hysterectomy, bilateral salpingo-oophorectomy, and omentectomy; establishes type, histologic grading and stage of tumor

        b. Goal to remove as much tumor as possible

    2. Radiation and/or chemotherapy

    3. Complete diagnostic evaluation of other organ systems to rule out metastases

Malignant Disease of the Vagina

- Definition: A malignant neoplasm of the vagina

- Etiology/Incidence

    1. Etiology unknown, but risk factors include cancer of cervix and vulva, and DES exposure

    2. Primary cancer represents less than 2% of gynecologic malignancies; usually represents metastases from another site

    3. Peak incidence 45-65 age group

    4. Most common site—upper $1/3$ of vagina

5. Progresses from vaginal intraepithelial neoplasm (VAIN) to invasive cancer

- Signs and Symptoms (usually asymptomatic)

    1. Abnormal vaginal bleeding or blood-tinged discharge

    2. If extensive, profuse, foul-smelling discharge causing vulvitis and pruritus

    3. Urinary distress, if bladder involved

    4. Visible or palpable mass/lesion

- Differential Diagnosis

    1. Benign tumors (Wolffian or Gartner's duct)

    2. Ulcerative lesion (Granuloma inguinale)

    3. Endometriosis

    4. Cancer of the urethra, bladder, rectum, or Bartholin's gland

- Physical Findings

    1. Mass may appear—fungate-like, cauliflower-like, flat and superficial, or deep and ulcerating

    2. May see pigmented lesion (suspect melanoma)

- Diagnostic Tests/Findings

    1. Cervical cytology

    2. Pap—if vaginal lesion present

    3. Colposcopic evaluation of vagina with directed biopsy of suspicious lesions

- Management/Treatment

    1. Determined by stage and extent of disease

    2. VAIN and precancerous lesions—local excision, cryosurgery, laser therapy, partial vaginectomy, chemotherapy and radiation

    3. Invasive cancer—radiation and/or radical pelvic surgery

Malignant Diseases of the Vulva

- Definition: Malignant neoplasms of vulva

- Etiology/Incidence
    1. Risk factors
        a. HPV types 16, 18 and 31, possibly 6 and 11
        b. Concurrent cancer (breast, endometrium, and cervical)
        c. History of chronic vulvar irritation
        d. Vulvar dystrophies
    2. Includes carcinoma in situ, extramammary Paget's disease, Bartholin's carcinoma, invasive cancer, melanomas, and metastatic cancers from other sites
    3. Most common in postmenopause, peak incidence in 60s; incidence increasing among younger women
    4. Most common site—labia majora
    5. Accounts for less than 5% of all gynecologic malignancies; 90% is invasive squamous cell carcinoma
- Signs and Symptoms
    1. May be asymptomatic
    2. Vulvar lesions(s) may be scaly, white, red, ulcerated or irregularly pigmented
    3. Extreme pruritus, sometimes burning
- Differential Diagnosis
    1. Ulcerative lesions secondary to HSV II, syphilis or granuloma inguinale
    2. Cervical cancer
    3. Condylomata lata or acuminata
    4. Chronic vulvar dermatitis; vulvar dystrophies
    5. Non-malignant nevi
    6. Endometrioma
    7. Lichen sclerosis
- Physical Findings
    1. White, red, pigmented or ulcerated lesion

2. Evidence of excoriation and irritation; patches of hyperkeratosis

3. Enlargement of the Bartholin's gland

4. Inguinal lymphadenopathy

- Diagnostic Tests/Findings

   1. Screening—visual detection

   2. Colposcopy and directed biopsy for diagnosis and disease staging

   3. Evaluation for cervical cancer

- Management/Treatment

   1. Local excision

   2. Simple or radical vulvectomy

   3. Topical treatment with chemotherapeutic or immunologic agents

   4. Recurrence is common; careful follow-up critical

Choriocarcinoma

- Definition: Rare, highly malignant tumor that may be primary in the ovary or a form of gestational trophoblastic neoplasia (GTN)

- Etiology/Incidence

   1. Nongestational—mixed germ cell tumor of ovary occurring in childhood and early adolescence; few in 20s and 30s

   2. Gestational trophoblastic tumors may follow any gestational event— intrauterine or ectopic pregnancy, or abortion (50%); hydatidiform mole (50%); malignant transformation occurs in the chorion

- Signs and Symptoms

   1. Non-gestational—high gonadotropin levels can induce precocious puberty, uterine bleeding and breast enlargement in postmenarchal girl; if ruptures, mimics ruptured ectopic

   2. Gestational trophoblastic tumor

      a. Irregular bleeding (intermittent to hemorrhage) continuing after immediate postpartum period with uterine subinvolution

      b. Abdominal pain suggestive of inflammation when parametrium affected

       c. Cough and bloody sputum with metastases

- Differential Diagnosis

  1. Intrauterine or ectopic pregnancy

  2. Invasive mole

  3. Benign ovarian tumor

  4. Other genital cancers

- Physical Findings

  1. Non-gestational may include—signs of precocious puberty; signs of abdominal mass and ascites; irregular bleeding

  2. Gestational trophoblastic tumor may include—vaginal or vulvar lesion (indicate metastases); irregular bleeding with enlarged, soft uterus

- Diagnostic Tests/Findings

  1. Complete medical and diagnostic work-up to confirm malignancy and metastases

  2. Will see abnormal beta hCG regression titers following hydatidiform mole

  3. Suggestive

     a. After evacuation of molar pregnancy, see rise in beta hCG for 2 successive weeks, or constant level for 3 successive weeks

     b. Beta hCG levels elevated at 15 weeks post evacuation

     c. Rising beta hCG titer after reaching normal level

- Management/Treatment

  1. If nonmetastatic—single agent chemotherapy or chemotherapy plus hysterectomy; prognosis excellent

  2. If metastatic—may use single agent chemotherapy for selected candidates or chemotherapy plus radiation; prognosis good to poor

Adenomyosis

- Definition: Presence of endometrial glands and stroma within uterine myometrium

- Etiology/Incidence
    1. Cause believed to be disruption of uterine wall during pregnancy, labor, and postpartum involution
    2. Peak incidence in parous women over 40; regresses after menopause
    3. Occurs in 2-30% of multiparous women in 30s and 40s
- Signs and Symptoms (often asymptomatic)
    1. Abnormal menstrual bleeding (menorrhagia)
    2. Dysmenorrhea; may be severe
    3. Infertility
- Differential Diagnosis
    1. Leiomyomas
    2. Endometriosis
    3. Pelvic adhesions
    4. Pregnancy
    5. Pelvic congestion
- Physical Findings
    1. Diffuse, globular enlargement of uterus
    2. Uterine tenderness during menses
    3. May see evidence of anemia
- Diagnostic Tests/Findings
    1. Bimanual exam just prior to menses—will reveal tenderness (Halban's sign)
    2. May perform endometrial biopsy to evaluate abnormal bleeding
    3. Vaginal ultrasound to rule out pelvic pathology
- Management/Treatment
    1. May require no intervention other than symptomatic relief
    2. Hysterectomy, if severe (is curative)

Endometriosis

- Definition: Presence of endometrial glands and stroma outside the uterus
- Etiology/Incidence
    1. Etiology poorly understood—possibilities include
        a. Retrograde menstruation
        b. Immunologic and hormonal factors
        c. Increased sensitivity to estrogen
        d. Genetic basis
    2. Occurs in 1% of women in childbearing years; some reports give 7-40% incidence
    3. May occur in any organ system; most common pelvic site is ovary; other sites include cul-de-sac, uterine broad ligaments, posterior uterus
- Signs and Symptoms (severity of symptoms do not always correlate with severity of disease)
    1. Increasing dysmenorrhea (onset precedes menses by 1-2 days)
    2. Dyspareunia and/or pelvic pain which may radiate to thigh
    3. Premenstrual spotting
    4. Dysuria, urgency, hematuria
    5. Dyschezia (painful defecation), rectal bleeding
- Differential Diagnosis
    1. Acute salpingitis
    2. Chronic PID
    3. Ectopic pregnancy
    4. Adenomyosis
    5. Benign or malignant ovarian neoplasm
- Physical Findings
    1. Tender nodule palpated at uterosacral ligament
    2. Generalized pelvic tenderness
    3. Tender and/or enlarged adnexa (endometrioma)

    4. Fixed, retroflexed uterus

    5. Pain on motion of pelvic structures just prior to and during menses

- Diagnostic Tests/Findings

    1. History and pelvic examination, including rectal

    2. Definitive diagnosis is made by laparoscopy and biopsy

    3. Elevated CA-125—correlates with degree of disease and treatment response

- Management/Treatment

    1. Goal—prevent disease progression, alleviate pain, and establish or restore fertility by interrupting cycle of stimulation and bleeding

    2. Analgesics for symptom control

    3. Continuous low dose monophasic OC to control symptoms

    4. Progestins—oral Provera and Depo Provera very effective for symptom control in mild to moderate disease

    5. Danazol—relieves pain, and prevents disease progression (creates high androgen, low estrogenic environment); 400 mg tablets twice daily for 6-9 months

    6. GnRh agonist to suppress ovarian function

    7. Laser surgery to remove endometrial implants; 60% pregnancy success rate; best chance to conceive 1st year after surgery

    8. Hysterectomy with bilateral salpingo-oophorectomy (curative)

    9. Complications of endometriosis

       a. Infertility

       b. Increased risk of spontaneous abortion

Reproductive Disorders

Ectopic Pregnancy

- Definition

1. Implantation of the blastocyst anywhere other than endometrial lining of uterine cavity; over 95% tubal

2. Sites

    a. Fallopian tube—ampulla (most frequent tubal site); isthmus (12%); interstitial (2%); fimbria (5%)

    b. Other sites—abdomen; ovary; broad ligament; combined or heterotypic (tubal plus intrauterine), very rare

- Etiology/Incidence

    1. Any condition that prevents fertilized ovum from reaching uterine cavity—salpingitis, peritubal adhesions, tubal abnormalities, previous ectopic, previous tubal surgery, current IUD use, tumors that distort tubes, external migration of ovum, menstrual reflux, and hormonal alteration of tubal motility

    2. Second leading cause of maternal mortality in U.S.

    3. Incidence is 1 per 100 pregnancies

- Signs and Symptoms

    1. Unruptured may include

        a. Lower pelvic and abdominal pain (often unilateral)

        b. Irregular vaginal bleeding (amenorrhea or spotting)

        c. Symptoms of pregnancy

    2. Ruptured may include

        a. Severe bilateral or generalized abdominal pain

        b. Neck or shoulder pain (due to diaphragmatic irritation from intraperitoneal hemorrhage)

        c. Vertigo/fainting/shock

- Differential Diagnosis

    1. Salpingitis

    2. Appendicitis

    3. Ruptured functional cysts

    4. Torsion of ovarian cyst or leiomyoma

- Physical Findings
    1. Abdominal tenderness
    2. Very tender adnexa
    3. Unilateral adnexal or cul-de-sac mass/fullness
    4. Normal or slightly enlarged uterus
    5. Pronounced cervical motion tenderness
- Diagnostic Tests/Findings
    1. Quantitative serum beta hCG (only confirms pregnancy, not whether intrauterine or extrauterine)—level will be low, usually < 5,000 mIU/mL
    2. Culdocentesis—positive if nonclotting blood obtained, indicates intraperitoneal bleeding and surgery required immediately; negative results do not rule out ectopic, further testing indicated
    3. Hemoglobin and hematocrit—normal unless significant hemorrhage
    4. Leukocyte count—may be normal or increased
    5. Transvaginal ultrasound to determine location of conceptus
    6. Surgery (laparoscopy, laparotomy)
- Management/Treatment
    1. Salpingectomy/salpingostomy
    2. Ipsilateral oophorectomy
    3. Tubal resection
    4. Methotrexate
    5. RhoGAM administration, if Rh negative

Gestational Trophoblastic Disease

- Definition
    1. Benign neoplasm of the chorion in which chorionic villi degenerate and become transparent "grape-like" vesicles containing clear fluid
    2. Two types of molar growth

a. Complete—characterized by large amount of edematous villi, no fetus or fetal membranes; carries risk of choriocarcinoma; generally have 46,XX karyotype

b. Incomplete (Partial)—some normal villi and fetal material or amniotic sac; less risk of choriocarcinoma; generally have triploid karyotype

- Etiology/Incidence

  1. Etiology unknown

  2. Varies from 1:1200 to 1:2000 pregnancies

  3. Higher among Asian women

  4. Increased frequency toward the beginning and end of childbearing years

- Signs and Symptoms

  1. Abnormal uterine bleeding (90%)

  2. Hyperemesis

  3. Abdominal cramps (secondary to uterine distension)

  4. May report passage of vesicular tissue

- Differential Diagnosis

  1. Spontaneous abortion

  2. Ectopic pregnancy

- Physical Findings

  1. Disproportionate uterine size (size > dates, size < dates)

  2. Absence of fetal heart tones at appropriate gestational age

  3. Signs of dehydration (with hyperemesis)

  4. Pregnancy-induced hypertension before 20 weeks is pathognomonic

  5. Signs of hyperthyroidism (8-10%)

  6. Palpable theca lutein cysts (50%)

  7. Evidence of vaginal bleeding

- Diagnostic Tests/Findings
    1. Ultrasound—multiple echoes with normal gestational sac; "snow-storm" pattern
    2. Quantitative hCG assay determination with values greater than 100,000 mIU/mL 100 days or more after last normal menstrual period (LNMP)
- Management/Treatment
    1. Evacuation of molar tissue
    2. Serial hCG titers performed weekly after evacuation; should fall to < 5 mIU/mL by 14 weeks post evacuation; persistent elevation may indicate choriocarcinoma; refer
    3. Gynecologic examination to evaluate uterine size, adnexal structures and external genitalia 1 week after evacuation; baseline chest x-ray
    4. Delay pregnancy for 1 year; may use OCs
    5. Approximately 100% survival rate

Induced Abortion

- Definition: Therapeutic or elective termination of pregnancy in first (conception through weeks 12-13 gestation) or second (weeks 13-14 through week 24) trimester
- Etiology/Incidence
    1. Approximately 1.6 million per year
    2. Fifty percent obtained by women younger than 25, peak age 18-19; incidence increasing among older women
- Diagnostic Tests/Findings
    1. Careful history and pregnancy test to accurately establish gestational age
    2. Vaginal ultrasound if unsure of gestational age
    3. Rh factor determination and blood type
    4. CBC
    5. Vaginitis/STD screening—chlamydia, GC, saline wet mount

- Management/Treatment

    1. Menstrual extraction—up to 6 weeks from LNMP; often before diagnosis of pregnancy confirmed

    2. Vacuum aspiration—most widely used procedure in U.S.; may be performed through 16 weeks gestation; likelihood of incomplete abortion if performed before 7 weeks

    3. Dilatation and evacuation—most common procedure done in second trimester; 13-20 weeks gestation

    4. Amnioinfusion—16-18 weeks gestation; prostaglandin solution, hypertonic saline or urea used

    5. Hysterotomy—surgical procedure to remove fetus and placenta after failed second trimester abortion; rarely used today

    6. Mifepristone (RU 486)—used in Europe for early pregnancy termination; not approved for use in U.S.

    7. Adjunctive techniques—laminarias, oxytocin and synthetic dilators may be used prior to second trimester procedures to assist cervical dilatation

- Postabortion (PAB) Care

    1. May give prophylactic antibiotics—doxycycline 100 mg, twice daily for 1-3 days

    2. Immunoprophylaxis with RhoGAM for Rh negative women

    3. Reinforce self-care and need for follow-up

    4. Counsel on signs of hemorrhage, uterine perforation, retained tissue, infection, subinvolution, Asherman's syndrome and missed pregnancy

    5. Recommend 2 week PAB visit

    6. Discuss contraceptive options

    7. Risk of continued pregnancy is greater after attempting termination of early pregnancy or when multiple or ectopic pregnancy present; careful tissue examination needed

    8. Support for possible feelings of ambivalence, depression, regret and/or sadness; single most important factor affecting a woman's reaction to her abortion is level of support received from significant others

Sexually Transmitted Diseases (STD)

Gonorrhea (GC)

- Definition: A classic bacterial STD that can be symptomatic or asymptomatic in men and women

- Etiology/Incidence

  1. Causative organism, *Neisseria gonorrhoeae,* a gram negative diplococcus; cultured from genitourinary tract, oropharynx and/or anorectum of men and women

  2. Estimated 1 million new infections in U.S. each year; greater than 80% occur in individuals younger than 30

  3. Incubation period 2-10 days

  4. Possible serious complications include PID, ectopic pregnancy, infertility, perihepatitis (Fitz-Hugh-Curtis Syndrome), conjunctivitis, disseminated gonococcal infection (DGI), bartholinitis, periurethral or tubo-ovarian abscess and epididymitis

  5. Pregnancy related complications include premature rupture of membranes, premature labor, chorioamnionitis, postpartum metritis, septic abortion and PAB metritis

  6. Neonatal complications may include ophthalmia neonatorum, pneumonia, and sepsis/meningitis

  7. Male-to-female transmission higher than female-to-male

  8. Ten to fifteen percent of women with endocervical GC will develop acute salpingitis

- Signs and Symptoms

  1. May be symptomatic, asymptomatic or complicated by infections at several sites

  2. Primary site in reproductive age women is endocervical canal

  3. Infection usually localized to vagina in prepubertal girls

  4. Infection of urethra, Skene's and Bartholin's duct is common; usually coexists with endocervical infection

5. Pharyngeal infection is transmitted through oral-genital contact with greater transmissibility from male-to-female

6. When symptoms present, include

   a. Purulent discharge from the cervix, Skene's gland or Bartholin's

   b. Intermenstrual bleeding

   c. Symptoms of anorectal infection may be absent, minimal or severe (pruritus, mucopurulent discharge, bleeding, pain, tenesmus, constipation)

   d. Sore throat (most pharyngeal infections are asymptomatic)

   e. Fever, chills, lower pelvic pain, dyspareunia and vaginal discharge (symptoms of salpingitis)

   f. Dysuria and frequency

- Differential Diagnosis

  1. Other STDs

  2. Vaginitis

- Physical Findings—may include

  1. Mucopurulent cervicitis

  2. Erythema, friability of cervix

  3. Bartholin's abscess

  4. Signs of other STDs

  5. Exudative pharyngitis

  6. Severely tender adnexa and cervical motion tenderness

- Diagnostic Tests/Findings (see Normal Women's Health Chapter)

- Management/Treatment

  1. For uncomplicated urethral, endocervical or rectal infections, the Centers for Disease Control and Prevention (CDC) recommends co-treatment for chlamydia and GC

     a. Ceftriaxone 125 mg IM. in single dose or

     b. Cefixime 400 mg orally in a single dose or

     c. Ciprofloxacin 500 mg orally in a single dose or

      d. Ofloxacin 400 mg orally in a single dose *plus*

      e. Doxycycline 100 mg orally 2 times a day for 7 days

      f. Spectinomycin 2 g IM. in single dose is recommended if cephalosporins or quinolones contraindicated

2. According to CDC, test-of-cure not essential if ceftriaxone and doxycycline used, unless symptoms persist

3. Examine and treat all sexual partners

4. Avoid intercourse until treatment of both partners completed

5. Evaluation for other STDs including serologic testing for HIV and syphilis recommended

6. Avoid quinolones and tetracyclines in pregnancy; current recommendation, ceftriaxone plus erythromycin

Chlamydia

- Definition: Common STD that produces cervicitis in women and urethritis in men

- Etiology/Incidence

  1. Causative organism—*Chlamydia trachomatis,* an obligate intracellular parasite regarded by many experts as modified bacteria; most common STD

  2. Estimated 4 million acute infections annually

  3. Highest rates are among 15-21 age group

  4. Conditions associated with chlamydia may include mucopurulent cervicitis; urethritis, Bartholinitis; salpingitis, endometritis; infertility; Fitz-Hugh-Curtis Syndrome

  5. Incubation period 10-30 days

  6. May cause conjunctivitis and/or pneumonia in newborn

- Signs and Symptoms (often asymptomatic)

  1. Mucopurulent discharge

  2. Intermenstrual or postcoital bleeding

  3. Suprapubic tenderness

4. Dysuria, hesitancy, frequency, often > 7-10 days duration

5. Symptoms of PID may include—fever, chills, nausea and vomiting, increased vaginal discharge, irregular bleeding, and symptoms of urinary tract infection (UTI)

- Differential Diagnosis

  1. Gonorrhea

  2. Salpingitis

  3. Urethritis

- Physical Findings

  1. Mucopurulent cervical discharge

  2. Tender, friable cervix

- Diagnostic Tests/Findings (see Normal Women's Health Chapter)

- Management/Treatment

  1. CDC recommended treatment for uncomplicated urethral, endocervical or rectal infection

     a. Doxycycline 100 mg orally 2 times a day for 7 days or

     b. Azithromycin 1 gram orally, single dose

     c. Alternative regimens

        (1) Ofloxacin 300 mg orally 2 times a day for 7 days or

        (2) Erythromycin base 500 mg orally 4 times a day for 7 days or

        (3) Erythromycin ethylsuccinate 800 mg orally 4 times a day for 7 days or

        (4) Sulfisoxazole 500 mg orally 4 times a day for 10 days

  2. Examine and treat all sexual partners

  3. Avoid intercourse during treatment or use condoms

  4. Test-of-cure not recommended after treatment with doxycycline or azithromycin unless symptoms persist

  5. Doxycycline and ofloxacin contraindicated in pregnancy; sulfisoxazole contraindicated near term and with lactation; safety and efficacy of

azithromycin in pregnancy and lactation unknown; recommend erythromycin base 500 mg orally 4 times a day for 7 days

Herpes Simplex Virus (HSV)

- Definition: A recurring viral STD that produces painful genital lesions
- Etiology/Incidence
  1. Causative organism—Herpes Simplex Virus (HSV)
  2. Two strains of herpes virus exist
     a. Type I (HSV I)—represents 5-10% of genital herpes lesions; primarily causes oral-labial lesions and resides in trigeminal ganglion
     b. Type II (HSV II)—causes 90-95% of all genital herpes lesions; lives in sacral dorsal root ganglia
  3. Total prevalence—20-30 million cases with 500,000 new cases per year
  4. Accounts for 50-70% of genital ulcerative disease
  5. Transmission through close contact of susceptible mucosal surface (oropharynx, cervix, or conjunctiva) or through crack in skin surface
  6. Incubation period—1-26 days
  7. Clinical classifications
     a. Primary, first episode (no previous circulating antibodies to HSV I or II)
     b. Nonprimary, first episode
     c. Recurrent
     d. Asymptomatic
  8. Serious complication is neonatal herpes
- Signs and Symptoms
  1. Primary, first episode
     a. Severely painful, usually multiple lesions on vulva, vagina, cervix, rectum, buttocks, penis, or scrotum

    b. Systemic symptoms usually present (fever, chills, malaise, headache)

    c. Vulvar pain, swelling

    d. Dysuria and urinary retention

    e. Duration of symptoms 12-20 days

    f. Mean duration of viral shedding approximately 12 days

  2. Recurrent genital herpes

    a. Have circulating antibodies to HSV

    b. May recur in absence of exposure

    c. Prodrome often precedes eruption (itching, burning, tingling)

    d. Shorter and less severe than primary, lasting 8-12 days with mean shedding time of 4 days

    e. Possible activators include illness, stress, menstruation, pregnancy, trauma and heat, HIV

- Differential Diagnosis

  1. Other causes of genital ulcerative disease (primary syphilis, chancroid, lymphogranuloma venereum)

  2. Erythema multiforme

  3. Neoplasm

- Physical Findings

  1. Multiple painful lesions appearing as papules, vesicles, or pustules with ulcerated areas

  2. Cervix—erythematous

  3. Profuse watery vaginal discharge—often present

  4. Inguinal lymphadenopathy, vulvar edema

  5. Low grade fever

- Diagnostic Tests/Findings (see Normal Women's Health Chapter)

- Management/Treatment

  1. No cure

2. Acyclovir (Zovirax), an antiviral agent; shortens the mean duration of primary eruptions and duration of viral shedding; may reduce systemic symptoms (not recommended for use during pregnancy)

   a. For primary infection—Acyclovir 200 mg orally 5 times a day for 7-10 days; recommend therapy be initiated within 6 days of lesion onset; Acyclovir ointment not as effective

   b. For recurrent therapy—Acyclovir 200 mg orally 5 times a day for 5 days

   c. Daily suppressive therapy reduces frequency of HSV recurrences by 75% among patients with frequent recurrences (6 or more/year)—Acyclovir 200 mg 2-5 times a day for up to 1 year; effective in reducing outbreaks only when taking medication; rebound effect possible when therapy discontinued

3. Patient counseling should include—abstain from intercourse from onset of prodrome until lesions healed; use condoms consistently because asymptomatic viral shedding possible; inform obstetrician or advanced practice nurse of HSV history due to potential life-threatening neonatal consequences; may need referral to support group; no cure for HSV

Condyloma Acuminata (Genital Warts)

- Definition: Viral STD causing either wart-like growths on the genitalia or subclinical infection

- Etiology/Incidence

  1. Caused by human papillomavirus (HPV); there are multiple species

  2. Among cases of abnormal cervical cytology, 80-96% are associated with HPV

  3. Estimated 3 million people infected annually

  4. High infectivity rate

  5. Present data shows positive association with high grade dysplasia and cervical cancer (especially types 16, 18, 31, and 33)

  6. Transmission

     a. Considered STD; fomite transmission possible

b. Unknown rate of subclinical infection

c. Incubation period 1-6 months or longer; virus may remain dormant for decades

- Signs and Symptoms

  1. Wart-like structures or "bumps" on vulva, perineum, penis, and perianal area

  2. Other less common symptoms—pain and burning with urination, pruritus, and postcoital bleeding

- Differential Diagnosis

  1. Condyloma lata

  2. Molluscum contagiosum

  3. Vulvar, vaginal, cervical carcinoma

- Physical Findings

  1. Single or multiple painless genital warts; may be flat, verrucous, inverted, or villiform (HPV 6 and 11 are most common; low oncogenic potential); appear as soft, pale, pink or flesh-colored, dry, irregular lesions on external genitalia

  2. Subclinical infections are common (normal appearing skin turns white after application of acetic acid due to cellular swelling of affected tissue)

  3. Warts may be as small as 1 mm or large enough to affect urination and defecation; may grow large enough in pregnancy to affect fetal descent

  4. Lesions may be visualized on cervix and in vaginal vault

  5. Large lesions may be cauliflower-like in appearance, and may be coalesced and friable

- Diagnostic Tests/Findings

  1. Application of acetic acid solution to establish subclinical infection

  2. Pap smear (reveals "koilocytosis," "parakeratosis")—diagnostic if lesion is sampled

  3. Colposcopy with biopsy and possible ECC

  4. DNA typing with HPV detection kits such as Virapap and ViraType to determine specific HPV strain

5. Additional diagnostic tests to rule out co-infection with other STDs

- Management/Treatment
  1. Goal of treatment is to remove warts; will not eliminate HPV
  2. If left untreated, genital warts may spontaneously resolve, remain unchanged or grow
  3. Inspection of vulva, vagina, perineum, anus and cervix, when lesion found at any location
  4. Chemical options
     a. Local application of 10-20% podophyllin in tincture of benzoin for external use only; (contraindicated during pregnancy, and with vaginal, cervical or oral warts)
     b. Podofilox 0.5% solution for self-treatment of genital warts twice daily for 3 days followed by 4 days of no therapy; repeat for 4 cycles; contraindicated in pregnancy
     c. Trichloracetic (TCA) acid 80-90% applied to vulvar, vaginal, or anal warts to decrease viral shedding; use talc or baking soda afterwards to remove excess acid
     d. 5-Fluorouracil for widespread vaginal warts and diagnosed sub-clinical infection; $1/3$ or $1/2$ applicator deep in vagina at bedtime 1 time weekly for 10 weeks; not a 1st choice
     e. Other interventions such as laser carbon dioxide vaporization, cryosurgery, surgical excision or interferon should be performed by specialist
     f. Normal Pap smear to be followed with repeat Pap smears every 6 months

Syphilis

- Definition: Systemic STD that progresses through distinct stages (primary, secondary, latent, and tertiary, if untreated)
- Etiology/Incidence
  1. Caused by *Treponema pallidum,* a spirochete organism that invades skin and mucous membranes through microscopic abrasions that occur secondary to direct sexual contact

2. Incubation period varies according to number of invading organisms; generally 10-90 days (average 21)

3. Transplacental transmission causes risks to fetus throughout pregnancy

4. More than 50,000 new cases reported annually in U.S.

- Signs and Symptoms

    1. Primary Syphilis

        a. Painless "sore" or lesion

        b. May be asymptomatic

    2. Secondary Syphilis

        a. Flu-like symptoms (low grade fever, malaise, headache, sore throat, arthralgias) and generalized lymphadenopathy

        b. Maculopapular rash on palms and soles of feet

        c. Condyloma lata (hypertrophic, flat, moist wart-like lesions)

        d. Patchy alopecia

        e. Roseola syphilitica—flat, erythematous, round to oval, rose to pale pink lesions on trunk

        f. Mucous patches (may be found on lips, tongue, palate, penis, vulva, vagina)

    3. Latent Syphilis—historical or serological evidence for syphilis; asymptomatic

        a. Early latency (less than 1 year's duration—may be infectious)

        b. Late latency (greater than 1 year's duration—not infectious)

    4. Tertiary Syphilis

        a. Destructive, non-infectious stage which may present with single or multisystem involvement

        b. Classic skin lesion—solitary gumma

        c. Neurosyphilis (diagnosed by examination of CSF)—optic, auditory, cranial nerve, meningeal symptoms most common

        d. Cardiovascular syphilis

- Differential Diagnosis

    1. Other STDs causing genital ulcerative disease—chancroid, lymphogranuloma venereum, HSV

    2. Other causes for skin rash

- Physical Findings

    1. Primary—classic chancre is painless, rounded, indurated ulcer with serous exudate; may be genital or extragenital and will heal in 3 to 6 weeks; may have regional lymphadenopathy

    2. Secondary—maculopapular rash covering entire body including palms of hands and soles of feet; roseola syphilitica; mucous patches, condylomata lata; spontaneous healing of all secondary manifestations

    3. Latent—asymptomatic

    4. Tertiary—symptoms expressed depend on which organ system affected

- Diagnostic Tests/Findings

    1. Positive dark-field microscopic examination is definitive test; if negative, repeat within 3 days

    2. Serologic testing when suspicious even if dark-field negative

    3. Primary—VDRL or RPR may be positive or negative; FTA-ABS or MHA-TP will be positive

    4. Secondary—all serologic tests positive

    5. Latent—serologic tests positive

- Management/Treatment

    1. For primary, secondary and early latent syphilis of less than 1 year's duration, CDC recommends

        a. Benzathine penicillin G 2.4 million units IM., single dose

        b. If penicillin allergy—doxycycline 100 mg 2 times a day for 2 weeks; however, penicillin is considered only adequate treatment; may be desensitized to penicillin

    2. For late latent, benzathine penicillin G 7.2 million units administered as 3 doses of 2.4 million units IM. given 1 week apart for 3 consecutive weeks

    3. Clinical and serologic follow-up at 3 and 6 months post-treatment

4. If symptoms persist or recur or sustained 4-fold increase in nontreponemal test titer compared to baseline or previous titer, either failed treatment or reinfection; re-treat after HIV testing

   a. Penicillin regimen appropriate for the stage of syphilis; some recommend second dose of benzathine penicillin G 2.4 million units 1 week after initial dose, especially in third trimester or with secondary syphilis

   b. If penicillin allergy, desensitize then treat with penicillin

Chancroid

- Definition: Ulcerative bacterial infection that is sexually transmitted
- Etiology/Incidence
  1. Caused by *Haemophilus ducreyi,* a gram negative bacillus
  2. Occurs most commonly in uncircumcised males, low incidence in women
  3. Well established as a co-factor for HIV transmission
  4. Incubation period is 4-7 days
  5. Rare in U.S.; estimated 3,000 reported cases annually
- Signs and Symptoms
  1. Men—ragged, painful ulcers around prepuce, on frenulum, or in coronal sulcus; inguinal tenderness
  2. Women—may have ulcer as above, be asymptomatic, or have nonspecific symptoms such as dysuria, discharge or dyspareunia
- Differential Diagnosis
  1. Genital herpes
  2. Syphilis
  3. Donovanosis
- Physical Findings
  1. Characteristic ulcerative lesions with bubo (50%) which can rupture
  2. Unilateral inguinal adenitis

- Diagnostic Tests/Findings

    1. Probable diagnosis if painful genital ulcer(s) present, no evidence of syphilis by darkfield examination or serologic test, and lesions are atypical for HSV

    2. Definitive diagnosis is made when *H. ducreyi* is isolated by culture

- Management/Treatment

    1. Regimens

        a. Azithromycin 1 g orally in single dose or

        b. Cetrixone 250 mg IM. in single dose or

        c. Erythromycin base 500 mg orally 4 times a day for 7 days

    2. Should be tested for HIV infection, and retested in 3 months for syphilis and HIV

    3. Follow-up—re-examine 3-7 days after therapy; if no improvement, reevaluate diagnosis and check compliance with medication

Lymphogranuloma Venereum (LGV)

- Definition: Bacterial STD that is rare in U.S.

- Etiology/Incidence

    1. Caused by *Chlamydia trachomatis* serovars L1, L2, and L3

    2. Infected men outnumber infected women 5:1

    3. Incubation period 3-12 days or longer

- Signs and Symptoms

    1. Usually asymptomatic

    2. May report genital ulcers and painful inguinal nodes

- Differential Diagnosis

    1. Chancroid

    2. Genital herpes

    3. Syphilis

- Physical Findings

1. Tender, unilateral inguinal lymphadenopathy (most common)

2. Other symptoms may include genital ulcer at site of inoculation, proctitis, and genital edema

- Diagnostic Tests/Findings

    1. Serologic testing

    2. Exclusion of other causes of inguinal lymphadenopathy or genital ulcers

- Management/Treatment

    1. If bubos present, may need to aspirate, incise and drain

    2. Preferred treatment—doxycycline 100 mg orally 2 times a day for 21 days

    3. Pregnant and lactating women should be treated with erythromycin 500 mg orally 4 times a day for 21 days

    4. Sexual contacts within last 30 days should be examined, tested and treated for chlamydia infection

Vaginal Infections

Bacterial Vaginosis (BV)

- Definition: Syndrome that results from homeostatic disruption in vagina; Lactobacilli, the predominant organism in normal vaginal flora, are absent or greatly reduced

- Etiology/Incidence

    1. Causative organism is *Gardnerella vaginalis,* which interacts with other anaerobes such as *Bacteroids* and *Mobiluncus* species

    2. Most prevalent form of vaginitis in reproductive aged women

    3. Not considered sexually transmitted; *G. vaginalis* may be found in low concentrations in 40-60% of normal vaginal cultures

- Signs and Symptoms

    1. May be asymptomatic

2. Malodor (often accentuated by coitus)

3. Abnormal vaginal discharge

- Differential Diagnosis

   1. Trichomoniasis

   2. Monilia vaginitis

- Physical Findings

   1. Large amount of homogeneous, whitish vaginal discharge

   2. Presence of foul odor

   3. Normal appearing vulva and vaginal mucosa

- Diagnostic Tests/Findings

   1. May be diagnosed by clinical or gram stain criteria

   2. Three of the following clinical criteria

      a. A homogeneous, white, non-inflammatory discharge that adheres to vaginal walls

      b. Presence of clue cells (stippled epithelial cells) on microscopic examination

      c. Vaginal pH $\geq$ 4.5

      d. Positive potassium hydroxide amine test ("whiff" test)

   3. May use gram stain to determine concentration of specific bacteria

   4. Culture not recommended as diagnostic tool

- Management/Treatment

   1. Routine treatment of asymptomatic women not recommended

   2. Recommended drug regimen—metronidazole (Flagyl) 500 mg orally b.i.d. for 7 days

   3. Alternatives

      a. Metronidazole 2 g orally in a single dose, or

      b. Metronidazole gel, 0.75%, one full applicator (5 g) intravaginally, b.i.d. for 5 days

      c. Clindamycin cream, 2%, one full applicator (5 g) intravaginally for 5 days

      d. Clindamycin 300 mg orally b.i.d. for 7 days

    4. Possible side effects of metronidazole

        a. Antabuse effect (vomiting and flushing)

        b. Possible alteration in depth perception

        c. Metallic after-taste

        d. Nausea, headache, dry mouth

        e. Ten percent incidence of monilia infection after 7 day course

        f. May prolong prothrombin time in patients taking oral anticoagulants

    5. Partner treatment recommended with recurrent infection; treatment identical to female

Trichomoniasis

- Definition: Form of vaginitis caused by a flagellated, anaerobic protozoan
- Etiology/Incidence

    1. Causative organism is *Trichomonas vaginalis*

    2. Usually sexually transmitted; men may be asymptomatic carriers; fomite transmission theoretically possible

    3. Estimated 6 million women and their partners infected annually

    4. Use of oral contraceptives and barrier methods decreases prevalence

- Signs and Symptoms

    1. Sites include vagina, urethra, endocervix and bladder, causing variable symptomatology

    2. May be asymptomatic

    3. When symptomatic, may have

        a. Copious vaginal discharge, may be malodorous

        b. Vaginal pruritus

        c. Dyspareunia

        d. Intermenstrual or postcoital spotting

e. Dysuria, urgency, frequency

f. Onset of symptoms often occurs after menses

- Differential Diagnosis

    1. Bacterial vaginosis

    2. Candidiasis

    3. Foreign body

- Physical Findings

    1. Homogeneous, watery, yellow, gray or green colored vaginal discharge that is frothy or bubbly

    2. pH $\geq$ 5

    3. Punctate lesions called colpitis macularis ("strawberry spots") of cervix and/or vagina

    3. May be erythema, edema, or excoriation of vulva

    4. Friable cervix

- Diagnostic Tests/Findings

    1. Saline wet mount

        a. Motile trichomonads

        b. Increased number of white blood cells

    2. Gram stains (without Giemsa, acridine orange, etc.)—no diagnostic advantage over wet mount

    3. Reports of trichomonads on Pap smear—sensitivity is low

    4. Culture—very sensitive and specific, but expensive and not widely available

- Management/Treatment

    1. Metronidazole (Flagyl) 2.0 g orally in single dose (treatment of choice)

    2. Alternative metronidazole regimens

        a. Metronidazole 2.0 g in divided doses within same day—less nausea, improved compliance

        b. Metronidazole 500 mg b.i.d. for 7 days

3. If treatment failure with 1. or 2.a., re-treat with metronidazole 500 mg b.i.d. for 7 days

4. If repeated failure, treat with single 2 g dose for 3-5 days

5. Recurrent trichomoniasis

   a. Usually due to reinfection

   b. If Skene's glands and/or urethra are infected, may have inadequate tissue levels of drug at these sites; may need to culture sites and change dose to achieve cure

Vulvovaginal Candidiasis (VVC or Monilia)

- Definition: Vaginal infection that occurs after alteration of vaginal flora has occurred

- Etiology/Incidence

  1. Most common candida species causing VVC is *Candida albicans,* followed by *C. tropicalis* and *C. glabrata*

  2. Predisposing factors

     a. Pregnancy

     b. Recent antibiotic

     c. Diabetes, HIV infection

     d. High carbohydrate intake

     e. Poor hygienc practices

     f. History of anal-oral contact

     g. Vaginal hypersensitivity/allergen response

  3. Not considered a STD, but can be transmitted between partners

  4. May be transmitted from infected mother to newborn at delivery

- Signs and Symptoms (vary from mild to severe)

  1. Vulvar pruritus

  2. Discharge

  3. Burning, irritation, soreness

  4. Dyspareunia and vulvar (external) dysuria

- Differential Diagnosis
  1. Allergic dermatitis
  2. Trichomoniasis
  3. Bacterial vaginosis
- Physical Findings
  1. Erythema of vaginal walls
  2. Thick, white discharge which adheres to vaginal walls
  3. Vulvar erythema and excoriation
- Diagnostic Tests/Findings
  1. pH—3.8-4.2
  2. Negative amine test
  3. Saline or 10% KOH wet mount—few WBCs, presence of pseudohyphae
  4. Culture—Sabouraud's agar, Nickerson's medium, or Microstick
  5. Gram stain—positive for spores and filaments
- Management/Treatment
  1. Intravaginal formulations—antimycotic agents
     a. Clotrimazole (Gyne-Lotrimin, Mycelex)—for acute and chronic infections
     b. Miconazole (Monistat)—for acute and chronic infections; may weaken latex condoms and diaphragms
     c. Terconazole (Terazole)—broad spectrum antifungal agent; more effective against non-albicans strains of candida
     d. Butoconazole—may weaken latex condoms and diaphragms
  2. Oral preparations
     a. Ketoconazole (Nizoral)
        (1) Effective for acute infection; very expensive
        (2) Causes hepatic toxicity in 5-10%; monitor liver function tests; reserve for long term suppression of chronic *C. albicans* infection

b. Other oral agents

(1) Fluconazole

(2) Itraconazole

3. Boric acid vaginal capsules may be effective; should not be used in pregnancy

4. Treat male partners if symptomatic

Urinary Tract Disorders

Urinary Tract Infection (UTI)

- Definition: Presence of 100,000 or more colonies/mL of a bacterial pathogen on 2 consecutive clean-catch midstream (CCMS) specimens, resulting in inflammation of urinary bladder (cystitis), distal urethra (urethritis), or kidney (acute pyelonephritis)

- Etiology/Incidence

  1. *Escherichia coli,* most common causative organism (80-90%) followed by *Staphylococcus saprophyticus*

  2. Ascent of bacteria—rectal flora to vaginal introitus to distal urethra to bladder and occasionally to kidney

  3. Risk factors depend on location of infection

     a. Cystitis—sexual activity (at risk for all UTIs), diaphragm use, childhood UTI

     b. Urethritis—sexual activity, new sexual partner, male partner with dysuria

     c. Pyelonephritis—childhood UTI, prior history pyelonephritis, 3 UTIs in last year, known structural abnormality or stone, immunosuppression, pregnancy, sickle cell trait/disease

  4. Approximately 10-25% of women will have lower UTI; may occur at any age; rate increases with age

- Signs and Symptoms

  1. Range from minimal to severe, depending on location of UTI

2. Cystitis—abrupt onset of dysuria, urgency, frequency, nocturia, suprapubic tenderness, painful bladder spasms, and gross blood in urine

3. Urethritis—gradual onset of dysuria; may be vaginal discharge with odor

4. Pyelonephritis—onset gradual; fever chills, nausea and vomiting; costovertebral angle tenderness (CVAT); may or may not have voiding symptoms

- Differential Diagnosis

    1. Urethritis, cystitis, or pyelonephritis

    2. Interstitial cystitis

    3. Renal calculi

- Physical Findings

    1. Acute pyelonephritis—may have symptoms of sepsis; dehydration; CVAT; elevated blood pressure and temperature

    2. Cystitis—suprapubic tenderness

    3. Urethritis—may have vaginal discharge, tenderness when urethra palpated

- Diagnostic Tests/Findings

    1. Microscopic evaluation of spun urine reveals > 6-8 WBC per high-power field, some RBCs and bacteria

    2. Urinalysis may show positive nitrites, 1+ or 2+ protein with lower UTI (3+ or 4+ may indicate kidney source), RBCs and growth of 10^5 bacteria per mm of urine

    3. Vaginal wet mount to rule out trichomoniasis, candida and bacterial vaginosis

    4. STD cultures to rule out gonorrhea and chlamydia

- Management/Treatment

    1. Routine pelvic examination to rule out vaginitis and STDs

    2. Pharmacotherapeutic therapy

        a. Uncomplicated first episode—trimethoprim/sulfamethoxazole, ampicillin, or nitrofurantoin effective against *E. coli;*

cephalosporins can also be used; single dose or 3 day therapy often effective

    b. Resistant cases, use aminoglycosides or quinolones

3. Prevention

    a. Void immediately after intercourse

    b. Adequate hydration

    c. Frequent bladder emptying

    d. Proper wiping technique (hygiene)

4. Bacterial persistence after full course of appropriate antibiotic indicates need for consultation; possible cystoscopy and intravenous pyelography to rule out structural abnormalities

Urinary Incontinence

- Definition

  1. Loss of normal urinary control

  2. Types

         a. Stress urinary incontinence—urinary leakage with coughing, laughing, sneezing

         b. Detrusor instability—uncontrolled bladder activity

         c. Detrusor hyperreflexia—detrusor muscle instability secondary to known neurologic disorder

- Etiology/Incidence

  1. Causes (alone or in combination) include

         a. Problems associated with aging—impaction, bed rest, certain drugs (antidepressants, diuretics, sedatives, antihistamines)

         b. Damage to urogenital structures

         c. Nerve damage from disease

         d. Bladder neoplasm, infection or fistula

  2. Incidence—50% of all women experience occasional incontinence, 10% regularly; incidence increases with parity and advancing age

- Signs and Symptoms
    1. History of urinary frequency and/or urgency
    2. Leaking urine with coughing, laughing, sneezing, exercising
    3. Nocturia
- Differential Diagnosis
    1. UTI
    2. Bladder prolapse
    3. Any mass that compresses the bladder
- Physical Findings
    1. Urine leakage with increased abdominal pressure
    2. Relaxed pelvic floor muscles
    3. Vaginal atrophy, perineal irritation
- Diagnostic Tests/Findings
    1. Urinary stress test—fluid instilled in bladder; leaking after coughing, straining while standing indicates poor anatomic support
    2. Neurologic examination—test reflexes, sensation and strength in lower extremities, perineum, and anal sphincter
    3. Radiographic studies
    4. Urinalysis and urine culture to rule out infection
    5. Cystometry, urethroscopy and cystoscopy helpful
- Management/Treatment
    1. Kegel exercises—strengthens pelvic floor
    2. Estrogen replacement—helpful if deficient
    3. Medications—specific drug therapy depends on diagnosis
    4. Behavior modification used to retrain bladder
    5. Surgery, type depending on diagnosis

Breast Disorders

Fibrocystic Breast Changes

- Definition: Physiologic change in breast tissue that occurs in response to endogenous hormone stimulation, particularly estrogen
- Etiology/Incidence
    1. Exact etiology unknown
    2. Most common between ages 35-50
    3. Occurs in 50% of all women
    4. Breast cancer risk increased only with diagnosed biopsy of lobular or epithelial hyperplasia
- Signs and Symptoms
    1. Bilateral breast pain and nodularity that begins prior to onset of menses
    2. Multiple, bilateral masses that increase in size, become tender prior to menses, regress after menses
- Differential Diagnosis
    1. Malignant breast mass
    2. Other benign breast conditions
- Physical Findings
    1. Multiple, usually cystic masses that are firm, well-defined and mobile
    2. Most common sites—upper outer quadrant and axillary tail
    3. May have clear or white nipple discharge
- Diagnostic Tests/Findings
    1. Mammography to identify and characterize any masses
    2. Fine needle aspiration, if dominant mass
    3. Excision and biopsy, if dominant mass
    4. Breast ultrasound

5. Simple mastectomy (rare), if woman has strong family history for breast cancer, strong fear of developing cancer, or extreme pain

- Management/Treatment

1. Mild analgesics, hot/cold compresses

2. Diuretics to reduce physiologic breast edema

3. Restriction of methylxanthines (caffeine, tea, cola, chocolate)

4. Good supportive brassiere

5. Danazol therapy, tamoxifen, bromocriptine, or OCs to reduce pain, tenderness, and nodularity

6. Vitamin E use to decrease pain and tenderness is controversial; if used, 50 to 600 IU daily recommended

Intraductal Papilloma

- Definition

1. Small wart-like growth in the lining of the mammary duct near the nipple

2. Commonly located in a major subareolar collection duct

- Etiology/Incidence

1. Caused by proliferation and overgrowth of ductal epithelial tissue

2. Peak age group 40-50

- Signs and Symptoms

1. Yellow or bloody discharge from nipple which may occur spontaneously

2. May have non-painful mass

3. Feeling of fullness or pain beneath areola (possible)

- Differential Diagnosis

1. Intraductal carcinoma

2. Multiple papillomatosis

- Physical Findings

1. Serosanguineous nipple discharge from a single duct—elicited when pressure applied over affected duct

2. Soft, poorly delineated mass may be palpated (usually too small)

- Diagnostic Tests/Findings

    1. May perform ductography

    2. Can perform Pap smear of breast fluid to screen for malignancy

    3. Biopsy is necessary

- Management/Treatment

    1. Refer for surgical excision

    2. Biopsy is curative

    3. After duct removal, may still breastfeed

Fibroadenoma

- Definition: Benign breast mass derived from specialized connective tissue

- Etiology/Incidence

    1. Cause thought to be hormonal

    2. Most common cause of dominant breast mass in younger women; peak incidence between ages 15-25; slow-growing

    3. Third most common breast lesion after fibrocystic changes and carcinoma

    4. No significant correlation to breast cancer

- Signs and Symptoms

    1. Painless mass, rounded to lobular in shape

    2. Does not change with menstrual cycle

- Differential Diagnosis

    1. Breast carcinoma

    2. Cystosarcoma phyllodes

- Physical Findings

1. Firm, well delineated, freely mobile, non-tender mass; usually unilateral

2. No nipple discharge

- Diagnostic Tests/Findings

  1. Fine needle aspiration to determine solid tumor, cyst, or cancer

  2. Mammography used to evaluate characteristics of mass

  3. Excisional biopsy and tissue examination

- Management/Treatment

  1. Observation, if diagnosis confirmed and younger than 25 years

  2. Surgical excision when palpable in women over 25

  3. Encourage monthly breast self-examination (BSE)

Breast Cancer

- Definition: A malignant neoplasm of the breast

- Etiology/Incidence

  1. Risk factors include

     a. Age (75% over 40)

     b. Mother or sister with breast cancer

     c. Personal history breast cancer (10-15% with cancer in one breast will develop in other)

     d. Nulliparity or first pregnancy after age 30

     e. Atypical hyperplasia of breast

  2. 1 in 9 will develop during lifetime

  3. Estimated 182,000 new invasive cases among women in the U.S. in 1995

  4. Incidence higher in African-American women

  5. Leading site of cancer in women, second to lung as leading cause of cancer death in women

- Signs and Symptoms

  1. Breast mass (upper outer quadrant most frequent location)

    2. Spontaneous, unilateral nipple discharge; may be clear, yellow, or bloody

    3. Nipple retraction/irritation

    4. Skin edema/dimpling

    5. Enlarged axillary or supraclavicular/infraclavicular lymph nodes

- Differential Diagnosis

    1. Benign breast neoplasm

    2. Mastitis

- Physical Findings

    1. A fixed, poorly defined mass; usually painless; palpable at 1 cm

    2. May have nipple discharge, irritation, retraction

    3. May have Peau d'orange skin (edema)

    4. Nodal involvement

- Diagnostic Tests/Findings

    1. Screening (see Normal Women's Health Chapter)

    2. Diagnosis

        a. Mammogram—may reveal mass or microcalcifications

        b. Ultrasound—to distinguish between cystic and solid mass

        c. Fine needle aspiration for cytologic evaluation

        d. Biopsy (needle or surgical)

        e. Lung, liver, bone scan

        f. Hormonal receptor assays to determine presence of estrogen receptors

- Management/Treatment

    1. Refer to oncology team

    2. Stage of disease determines treatment

    3. Surgical options include local incision to total mastectomy

    4. Premenopausal—chemotherapy with tamoxifen

    5. Radiation in combination with lumpectomy for early stage

6. Postmenopausal

a. Tamoxifen for estrogen receptor positive tumors

b. Chemotherapy for estrogen receptor negative tumors

7. Nursing intervention/emotional support

Congenital and Chromosomal Abnormalities

Müllerian Abnormalities

- Definition

  1. Abnormalities of fallopian tubes, uterus and upper vagina that occur in fetal development

  2. Results from genetic patterns of inheritance

- Etiology/Incidence

  1. Tubes, uterus, and upper portion of vagina created by fusion of Müllerian system by the 10th week of gestation

  2. Abnormalities found in 5-10% of infertile women and in up to 15% of women with recurrent abortions

- Signs and Symptoms

  1. History of infertility or pregnancy loss

  2. Dyspareunia

  3. Amenorrhea/dysmenorrhea

- Differential Diagnosis

  1. Congenital anomalies

  2. Urinary tract anomalies

  3. Primary amenorrhea

- Physical Findings

  1. Common for ovaries to be normal and have well-developed secondary sex characteristics

  2. Part or all of vagina may be absent; uterus often absent

3. Common to have transverse vaginal septum; may be complete or incomplete

4. May have double vagina and uterus; often one side fully developed, other rudimentary development

- Diagnostic Tests/Findings

    1. Ultrasound, hysterosalpingogram, and laparoscopy often used to detect structural abnormalities

    2. May perform karyotyping to rule out chromosomal abnormality

- Management/Treatment

    1. Refer to reproductive endocrinologist

    2. Laparoscopy/hysteroscopy for corrective intervention

Testicular Feminization

- Definition

    1. Maternal X-linked recessive disorder

    2. Person with testes and a 46,XY karyotype but phenotypically female (male pseudohermaphrodite)

    3. Referred to as androgen insensitivity syndrome (produces testosterone without androgen response); individuals are infertile

- Etiology/Incidence

    1. A congenital insensitivity to androgens, whereby Wolffian duct development does not occur

    2. Sisters of affected individuals have a 1 in 3 chance of being XY, and female offspring of a normal sister of affected person, have a 1 in 6 chance of being XY

    3. Accounts for 10 percent of all cases of amenorrhea

- Signs and Symptoms

    1. May appear normal at birth with subsequent normal growth and development

    2. Usually presents at time of expected puberty, with amenorrhea, scanty or absent pubic and axillary hair; abnormal or no breast development

- Differential Diagnosis
    1. Müllerian agenesis
    2. Incomplete androgen insensitivity
- Physical Findings
    1. Breasts may have scant glandular tissue, small nipples, pale areolae
    2. Underdeveloped labia minora; shallow, blind vagina
    3. Absent cervix and uterus
    4. Primary amenorrhea
    5. Testes may be present in inguinal canal (at risk for neoplastic changes; gonadal removal required)
    6. Horseshoe kidneys reported in some cases
- Diagnostic Tests/Findings
    1. Genetic screen reveals normal female phenotype with 46,XY karyotype
    2. Hormone profile reveals high LH, normal to slightly elevated male testosterone levels, high estradiol levels, and normal to elevated FSH
- Management/Treatment
    1. Gonadectomy at about age 16-18
    2. Careful evaluation for other affected family members

Turner Syndrome

- Definition: Congenital absence of ovaries with bilateral rudimentary streak gonads due to an abnormality or absence of one of the X chromosomes
- Etiology/Incidence
    1. About 60% of Turner patients have total loss of one X chromosome; the remainder have structural abnormality in the chromosome or mosaicism with an abnormal X
    2. Approximately 98% of conceptions with only one X chromosome abort; total incidence is 1 in 2,000-5,000 liveborn girls

- Signs and Symptoms

  1. Short stature with webbed neck

  2. Amenorrhea, lack of breast development, scant axillary and pubic hair

- Differential Diagnosis includes other forms of gonadal dysgenesis

- Physical Findings

  1. Short stature, sexual infantilism, streak ovaries

  2. Congenital problems—webbed neck; high, arched palate; broad, shield-like chest; low hairline on the neck; short fourth metacarpal bones; short legs; renal abnormalities.

  3. Autoimmune disorders are common—Hashimoto's thyroiditis, Addison's disease, alopecia, and vitiligo

  4. Some may have hypothyroidism, hearing loss and mild insulin resistance

  5. Normal intelligence

- Diagnostic Tests/Implications

  1. Karyotyping—phenotypically female

  2. Measurement of gonadotropins (very high FSH/LH)

  3. Testosterone levels will be normal or elevated

- Management/Treatment

  1. Refer to reproductive endocrinologist for evaluation and management

  2. After diagnosis, additional studies to detect cardiac and renal malformations

Additional Gynecologic Disorders

Pelvic Inflammatory Disease (PID, Salpingitis)

- Definition: Acute or chronic bacterial infection capable of ascending from lower to upper genital tract to cause endometritis, salpingitis, tubo-ovarian abscess and pelvic peritonitis

- Etiology/Incidence
  1. Most frequent causative organisms are *N. gonorrhoeae* and *C. trachomatis*
  2. Other etiologic agents include
     a. Anaerobes
     b. Gram-negative rods
     c. Streptococci
     d. *G. vaginalis*
     e. Mycoplasma
  3. Risk factors include
     a. Previous episodes of PID
     b. Multiple sexual partners
     c. IUD use
     d. Age—less than 25 years old
  4. Possible sequelae—infertility, ectopic pregnancy, and chronic pelvic pain
- Signs and Symptoms (may be acute or mild)
  1. Lower abdominal pain/tenderness
  2. Irregular bleeding; 30% have spotting
  3. Fever/chills, nausea and vomiting
  4. Vaginal discharge; symptoms of UTI
- Differential Diagnosis
  1. Ectopic pregnancy
  2. Appendicitis
  3. Ruptured functional cyst
  4. Torsion of adnexal mass
  5. Ulcerative colitis
  6. Endometriosis

7. Degenerative leiomyoma

- Physical Findings

    1. May have > 38°C temperature

    2. May have bilateral adnexal tenderness and mass

    3. Cervical motion tenderness/uterine tenderness

    4. Purulent vaginal discharge

    5. Possible hydrosalpinx; friable, hypertrophic cervix

- Diagnostic Tests/Findings

    1. Assessment of LNMP, STD history, contraceptive use and sexual history

    2. Complete gynecologic examination, including rectal

    3. Erythrocyte Sedimentation Rate (ESR) > 50 mm/hr

    4. CBC with differential—leukocytosis and "shift to the left" consistent with diagnosis

    5. Cultures for GC and CT

    6. Sonography helpful to rule out abscess/ectopic pregnancy

    7. Pregnancy test to rule out intrauterine and ectopic pregnancy

    8. Routine criteria for diagnosis includes—oral temperature > 38.3°C, abnormal cervical or vaginal discharge, elevated ESR, elevated C-reactive protein, and/or laboratory documentation of GC or CT

    9. Criteria for positive diagnosis includes histopathologic evidence of endometritis on endometrial biopsy, tubo-ovarian abscess on ultrasound, and laparoscopic abnormalities consistent with PID

- Management/Treatment

    1. Treat empirically if following 3 criteria are present and no other condition is established—lower abdominal tenderness, adnexal tenderness, cervical motion tenderness

    2. Outpatient Treatment

        a. Regimen A

            (1) Cefoxitin 2 g IM. plus probenecid, 1 g orally in single dose concurrently, or ceftriaxone 250 mg IM. *plus*

      (2) Doxycycline 100 mg orally 2 times a day for 14 days

  b. Regimen B

     (1) Ofloxacin 400 mg orally 2 times a day for 14 day plus

     (2) Either clindamycin 450 mg orally 4 times a day, *or* metronidazole 500 mg orally 2 times a day for 14 days

  c. Patient must be re-examined in 72 hours; if symptoms not resolved or markedly improved, needs hospitalization and IV. antibiotics

3. Recommend hospitalization when

  a. Woman is pregnant, adolescent, HIV-infected, immunosuppressed, has severe illness, nausea and vomiting, or abscess is suspected

  b. Diagnosis uncertain and cannot rule out ectopic or appendicitis

  c. Unable to follow or tolerate outpatient regimen

  d. Failed to respond to outpatient therapy within 72 hours or no follow-up can be arranged within 72 hours of initiating antibiotic

4. All treatments include

  a. Notification and treatment of sexual partners

  b. Screen for other STDs and HIV; counsel on safe sex practices

  c. Test of cure within 7 days of completing therapy; rescreening in 4-6 weeks

  d. Removal of IUD, if in-situ

Chronic Pelvic Pain

- Definition: Episodic or continuous pain for 6 months or longer severe enough to affect daily functioning; diagnosis is difficult

- Etiology/Incidence

  1. Cause may be functional or organic; may involve bowel, urinary tract or musculoskeletal system; may be psychosexual in origin

  2. Accounts for up to 10% of outpatient gynecologic visits per year

  3. Cause of 70,000 hysterectomies annually

4. Endometriosis most common cause; others include—adenomyosis, sacral ache, pelvic adhesions, pelvic relaxation, irritable bladder

- Signs and Symptoms
  1. Pain for greater than 6 months unrelieved by previous treatment, usually not present on awakening
  2. May complain of impaired functioning, weight loss, anorexia
  3. May have history of abuse, incest, rape, substance abuse or current sexual dysfunction
  4. May complain of depression

- Differential Diagnosis
  1. Gastrointestinal disorders—irritable bowel syndrome, ulcerative colitis, diverticulosis
  2. UTI
  3. Depressive disorders

- Physical Findings
  1. If psychogenic, pain is not reproduced by pelvic manipulation
  2. Fever, tender pelvis or adnexa may indicate inflammation
  3. Cul-de-sac fullness or adnexal mass may indicate endometriosis
  4. Adnexal fullness or fixed structures, possible adhesions

- Diagnostic Tests/Findings
  1. Ultrasound
  2. Hysterosalpingogram
  3. Appropriate tests/cultures to rule out vaginitis, STDs
  4. Stool guaiac to rule out gastrointestinal disorder
  5. Urinalysis to rule out UTI
  6. If all diagnostic tests are normal, suspect psychosexual origin

- Management/Treatment
  1. Careful evaluation of complaint
  2. Complete physical examination

3. If organic pathology identified, refer for appropriate treatment

4. If suspect psychological origin, refer for evaluation and therapy

5. NSAIDS for pain relief; use of tricyclic antidepressants may enhance effectiveness of regimen

6. OCs helpful with cyclic pain

7. Alternative treatments included biofeedback, acupuncture, transcutaneous nerve stimulation

8. Laparoscopy may be diagnostic and therapeutic

Pelvic Relaxation

- Definition: Failure of pelvic musculature to maintain support and position of pelvic organs; includes

    1. Rectocele—bulging of the bowel through the posterior vaginal wall

    2. Cystocele—prolapse of the posterior bladder wall through the anterior vaginal wall

    3. Urethrocele—bulging of the urethra through the anterior vaginal wall; usually occurs with cystocele

    4. Enterocele—bulging of the bowel through the posterior cul-de-sac and vaginal wall; may be part of a rectocele

    5. Uterine prolapse—descent of the uterus through the pelvic floor and into the vaginal canal

- Etiology/Incidence

    1. Causes include—childbirth; conditions that increase intra-abdominal pressure (straining with defecation, obesity, heavy lifting, and respiratory conditions); effects of gravity on posture; tissue atrophy secondary to estrogen deficiency; congenital weakness

    2. Majority of parous women have some degree of pelvic relaxation; 10-15% will require surgery

- Signs and Symptoms

    1. Cystocele, urethrocele, prolapse—sensation of vaginal fullness and incomplete emptying of bladder; urinary incontinence; presence of mass bulging into the anterior vagina

2. Rectocele and enterocele—difficult evacuation of feces; sensation of vaginal fullness; presence of mass bulging into lower half of posterior vagina

- Differential Diagnosis

    1. Pelvic or abdominal tumor

    2. Tumor of rectovaginal septum

    3. Urethral diverticulum

- Physical Findings

    1. Soft, reducible mass bulging into lower half of posterior vagina or anterior vagina

    2. Leaking of fluid with coughing

    3. Lack of strength with contraction of pubococcygeal muscle

- Diagnostic Tests/Findings

    1. Complete gynecologic exam to visualize relaxed structures

    2. Valsalva maneuver to determine which organs prolapse and the degree of prolapse

- Management/Treatment

    1. Estrogen replacement therapy to improve tone and vascularity of supportive tissues for perimenopausal and menopausal women

    2. Analgesics for relief of associated discomfort (Acetaminophen or NSAID)

    3. Nutrition counseling to prevent constipation and straining

    4. Kegel exercises to strengthen and restore vaginal tone

    5. Vaginal pessary, cones, or tampons to provide support

    6. Surgical intervention for severe cases

Toxic Shock Syndrome (TSS)

- Definition

    1. Acute and severe multisystem disorder caused by toxin(s) produced by *Staphylococcus aureus* bacteria

    2. Occurs in menstruating women using tampons, menstruating women not using tampons, nonmenstruating women, and in men

    3. Three conditions are required for TSS

       a. Must be colonized or infected with *S. aureus*

       b. Staphylococci must be capable of producing toxins

       c. Must be portal of entry for toxin

- Etiology/Incidence

    1. White, menstruating women using tampons at greatest risk

    2. Incidence is 1-2 per 100,000 per year in women using tampons or barrier contraceptives

- Signs and Symptoms (case definition of TSS)

    1. Sudden onset with rapid progression to hypotensive shock

    2. Fever > 38.9°C (102°F)

    3. Diffuse sun-burn like rash over face, trunk, extremities

    4. Skin desquamation 1-2 weeks after illness onset

    5. Hypotension or orthostatic syncope

- Differential Diagnosis

    1. Rocky Mountain Spotted Fever

    2. Septic abortion

    3. Meningococcal meningitis

    4. Kawasaki disease

    5. Scarlet fever

    6. PID

    7. Viral gastroenteritis

- Physical Findings

    1. Temperature of 102°F or greater, low systolic blood pressure (less than 90 mm Hg)

    2. Sunburn-like rash; evidence of desquamation on palms and soles; conjunctival hyperemia; oropharyngeal erythema; strawberry tongue; vaginal hyperemia

3. Nonspecific abdominal tenderness

4. May be disoriented without neurological findings

5. Multisystem involvement, at least 3 of following

    a. Gastrointestinal (nausea and vomiting)

    b. Muscular (myalgia)

    c. Mucous membrane (hyperemia of vagina, oropharynx or conjunctiva)

    d. Renal (increased BUN or creatinine level)

    e. Hepatic (enzyme abnormalities)

    f. Hematologic ($\leq$ 100,000/mm^3 platelets)

    g. Central nervous system (disorientation)

    h. Cardiopulmonary (Adult respiratory distress syndrome [ARDS], pulmonary edema, heart block)

- Diagnostic Tests/Findings

1. CBC with differential—platelet count will be $\leq$ 100,000/mm^3

2. SMA24

3. VDRL to rule out syphilis

4. Culture—wound, throat, vagina, cervix, blood, cerebrospinal fluid

5. No definitive diagnostic or confirmatory laboratory test

- Management/Treatment

1. Immediate hospitalization with aggressive medical intervention

2. With history of TSS, should not use tampons, cervical cap, diaphragm or contraceptive sponge

3. If tampons used, use low-absorbency and alternate with pads; if fever, chills, nausea and vomiting occur during menstruation, discontinue tampon use and seek medical evaluation immediately

DES Exposure in utero

- Definition: Diethylstilbestrol (DES), a synthetic, potent estrogen, was prescribed to pregnant women for threatened abortion, prematurity, toxemia, and postmaturity between 1948 and 1971

- Etiology/Incidence
    1. Documented sequelae for female offspring
        a. Increased risk for clear cell adenocarcinoma of vagina and cervix (1:1000 under age 25)
        b. Cervical and uterine abnormalities
        c. Infertility
    2. Estimated 3 million women treated with DES

- Signs and Symptoms
    1. DES-exposed daughters
        a. History of maternal ingestion of DES
        b. May report infertility, history of poor pregnancy outcome (ectopic, spontaneous abortion, premature delivery), or menstrual irregularities
        c. May have history of abnormal Pap smear result
    2. DES-mothers—studies inconclusive regarding increased risk for breast or endometrial cancer

- Differential Diagnosis
    1. Congenital anomalies
    2. Genetic disorder

- Physical Findings
    1. Vaginal adenosis (most common)
    2. Cervical or vaginal nodularity (may indicate adenocarcinoma)
    3. Cervical abnormalities may be present (ridges, cockscomb, collar, hood, pseudopolyps, hypoplasia)
    4. Transverse or longitudinal vaginal septum

5. Uterine abnormalities (may include T-shaped uterus, bicornuate or didelphys uterus, septate uterus)

- Diagnostic Tests/Findings

  1. Careful gynecologic exam and history to identify risk

  2. Careful inspection and palpation of vulva, vaginal fornices, and cervix

  3. Pap smear of vaginal fornices, cervix and areas of adenosis

  4. Colposcopy and iodine staining of cervix and vagina followed by biopsy of any suspicious areas

- Management/Treatment

  1. Annual exams with Pap smear recommended

  2. Treat abnormal Pap results, infertility, or pregnancy complications

Infertility

- Definition: Inability to conceive after a year of regular unprotected intercourse or to carry a pregnancy to a live birth

  1. Primary—couple has never established a pregnancy

  2. Secondary—couple has conceived previously, but is unable to establish a subsequent pregnancy

  3. Fecundability—probability of conceiving during a monthly cycle; for healthy couples, probability is 20-25% each month

- Etiology/Incidence

  1. Approximately 10-20% of U.S. couples are infertile; fertility rate decreases with age; $1/3$ of women attempting pregnancy in mid-to-late 30s will experience infertility problem

  2. Ten percent of infertility cases are caused by unknown or unidentified factors

  3. Male factors causing infertility account for 35-40% of cases and include

     a. Oligospermia

     b. High viscosity of semen

     c. Varicocele

        d. Retrograde ejaculation

    4. Female factors represent 35-40% of causes and include

        a. Ovulatory factors (PCO, primary ovarian failure)

        b. Tubal factors (salpingitis, adhesions)

        c. Endometriosis

        d. Cervical factors (immunologic response, abnormal sperm-mucus interaction, cervicitis)

        e. Other causes include congenital anomalies, neoplasms, fibroids

        f. Multiple factors represent 25-35% of causes

- Signs and Symptoms—inability to conceive as described previously

- Differential Diagnosis includes all conditions listed previously

- Physical Findings—routine examination within normal limits, unless underlying condition discovered

- Diagnostic Tests/Findings

    1. Variety of tests available; evaluation is based on couple's history

    2. Routine infertility assessment includes

        a. Basal Body Temperature (BBT) Chart to determine ovulatory status; will see sustained temperature rise after ovulation

        b. Postcoital Test (PCT) to evaluate receptivity of cervical mucus and sperm viability; normal test shows clear cervical mucus with spinnbarkeit, positive ferning pattern, 5-10 motile sperm per high power field

        c. Semen Analysis—if abnormal, repeat in 4-6 weeks; normal results include

            (1) Volume—2-5 mL

            (2) Viscosity—liquefaction occurs within 1 hour

            (3) pH—7-8

            (4) Count—20-250 million/mL

            (5) Motility—more than 50% with forward progression, or more than 25% with rapid progression within 60 minutes of ejaculation

(6) Morphology—more than 50% normal forms

(7) White Blood Cell Count—less than 1 million per mL

(8) Semen Ureaplasma/Mycoplasma—negative

d. Hysterosalpingogram (HSG) performed after menses and before ovulation to determine patency of fallopian tubes

e. Endometrial biopsy performed after BBT-documented temperature rise to document ovulation and adequacy of hormone production

f. Laparoscopy to directly visualize pelvic structures

3. Additional tests may include

a. Hysteroscopy with laparoscopy, if HSG revealed uterine anomalies

b. Pap smear to rule out cervical cancer and inflammation

c. Serum progesterone to confirm ovulation (> 10 ng/mL adequate)

d. Tests for antisperm antibodies if PCT reveals nonmotile spermatozoa

e. Hamster Egg Penetration Test to assess spermatozoa capacitation and fertilization ability

f. Cervical tests/cultures to rule out *Chlamydia trachomatis* and *Ureaplasma urealyticum*; thyroid function tests, and prolactin level

g. More extensive evaluation is indicated when results of initial evaluation are abnormal; additional testing often required after results of initial evaluation

- Management/Treatment

  1. Treatment is dependent on underlying condition

     a. Male factors

        (1) Treat antisperm antibodies—sperm washing, immunosuppressive drug therapy

        (2) Repair of varicocele

        (3) Vasectomy reversal (50-60% success rate)

           (4)   Assisted reproductive techniques for nonreversible conditions

      b. Female factors

           (1)   Ovulation-induction therapy for ovulatory dysfunction disorders

           (2)   Progesterone therapy for luteal phase defect

           (3)   Appropriate treatment for underlying infections or endometriosis

           (4)   Surgery may be indicated as treatment for conditions, e.g., tubal occlusion, tubal adhesions, endometriosis

2. Management of infertility may include the following assisted reproductive technologies

      a. In Vitro Fertilization-Embryo Transfer (IVF-ET)—controlled ovarian hyperstimulation, egg retrieval, in vitro fertilization, embryo transfer to uterus; 15-20% pregnancy rate

      b. Gamete intrafallopian transfer (GIFT)—controlled ovarian hyperstimulation, egg recovery followed by transfer of sperm and oocytes into the fallopian tube(s), in vivo fertilization; about 25% success rate

      c. Zygote intrafallopian transfer (ZIFT)—same as GIFT but fertilization is in vitro

      d. Oocyte donation—used primarily for agonadal women; donated embryo transferred to woman's uterus at appropriate time in menstrual cycle; about 30% success rate

3. Infertile couples often experience intense psychological, physical and financial stress; a significant contribution to management is anticipatory guidance and support including discussions about alternatives to pregnancy (adoption, child-free living, surrogacy)

Common Disorders of Menopause

Dyspareunia

- Definition: Painful vaginal intercourse with entry or deep penetration of the penis
- Etiology/Incidence
    1. The most common cause in the menopausal woman is estrogen deficiency with resulting atrophy of pelvic structures
    2. Incidence is unknown
- Signs and Symptoms
    1. Vaginal dryness
    2. Postcoital bleeding
    3. Introital pain or pain with deep penetration during intercourse
- Differential Diagnosis
    1. Vulvovaginitis/atrophic vaginitis
    2. Pelvic relaxation disorders
- Physical Findings
    1. If estrogen deficient—thin, dry, pale, friable vaginal epithelium; shortened vagina; atrophy of genital structures
    2. Thin, watery, yellowish vaginal discharge, if atrophic vaginitis present
    3. Evidence of cystocele, urethrocele, rectocele, uterine prolapse, or enterocele
- Diagnostic Tests/Findings
    1. Speculum examination may reveal above findings
    2. Saline wet mount may reveal white blood cells, indicating vaginitis
    3. Vaginal pH—alkaline
- Management/Treatment
    1. Routine sexual activity with lubricants may be helpful

2. Evaluate for use of oral hormone replacement therapy or vaginal estrogen cream; if uterus intact, progestin should be added

3. Kegel exercises to strengthen vaginal tone if relaxation present

4. Treat underlying vaginal infection

Vaginal Dryness

- Definition: Decreased amount of normal vaginal secretions
- Etiology/Incidence
    1. In menopausal woman, most common cause is estrogen deficiency
    2. Incidence is unknown
- Signs and Symptoms
    1. Signs of estrogen deficiency—thin, dry, pale, and friable vaginal epithelium; decreased or absent vaginal discharge; sparse pubic hair; atrophy of genital structures
    2. May complain of dyspareunia; postcoital spotting
- Differential Diagnosis: Vulvovaginitis
- Physical Findings
    1. Thin, pale vagina with decreased rugae
    2. Dry vaginal vault and external genitalia
- Diagnostic Tests/Findings
    1. Vaginal pH—alkaline
    2. Speculum examination reveals signs of estrogen deficiency
- Management/Treatment
    1. Routine intercourse with use of lubricants may be helpful
    2. Evaluate for use of oral hormone replacement therapy or vaginal estrogen therapy; if intact uterus, progestin therapy also indicated

Vasomotor Instability

- Definition: Referred to as "hot flash/flush," a sudden, transient sensation ranging from warmth to intense heat that spreads over the body, especially the head, neck, and chest, lasting an average of 45 seconds, and often accompanied by flushing, profuse perspiration, chills

- Etiology/Incidence
    1. Caused by loss of estradiol and resulting decreased ovarian function
    2. Onset begins in perimenopausal years, continues through menopause
    3. Most common symptom associated with menopause; affects about 85% of women not on hormone replacement therapy
    4. Frequency, intensity and duration varies within and among individuals
- Signs and Symptoms
    1. Sudden onset of pressure sensation in head progressing to hot flush, then profuse perspiration; may have palpitations
    2. Night sweats and insomnia common
    3. May occur during day or night
- Differential Diagnosis
    1. Hypothalamic/pituitary tumor
    2. Thyroid disorder
    3. Systemic infection (tuberculosis, HIV)
- Physical Findings—consistent with estrogen deficiency
- Management/Treatment
    1. Hormonal
        a. May evaluate for estrogen replacement therapy; effective in 90% of women; if intact uterus, progestin therapy indicated
        b. Use of progestins alone may occasionally be used if estrogen use contraindicated
        c. Bellergal and Clonidine may provide relief for some women
    2. Nonhormonal
        a. Limit caffeine and alcohol intake
        b. Encourage regular exercise and adequate nutrition

Osteoporosis

- Definition: An imbalance between bone formation and bone resorption associated with skeletal fractures; 2 distinct types

    1. Type I—occurs mostly in women within 15-20 years after menopause; primarily involves trabecular bone loss; most common fracture sites include vertebrae and distal radius

    2. Type II—occurs in men and women in their 70s; primarily cortical bone; most common fracture site is hip

- Etiology/Incidence

    1. Most bone loss occurring during postmenopausal years is caused by estrogen deficiency; preventable with estrogen replacement therapy

    2. Risk factors include

        a. Age, female, early menopause

        b. Caucasian or Asian descent

        c. Sedentary lifestyle, smoking

        d. Chronic low dietary intake of calcium throughout reproductive years

        e. Small boned, underweight

        f. Family history of osteoporosis

- Signs and Symptoms

    1. May be asymptomatic

    2. May report history of back pain, loss of height, multiple fractures

- Differential Diagnosis

    1. Rheumatoid arthritis

    2. Cushing's syndrome

- Physical Findings

    1. Documentation of loss of height

    2. May have curvature of cervical and upper portion of spine (dowager's hump)

- Diagnostic Tests/Findings

1. Bone density tests determine decreased bone mass

2. Often undiagnosed until fracture occurs

- Management/Treatment

    1. Estrogen replacement therapy to treat and prevent further progression; minimum dose without calcium supplementation, Premarin 0.625mg; add progestin with intact uterus

    2. Adequate calcium intake to maintain positive calcium balance; recommended daily dosage 1000 mg prior to menopause, 1500 mg daily postmenopause if not on ERT; 1000 mg daily if on ERT

    3. Calcitonin and Fluoride for some individuals; efficacy not well-established

    4. Weight-bearing exercise program, about 30 minutes 3 times per week

    5. Eliminate smoking (increases liver metabolism of estrogen), decrease caffeine

Depression/Mood Swings

- Definition: Alterations in mood that affect daily activities

- Etiology/Incidence

    1. Often biological—a chemical imbalance in serotonergic, dopaminergic, and adrenergic neurotransmitters in the brain

    2. Decreased estrogen levels may trigger nocturnal hot flashes and subsequent sleep deprivation which can contribute to mood disturbances

    3. Other causes include—physical/chronic illness, medications, general stress of aging, feelings of isolation and bereavement

    4. Mean incidence for depression is around age 40

- Signs and Symptoms

    1. Depression can be a normal reaction to events that occur in everyday life

    2. Frequently presents with somatic complaints such as headaches, constipation, sleep disturbance, loss of energy, change in appetite, decreased libido, and chronic pain

3. May also report feelings of sadness, guilt, worthlessness, hopelessness, and thoughts of suicide

- Differential Diagnosis
    1. Chronic illness
    2. Hypothyroidism
    3. Substance abuse
    4. Medication side effects

- Physical Findings
    1. Evidence of emotional distress
    2. Physical exam will be within normal limits unless underlying cause detected

- Diagnostic Tests/Findings
    1. No specific tests available
    2. Appropriate tests to rule out hypothyroidism and substance abuse, if suspected

- Management/Treatment
    1. Thorough medical evaluation to rule out underlying physical or emotional disorder
    2. May require consultation and evaluation with mental health specialist and initiation of antidepressants
    3. Relaxation techniques, diet modifications, and regular exercise may be helpful
    4. Estrogen replacement therapy may reduce frequency of nocturnal hot flashes, thereby improving quality of sleep which may have indirect effect of altering mood response

Cardiovascular Disease

- Definition: Diseases of the heart which include coronary heart disease, cerebral vascular disease, hypertension, and peripheral vascular disease
- Etiology/Incidence

1. Lipid changes in menopause favor development of atherosclerosis in major vessels—increased low-density lipoproteins (LDL); increased total cholesterol; unchanged or decreased high-density lipoproteins (HDL)

2. Risk factors in women include—obesity, abnormal lipid profile, hypertension, diabetes mellitus, cigarette smoking, sedentary lifestyle, and estrogen deficiency

3. Most common cause of death in the U.S.; leading cause of death in women; responsible for 500,000 deaths in women each year

- Signs and Symptoms

   1. In addition to menopausal status, history may contain risk factors for cardiovascular disease

   2. May be asymptomatic, with no risk factors

   3. May have symptoms of acute cardiovascular condition—chest pain, shortness of breath, and hypertension

- Differential Diagnosis

   1. Coronary artery disease

   2. Hypertension

   3. Hyperlipidemia

   4. Peripheral vascular disease

- Physical Findings

   1. In acute process, signs of cardiac distress

   2. May be asymptomatic

- Diagnostic Tests/Implications

   1. Lipid profile may reflect normal physiologic changes consistent with aging—increased LDL, increased total cholesterol, and unchanged or decreased HDL, or serious alterations which reflect cardiovascular problems

   2. May see alterations in measurements of glucose tolerance and blood pressure readings

- Management/Treatment

1. Maintenance of ideal body weight with balanced diet and active lifestyle

2. Maintain total cholesterol level ≤ 200 mg/dL; HDL ≥ 55 mg/dL; LDL at or below 130 mg/dL, with low-fat diet, weight control, and if necessary, lipid-lowering medications

3. Maintain normotensive status with weight control, salt-restriction, and if necessary, antihypertensive drug therapy

4. Monitor for early signs of glucose intolerance; if develop, control with weight and diet modifications and if necessary, hypoglycemic therapy

5. Eliminate cigarette smoking

6. Estrogen replacement therapy is single most significant factor in prevention of cardiovascular disease in women; oral estrogen increases HDL, lowers LDL, and lowers total cholesterol

7. Studies indicate combination estrogen and progestin replacement therapy has an overall protective effect

QUESTIONS

Select the best answer.

1. A 30 year-old G2P1 presents with a previous history of regular, predictable menses, but now reports amenorrhea for the last six months. She has a 2 year-old whom she breastfed for four months, and she had a spontaneous abortion with a D & C six months ago. She has always used a diaphragm successfully. Today her beta hCG is negative, and her uterus is normal size. Your initial diagnostic plan includes a:

   a. FSH and LH level
   b. Prolactin level
   c. Progestin challenge

2. A 47 year-old G2P2 reports that for the last six months her menses have become unpredictable in onset, amount and duration. She is not sexually active. A tentative diagnosis, pending complete evaluation is

   a. Dysfunctional uterine bleeding
   b. Hypomenorrhea
   c. Oligomenorrhea

3. Endometrial hyperplasia can be expected in which of the following conditions?

   a. Chronic anovulation
   b. Endometriosis
   c. Leiomyomas

4. A 1 cm x 1 cm round, smooth, firm, nontender, movable mass is palpated in the breast of a 20-year old. This is most probably a(n):

   a. Fibroadenoma
   b. Fibrocystic changes
   c. Intraductal papilloma

5. The greatest number of women die from which of the following cancers?

   a. Breast
   b. Lung
   c. Ovarian

6. The most common method available for detection of ovarian cancer is:

    a. Hysteroscopy
    b. CA-125 assay
    c. Pelvic examination

7. The Bethesda system equivalent for a Class III, moderate dysplasia pap smear is:

    a. Atypical cells of undetermined significance
    b. High grade squamous intraepithelial lesion
    c. Carcinoma in situ

8. The origin of cervical polyps must be confirmed by pathology because:

    a. Endocervical polyps are often malignant
    b. Endometrial polyps may indicate malignancy
    c. The origin determines the stage of malignancy

9. Symptomatic adenomyosis is characterized by:

    a. Amenorrhea
    b. Anovulation
    c. Dysmenorrhea

10. Which of the following is a normal index of sperm motility/morphology?

    a. 20%
    b. 40%
    c. 60%

11. An individual with Turner syndrome may have:

    a. Streak ovaries
    b. Vaginal agenesis
    c. Secondary amenorrhea

12. The gonads must be removed in an apparently female individual with a 46,XY karyotype to prevent:

    a. Hirsutism
    b. Delayed menarche
    c. Cancer

13. Which of the following findings is commonly found with an unruptured ectopic?
    pregnancy

    a. Abdominal rigidity
    b. Irregular vaginal bleeding
    c. Shoulder pain

14. Signs and symptoms of molar pregnancy include:

    a. Hypothyroidism
    b. Pregnancy Induced Hypertension
    c. Polyhydramnios

15. Spinnbarkeit describes the:

    a. Color of cervical mucus
    b. Elasticity of cervical mucus
    c. Ferning pattern of cervical mucus

16. Which of the following may artificially elevate a serum prolactin level?

    a. Clinical breast exam
    b. Vitamin supplements
    c. Hyperthyroidism

17. Which of the following is always true regarding the primary stage of syphilis?

    a. An infectious lesion will be present
    b. Results of RPR will be positive
    c. Result of VDRL will be positive

18. The high level of unopposed estrogen present with polycystic ovaries may
    increase the risk for:

    a. Breast cancer
    b. Liver disease
    c. Ovarian cancer

19. A common cause for dysfunctional uterine bleeding is:

    a. Progesterone excess
    b. Anovulation
    c. Hyperprolactinemia

20. Herniation of the bladder into the vagina is called:

    a. Cystocele
    b. Urethrocele
    c. Enterocele

21. An ovulatory woman reports symptoms of severe bloating each month beginning about one week before menses. An appropriate therapy for the symptom is:

    a. Progesterone suppository
    b. Low doses of Danazol
    c. Spironolactone

22. In postmenopausal women, estrogen replacement lowers cardiovascular risk by increasing:

    a. High density lipoproteins
    b. Low density lipoproteins
    c. The HDL:LDL ratio

23. The following values were obtained from an initial semen analysis:

    Count 10 million/mL or greater
    Volume 2-5 mL per ejaculate
    Motility 50-60%, with good forward progression
    Morphology 30% normal

    Based on these results, management should be to:
    a. Repeat the test
    b. Obtain semen culture
    c. Refer to specialist

24. A major health risk for a menopausal age woman not on estrogen replacement therapy is:

    a. Endometrial hyperplasia
    b. Breast cancer
    c. Cardiovascular disease

25. In a woman with suspected polycystic ovaries, the expected laboratory value for LH is:

    a. High
    b. Low
    c. Normal

26. A common adnexal mass found in reproductive aged women is:

    a. Dermoid cyst
    b. Endometrioma
    c. Fibroma

27. The most widely used abortion procedure in the U.S. today is:

    a. Dilatation and evacuation
    b. Vacuum aspiration
    c. Amnioinfusion

28. Effective treatment for primary dysmenorrhea is:

    a. Prostaglandin synthetase inhibitors
    b. GnRH analogues
    c. Progestins

29. A patient with latent syphilis may present with:

    a. A maculopapular rash
    b. An indurated, painless sore
    c. No signs of infection

30. A major risk factor for ectopic pregnancy is:

    a. Previous ectopic pregnancy
    b. DES-exposure
    c. Recurrent vaginitis

ANSWERS

1. c	11. a	21. c
2. a	12. c	22. a
3. a	13. b	23. a
4. a	14. b	24. c
5. b	15. b	25. a
6. c	16. a	26. a
7. b	17. a	27. b
8. b	18. a	28. a
9. c	19. b	29. c
10. c	20. a	30. a

BIBLIOGRAPHY

American Cancer Society. (1995). *Cancer facts and figures-1995*. Atlanta: American Cancer Society.

American College of Obstetricians and Gynecologists. (1993). *Cervical cytology: Evaluation and management of abnormalities*. ACOG Technical Bulletin, No. 183. Washington, DC: ACOG.

Berkow, R. (1987). *The Merck manual of diagnosis and therapy: Vol. 1* (15th ed.). Rathway, NJ: Merck, Sharpe, & Dohme Research Laboratories.

Centers for Disease Control. (1993). Sexually transmitted diseases treatment guidelines. *MMWR, 38* (No. S-8).

Cibley, L.J., & Cibley, L.J. (1991). Cytologic vaginosis. *American Journal of Obstetrics and Gynecology, 165,* 1235-1248.

Combined therapy helps cure trichomoniasis. (1991, February). *Contraceptive Technology Update STD Quarterly,* 27-83.

Copeland, L. (1993). *Textbook of gynecology*. Philadelphia: W.B. Saunders.

Freeman, S. (1991). Management of perimenopausal symptoms. In C. Garner (Ed.), *NAACOG's clinical issues in perinatal and women's health nursing: Midlife women's health* (pp. 429-439). Philadelphia: J.B. Lippincott.

Fischback, F. (1992). *A manual of laboratory and diagnostic tests* (4th ed.). Philadelphia: J.B. Lippincott.

Fogel, C., & Woods, N. (1995). *Women's health care: A comprehensive handbook*. Thousand Oaks, CA: Sage Productions.

Herbst, A.L., Mishell, D.R., Stenchever, M.A., & Droegemueller, W. (1992). *Comprehensive gynecology* (2nd ed.). St. Louis: Mosby-Year Book.

Horowitz, B. (1991). Mycotic vulvovaginitis: A broad overview. *American Journal of Obstetrics and Gynecology,* 1188-1191.

Lehne, R. (1994). *Pharmacology for nursing care* (2nd ed.). Philadelphia: W.B. Saunders.

Lobo, R. (Ed.). (1994). *Treatment of the postmenopausal woman: Basic and clinical aspects*. New York: Raven Press.

Mishell, D., & Brenner, P. (1994). *Management of common problems in obstetrics and gynecology* (3rd ed.). Boston: Blackwell Scientific Publications.

Pernoll, M.S. (1991). *Current obstetric and gynecologic diagnosis and treatment* (7th ed.). Norwalk, NJ: Appleton & Lange.

Seltzer, V., & Pearse, W. (1995). *Women's primary health care.* New York: McGraw-Hill.

Sparks, J. (1991). Vaginitis. *The Journal of Reproductive Medicine, 36,* 745-752.

Speroff, L., Glass, R., & Kase, N. (1994). *Clinical gynecologic endocrinology and infertility* (5th ed.). Baltimore, MD: Williams & Wilkins.

Stenchever, M.A. (Ed.). (1992). *Office gynecology.* St. Louis: Mosby-Year Book.

Wilson, J.R., & Carrington, E.R. (Eds.). (1992). *Obstetrics and gynecology* (9th ed.). St. Louis: Mosby-Year Book.

Youngkin, E., & Davis, M. (1994). *Women's health: A primary care clinical guide.* Norwalk, CT: Appleton & Lange.

Pregnancy

Barbara Peterson Sinclair
Jane G. Conner
Jane E. Heath

Physiology of Pregnancy

- Physiologic maternal changes
    1. General appearance
        a. Varies with age, general health and socioeconomic status
        b. Observations:
            (1) Appropriateness of appearance for age
            (2) General health status
            (3) General nutritional status
            (4) Grooming and hygiene
            (5) Posture, gait, and body movements
            (6) Mental and emotional state
    2. Cardiovascular
        a. Enlarging uterus displaces heart upward and to the left
        b. Blood volume increases 30-50% by term
        c. Cardiac output increases up to $1/3$ in last 2 trimesters
        d. Pulse rate may increase up to 10-15 beats per minute
        e. Blood pressure may remain unaltered or may decrease in second trimester and slowly rise to pre-pregnant levels by term
        f. Changes in heart sounds may include
            (1) Increased loudness of systolic and diastolic components with an easily heard third sound
            (2) Exaggerated split S_1
            (3) Systolic murmur due to increased blood volume
        g. When lying supine, hypotension occurs as uterus compresses vena cava producing low blood pressure, dizziness and pallor
        h. Decreased blood return from lower extremities and increased fluid volume contribute to dependent edema and tendency to varicosities

3. Respiratory

    a. Rate is relatively unchanged but tidal volume is increased resulting in total oxygen increase of 15-20%

    b. Diaphragm is elevated and lower rib cage is flared

    c. Increased sensitivity to CO_2 may result in shortness of breath upon exertion

4. Hematologic

    a. Red blood cell volume increases by 30% but plasma volume increases by 50%, often resulting in a physiologic anemia

    b. True anemia occurs with hemoglobin of less than 11 g/dL and hematocrit of less than 33%

    c. Leukocytes may physiologically increase to 10,000-11,000/mm³

    d. Fibrin, fibrinogen and blood factor VII, IX, and X are increased but clotting time remains same

5. Gastrointestinal

    a. Human chorionic gonadotropin (hCG) associated with early nausea and vomiting

    b. Estrogen causes hypertrophy and bleeding of gums

    c. Sense of taste is dulled, cravings for certain foods may occur

    d. Ptyalism (excessive salivation) may occur

    e. Displacement of intra-abdominal organs due to enlarging uterus and general decrease in smooth muscle tone and motility due to progesterone result in

        (1) Delayed gastric emptying

        (2) Relaxation of cardiac sphincter, leading to gastric reflux and heartburn

        (3) Diminished intestinal peristalsis

    f. Prolonged gallbladder emptying time increases risk for gallstones

6. Urinary

    a. Relaxation of smooth muscles and compression by uterus leads to dilation of ureter and kidney (especially on right) and decreased bladder tone creating risk for urinary stasis and infection

 b. Glomerular filtration rate and renal plasma flow increase

 c. Urinary frequency is seen early and again late in pregnancy due to uterine pressure on the bladder

7. Endocrine

 a. Thyroid gland enlargement may occur due to hyperplasia and increased vascularity; protein-bound iodine (PBI) and basal metabolism rate (BMR) increase

 b. Adrenal cortex hypertrophies; increase in circulating cortisol which regulates carbohydrate and protein metabolism

 c. Insulin needs increase due to diabetogenic action of placental lactogen (hPL); blood glucose levels are low in response to fetal demands for fuel; gestational diabetes can be precipitated

8. Musculoskeletal

 a. Progesterone-induced relaxation of joints, e.g., sacroiliac, sacrococcygeal, and symphysis pubis, results in discomfort and walking difficulties

 b. Enlarging uterus causes the center of gravity to shift

  (1) Exaggerated lumbar curvature (lordosis) and posture change

  (2) Low backache and fatigue are common

 c. Separation of rectus abdominis muscles (diastasis recti) possible

9. Integumentary

 a. Estrogen-related changes

  (1) Increased pigmentation—chloasma, linea nigra, and areola

  (2) Striae gravidarum

  (3) Vascular spider nevi and palmar erythema

 b. Progesterone-related changes—increased sebaceous and sweat gland activity

10. Reproductive

    a. Uterus

        (1) Increases in size and weight due to hypertrophy and hyperplasia in response to estrogen

        (2) Blood supply greatly increased

        (3) Braxton-Hicks contractions as early as 16 weeks

        (4) Softening of lower uterine segment (Hegar Sign)

    b. Cervix

        (1) Increased vascularization causes softening and bluish color (Chadwick Sign)—6-8 weeks gestation

        (2) Increased mucus with plug blocking endocervical canal

        (3) Softening (Goodell Sign)—as early as 4 weeks gestation

    c. Vagina

        (1) Increased vascularity causes bluish color

        (2) Mucosa thickens and supportive tissue relaxes

        (3) Secretions increase (leukorrhea)

    d. Ovary

        (1) Corpus luteum lasts for 10-12 weeks; produces progesterone to sustain pregnancy until placenta develops

        (2) Regular ovarian function ceases during pregnancy

    e. Breasts (changes most noticeable in primiparas)

        (1) Early increase in size, nodularity, and tenderness

        (2) Veins prominent

        (3) Areolae darken and nipples become erect

        (4) Montgomery follicles hypertrophied

        (5) Striae may occur

        (6) Colostrum in last trimester

- Maternal psychological changes—developmental tasks of pregnancy

    1. Acceptance of pregnancy by self, partner; ambivalence common at first—"Who me?, Not now!"

2. Adjustment to changes in self

    a. Emotional changes—increased introversion, dependence, mood swings, dreams and fantasies

    b. Physical changes—adjustment to changing body image

3. Prenatal attachment to fetus

    a. Fetal incorporation—acceptance of newcomer

    b. Recognition of fetus as separate individual

        (1) Traditionally occurs with quickening; frequently develops earlier with viewing of real time ultrasound

        (2) Recognition of fetal movements and "communication" with fetus

4. Preparation for maternal role

    a. Reviewing relationship with own mother and observing other women

    b. Identifying maternal behaviors she chooses for self

    c. Grief work for roles which will change or be lost

5. Preparation for fetal separation and birth process

    a. Preparation of home, self and family

    b. Eager/anxious regarding end of pregnancy

- Signs and Symptoms of Pregnancy

1. Presumptive evidence

    a. Amenorrhea

    b. Breast changes

    c. Nausea with or without vomiting

    d. Urinary frequency

    e. Vaginal mucosa and skin changes

    f. Fatigue

    g. Mother's perception of fetal movement (quickening) between 14 and 26 weeks (usually 18-22 weeks)

2. Probable evidence

    a. Softening of cervix (Goodell sign) and lower uterine segment (Hegar sign)

    b. Cyanosis of cervix and vagina (Chadwick sign)

    c. Enlargement of uterus and abdomen

    d. Braxton-Hicks contractions

    e. Ballottement

    f. Palpation of fetal outline by examiner

    g. Pregnancy tests (endocrine tests for hCG in maternal urine or blood, e.g., agglutination, radioimmunoassay, ELISA, monoclonal antibodies)

3. Positive evidence

    a. Fetal heartbeat

    b. Palpation of fetal movements by examiner

    c. Visualization of fetus, e.g., ultrasonography

- Placental Function and Anatomy

  1. Maternal contribution is decidua basalis and its circulation

  2. Chorionic villi invade and attach to decidua basalis

  3. In week 2, amnion forms around embryo and fills with amniotic fluid; outer membrane (chorion) lays against decidua

  4. Amniotic fluid maintains fetus at even temperature, cushions against injury, permits movement, and fetus swallows and breathes it

  5. Placenta is complete by 12th week and has 15-20 segments (cotyledons), in which exchange of gases and nutrients occur

  6. Umbilical cord connects fetus to placenta; has 2 arteries (deoxygenated fetal blood to placenta), 1 vein (oxygenated blood to fetus), no nerves, is 45-60 cm long and is covered with gelatinous, protective substance (Wharton's jelly)

  7. Placental hormones

    a. Human chorionic gonadotropin (hCG) is secreted by early trophoblasts and stimulates corpus luteum to produce estrogen and progesterone until placenta takes over at about 8 weeks

    b. Estrogen causes hypertrophy and hyperplasia of uterus, increases uteroplacental blood flow, and stimulates development of the ductal system of breasts

    c. Progesterone causes qualitative changes in endometrium, reduces uterine contractility, and relaxes smooth muscle; influences lobuloalveolar development in breasts

    d. Human placental lactogen (hPL) is involved with metabolism of fatty acids, glucose, and amino acids; aids in growth of breasts and other maternal tissues

    e. Relaxin aids in softening smooth muscle and connective tissue

8. Functions of placenta

    a. Metabolic

    b. Transport

    c. Endocrine

    d. Immunologic

- Growth and Development of Fetus

  1. Calculating from last menses, pregnancy is 10 lunar months, 40 weeks, or 280 days; "fetal" calculation is from conception, or 38 weeks or 266 days

         a. Preimplantation—weeks 1 and 2

         b. Embryonic period—weeks 3-8

         c. Fetal period—begins week 9

  2. Implantation complete by end of week 2

  3. Week 3—several organs forming, e.g., heart and kidneys

  4. Week 6

         a. Face is forming, also eyes and ears

         b. Arms and legs have digits

         c. Blood cells produced by liver and spleen begin circulating

  5. Week 8

         a. Embryo is 3 cm long and weighs 2 g, head is 50% of body

  b. Organogenesis is completed

  c. Less susceptible to teratogens

  d. Ossification begins

  e. End of "embryonic" period

6. Week 12

  a. Spontaneous movement

  b. Urine formation established

  c. Sex distinguishable

  d. Is 8 cm long and weighs 45 g

  e. Fetal heart should be heard with doppler (may be heard at 10 weeks)

7. Week 16

  a. Active movements present

  b. Swallows amniotic fluid and produces meconium

  c. Scalp hair and some lanugo present

  d. Ovaries differentiated

8. Week 20

  a. Quickening felt

  b. Fetal heart tones (FHT) heard with stethoscope

  c. Lanugo covers body

  d. Brown fat forms

  e. Alveoli of lungs completed

  f. Fetal antibodies present

  g. Fetus is 20 cm long and weighs 435 g

9. Weeks 28-40—period of maturation and weight gain

  a. Vernix slowly increases and lanugo decreases

  b. Nails, eyebrows and lashes at 28 weeks; testes descend

  c. Eyelids open by 32 weeks

      d. Nervous system begins regulation of body functions

      e. Lecithin/sphingomyelin (L/S) ratio approaches 2:1 at 38 weeks; cartilage forms in ear lobes

      f. Amniotic fluid diminishes as fetus fills uterine cavity

10. Risk factors for abnormal growth

      a. Genetic factors/chromosomal abnormalities

      b. Maternal malnutrition

      c. Maternal substance use, e.g., cigarettes, alcohol, drugs

      d. Maternal disease, e.g., hypertension, diabetes, cardiac disease

      e. Multiple gestation

Prenatal Care

- Definition: Preventive care to help mother maintain well-being and achieve a healthy outcome for herself and her infant

  1. Early and adequate prenatal care reduces maternal and fetal morbidity and mortality

  2. Ideally, potential parents should consult health care provider prior to conception in order to correct problems and minimize risk in critical early weeks of gestation

  3. Women should be encouraged to seek care soon after first missed menstrual period

- Components

  1. Assessment for normal development and signs of complications

  2. Fetal surveillance

  3. Laboratory tests

  4. Education for self-care

     a. Nutrition

     b. General health promotion

     c. Common discomforts

     d. Danger signals

      e. Preparation for childbirth and parenting

  5. Social services

● Comprehensive Assessment

  1. Initial visit

      a. Laboratory confirmation of pregnancy if not previously obtained

      b. Routine laboratory screening

        (1) CBC

        (2) Blood type and Rh

        (3) Antibody screen and titer

        (4) Hepatitis B surface antigen

        (5) Syphilis screen (VDRL or RPR)

        (6) Chlamydia/Gonorrhea screen

        (7) Rubella immune status

        (8) Urinalysis (and culture, if indicated)

        (9) Offer HIV antibody testing

        (10) Tuberculin testing in high risk populations

        (11) Pap smear

        (12) Other tests as indicated by risk status of individual or general patient population, e.g., sickle cell screen

      c. Complete health history with emphasis on factors which may influence maternal or fetal outcomes during pregnancy

        (1) Maternal age

        (2) Family history of multiple gestation, congenital anomalies or inherited diseases

        (3) Maternal family history of diabetes, hypertension, cancer

        (4) Maternal history of allergy, significant illness

        (5) Medications

        (6) Previous reproductive history

          (a) History of infertility

    (b) History of complications with previous pregnancies, e.g., preterm labor, gestational diabetes, hypertension, placenta previa, postpartum hemorrhage or psychiatric problems

    (c) Previous pregnancy loss, including gestational age at time of loss, related factors

    (d) Previous cesarean birth; indication and type of uterine incision

  (7) Use of tobacco, alcohol, or other drugs

  (8) Occupation, physical activity, lifestyle

 d. Complete physical assessment

  (1) Rule out pre-existing medical conditions

    (a) Diastolic or other abnormal heart murmur

    (b) Thyroid nodule or enlargement

    (c) Severe varicosities

    (d) Chronic hypertension

    (e) Nutritional status—significantly over- or underweight, anemia

  (2) Confirm pregnancy and determine gestation based on uterine size and other changes

    (a) Uterine size fairly accurately reflects gestational age up to 12 weeks

      i) 8 weeks—about 9 cm

      ii) 10 weeks—about 12 cm, or double pre-pregnancy size

      iii) 12 weeks—at symphysis pubis

    (b) Crown-rump length by ultrasound is most accurate between 7 and 14 weeks gestation

    (c) Goodell sign—as early as 4 weeks

    (d) Chadwick sign—6-8 weeks

    (e) Hegar sign—6-8 weeks

      (3)   Evaluate pelvic dimensions

          (a)   Inlet: Diagonal conjugate 12.5 cm

          (b)   Midplane: Note contour and prominence of ischial spines

          (c)   Outlet: Angle of pubic arch $\geq$ 90 degrees; intertuberous diameter $\geq$ 8.5 cm

          (d)   Flexibility of coccyx

      (4)   Obtain Pap smear and cervical cultures as indicated

      (5)   Perform vaginal smear of abnormal discharge

      (6)   Assess breasts/nipples in relation to lactation

      (7)   Doppler auscultation of fetal heart and/or ultrasound per agency protocol (FHT usually audible by 10-12 weeks with doppler)

  e. Psychosocial assessment

      (1)   Response to pregnancy

      (2)   Social support

      (3)   Expectations related to pregnancy and childbirth

          (a)   Cultural beliefs

          (b)   Previous experience

      (4)   History or risk of physical or sexual abuse

  f. Establish physical and psychosocial risk status and plan for further prenatal care according to individual's needs and preferences

      (1)   Routine monthly visits up to 28 weeks, every 2-3 weeks until 36 weeks, then weekly until delivery

      (2)   Genetic counseling referral if indicated

          (a)   Maternal age 35 or greater by time of delivery

          (b)   Family history of congenital anomaly

          (c)   History of $\geq$ 3 successive spontaneous abortions

          (d)   Previous unexplained pregnancy loss

        (e) Parents possible carriers of sickle cell, Thalassemia or Tay-Sachs

        (f) Teratogen exposure

    (3) Preterm labor risk assessment (PTL)

        (a) Demographic factors, e.g., age < 17 or > 35, African-American race, low socioeconomic status

        (b) Behavior factors, e.g., smoking, substance use/abuse, poor nutrition/weight gain, excessive physical activities, psychological stress

        (c) Medical/obstetrical factors, e.g., prior preterm labor, DES exposure, multiple gestation, leiomyomata, vaginal/cervical/intrauterine infection, cervical effacement or dilation, poly/oligohydramnios, bacteriuria or pyelonephritis, hypertension, diabetes

        (d) Repeat assessment at 24, 28 and 32 weeks

2. Interval Visits

    a. Components of routine visits

      (1) Measure weight, blood pressure

      (2) Test urine for protein and glucose; nitrites and ketones may be included

      (3) Obtain interval history of risk-related symptoms

      (4) Measure uterine growth

        (a) Up to 14 weeks bimanual exam is most accurate

        (b) Abdominal measurement of fundal height

            i) Consistency in system of measurement is important

            ii) Measure from top of symphysis pubis to top of uterine fundus

                a) Paper or other flexible tape most commonly used

                b) Calipers most accurate (avoids differences related to maternal obesity)

         c) McDonald's rule—between 16 and 34 weeks, height of fundus in centimeters equals weeks gestation

  (5) Obtain screening tests as indicated by gestational age or patient history

  (6) Answer questions and provide anticipatory guidance regarding nutrition, common discomforts, general health promotion, PTL, and childbirth education

b. Specific needs as indicated by gestation

  (1) First trimester/first visit

    (a) Overview of pregnancy and prenatal care

    (b) Impact of pregnancy—psychological and physical responses

    (c) Habits

    (d) Avoidance of teratogens

    (e) Nausea

    (f) Sexuality

    (g) Introduce discussion of breastfeeding during breast examination

    (h) Warning signs of early complications, e.g., threatened abortion

    (i) Support system

  (2) 14-18 weeks

    (a) Alphafetoprotein/Triple Marker Down Syndrome— screen at 15-19 weeks

    (b) Diet and weight gain

    (c) Activity and rest

    (d) Remind patient to note date of quickening

  (3) 18-22 weeks

    (a) Screening may include ultrasound for dating and fetal anatomical survey if indicated

        (b) FHT audible with fetoscope

    (4) 22-26 weeks

        (a) Sign up for childbirth education classes

        (b) Avoid supine position for sleep or exercise

        (c) Preterm birth prevention—teach signs and symptoms; instruct patient to seek care promptly

    (5) 26-30 weeks

        (a) 50 gram glucose challenge

        (b) Baseline evaluation of cervix, review information regarding PTL

        (c) Rh negative patient receives RhoGAM

        (d) Repeat hemoglobin and VDRL

        (e) Common complaints and discomforts

        (f) Sexuality

        (g) Warning signs of later complications

        (h) Fetal movement (kick count) instruction

    (6) 30-36 weeks

        (a) Leopold's maneuvers to note fetal position

        (b) Repeat indirect Coombs in Rh sensitized mother

    (7) 36-40 weeks

        (a) Labor instructions

        (b) Information regarding hospitalization

        (c) Newborn feeding preference

        (d) Discussion of postpartum contraception needs

3. Nutrition in pregnancy

    a. Caloric intake and weight gain

        (1) Recommended gain: Woman of normal weight—22-27 pounds (10-12 kg); obese (> 120% of ideal body weight)—15-20 pounds (6-9 kg); underweight (< 85% of

ideal body weight)—gain up to ideal weight plus 22-27 pounds

(a) Inadequate weight gain is associated with small for gestational age infant and PTL

(b) Excessive weight gain is associated with fetal macrosomia

(c) Discourage weight loss during pregnancy

(2) Pattern of weight gain

(a) First trimester—0-3 pounds

(b) Second and third trimesters—approximately 0.8-1 lb/week

(3) Nutritional requirements

(a) Calories—increase by 300 kilocalories/day

(b) Calcium—1200 mg/day

(c) Protein—60 grams/day

(d) Carbohydrates—100 g/day will prevent ketosis

(e) Fat—not more than 20-30% of caloric intake

(f) Iron—30-60 mg supplement/day

(g) Folic acid—0.8-1 mg/day

(h) Other vitamin and mineral needs can be met from balanced diet; avoid excessive vitamin supplementation

(i) Fiber—encourage adequate fiber to prevent constipation

(j) Fluids—maintain 8-10 glasses of fluids/day

(4) Counseling

(a) Review 24-hour diet recall

(b) Evaluate adequacy of major food groups using food pyramid recommended daily allowances

(c) Special considerations

i) Adolescent

    a) Younger than 16 years may still be growing

    b) Higher needs for protein, calories and calcium

    c) Tendency toward poor nutrition

    d) High incidence of eating disorders

ii) Vegetarian—needs special counseling to assure adequate protein and calcium intake

iii) Pica—of particular concern if displaces intake of nutritious food or contains harmful elements

(d) Socioeconomic considerations—refer low-income patient to Women, Infants and Children (WIC) program and other sources of assistance, e.g., food banks

4. Common Discomforts of Pregnancy

  a. Backache

    (1) Etiology: Relaxin causes softening and relaxation of pelvic joints; increased lordosis of spine as uterus enlarges

    (2) Management

      (a) Rule out labor, pyelonephritis, and musculoskeletal disease

      (b) Teach pelvic tilt to restore body alignment

      (c) Use of proper posture and good body mechanics

      (d) Abdominal support garment for pendulous abdomen

      (e) Discourage wearing high heeled shoes

      (f) Walking or stretching exercises

  b. Constipation

    (1) Etiology

      (a) Progesterone causes decreased intestinal motility

        (b) Displacement of intestines by enlarging uterus

        (c) Oral iron supplements

    (2) Management

        (a) Increase dietary fiber and fluid intake

        (b) Adequate daily exercise

        (c) Bulk laxative, e.g., psyllium as needed

c. Dizziness

    (1) Etiology

        (a) Postural hypotension

        (b) Blood pooling in lower extremities causing transient cerebral ischemia

    (2) Management

        (a) Rule out hypoglycemia, hyperventilation, nausea and vomiting, substance use/abuse, illness

        (b) Wear prenatal support stockings

        (c) Avoid prolonged periods of sitting or standing

        (d) Change slowly from supine to seated to standing position

        (e) Avoid vena cava compression; rest on side rather than back

        (f) Avoid activities where loss of balance is likely to occur

        (g) Isometric exercises

d. Dyspnea

    (1) Etiology

        (a) Progesterone effect causes increased sensitivity to lower levels of CO_2

        (b) Increase in tidal volume

        (c) Displacement of diaphragm by enlarging uterus

(2) Management

    (a) Rule out respiratory infections, asthma, cardiovascular disease

    (b) Teach proper posture and body alignment

    (c) Sleep with head elevated

    (d) Control hyperventilation by conscious effort to slow breathing rate or breathe in paper bag

e. Edema

  (1) Etiology

    (a) Increased intracellular fluid retention

    (b) Pressure on vena cava from uterus impedes venous return

  (2) Management

    (a) Assess for Pregnancy Induced Hypertension (PIH)

    (b) Elevate legs several times during day

    (c) At night and several time during day, lie on left side with legs slightly elevated to promote venous return

    (d) Avoid constrictive clothing

    (e) Avoid long periods of standing

f. Epistaxis

  (1) Etiology

    (a) Estrogen causes engorgement of nasal mucosa

    (b) Superficial capillary plexus in anterior nares engorged and bleeds easily with minimal trauma

  (2) Management

    (a) Rule out sinusitis, polyps, allergic rhinitis, and PIH

    (b) Avoid trauma, i.e., vigorous blowing or picking of nose

    (c) Cool steam vaporizer or saline nose drops to prevent drying of nasal mucosa

g. Headache

  (1) Etiology

  (a) Increased circulating blood volume and heart rate

  (b) Vascular congestion

  (c) Emotional tension with spasm of neck muscles

  (d) Ocular changes of pregnancy may lead to refractive changes

  (e) Possible hypoglycemia

  (2) Management

  (a) Assess for PIH

  (b) Acetaminophen

  (c) Increased rest

  (d) Stress reduction/relaxation techniques

  (e) Frequent small meals rich in complex carbohydrates

  (f) Massage, moist heat/cold compresses

  (g) Delete foods and beverages from diet if strongly associated with symptom recurrence, e.g., nitrites, MSG, chocolate

h. Hemorrhoids

  (1) Etiology

  (a) Genetic predisposition to varicosities

  (b) Pressure of enlarging uterus

  (c) Constipation

  (2) Management

  (a) Prevent or treat constipation; increase fluids, exercise

  (b) Ice packs

  (c) Warm soaks "sitz baths"

  (d) Topical anesthetic ointment

  (e) Manual reduction if necessary

     (f) Refer for medical evaluation if severe bleeding or thrombosis occurs

   i. Insomnia

    (1) Etiology

     (a) Most common in third trimester due to enlarged abdomen, fetal activity and other discomforts

     (b) May be related to anxiety or depression

    (2) Management

     (a) Treat physical discomforts

     (b) Pillows to support back, between legs; upper arm in side-lying position

     (c) Warm drinks, especially milk; avoid caffeinated beverages

     (d) Relaxation techniques—warm baths, back rubs, guided imagery

   j. Leg Cramps

    (1) Etiology

     (a) Pressure of growing uterus on pelvic nerves and blood vessels

     (b) Fatigue

     (c) Poor circulation

     (d) Inadequate calcium intake

     (e) Excessive dairy product intake leading to calcium/phosphorus imbalance

    (2) Management

     (a) Rule out thrombophlebitis and musculoskeletal disease

     (b) Dorsiflexion of foot to relieve cramp in calf; avoid pointing toes when stretching

     (c) Diet evaluation and supplementation as needed to reach recommended calcium intake

(d) Antacids to bind phosphorus and free calcium ions; advise sodium free antacids

(e) Heat and massage to affected muscles

k. Leukorrhea

(1) Etiology: Estrogen-induced hyperplasia of vaginal mucosa and increased production of mucus by endocervical glands

(2) Management

(a) Rule out infection—wet mount or cultures as indicated

(b) Wear cotton underwear and loose clothes

(c) Do not douche

(d) Keep vulva clean and dry

l. Nausea and Vomiting

(1) Etiology

(a) Most common in first trimester related to high levels of hCG; may persist in some individuals

(b) Changes in carbohydrate metabolism

(c) Slowed gastric emptying (progesterone effect)

(d) Emotional factors

(2) Management

(a) Rule out hyperemesis gravidarum—signs include marked weight loss, dehydration, ketosis, electrolyte imbalance

(b) Rule out pyelonephritis

(c) Small frequent high carbohydrate meals, avoid empty and overdistended stomach

(d) Avoid high fat or spicy meals

(e) Take fluids separate from meals

(f) Eat dry soda crackers before arising

(g) Sip carbonated beverages

(h) Mint or raspberry herbal teas

(i) Emetrol or Coca Cola syrup

m. Heartburn

(1) Etiology

(a) Progesterone causes relaxation of cardiac sphincter

(b) Delayed gastric emptying

(c) Pressure on stomach from enlarging uterus

(2) Management

(a) Rule out gallbladder disease, peptic ulcer, and PIH

(b) Frequent small meals

(c) Take fluids between meals, not with meals

(d) Do not lie down for at least one hour after eating

(e) Decrease fatty food intake

(f) Antacid preparations (low sodium)

(g) Systemic antacids, e.g., bicarbonate of soda, are contraindicated

(h) Elevate head of bed

n. Round ligament pain

(1) Etiology

(a) As pregnancy progresses, uterus rises into abdomen and dextrorotates

(b) Uterine ligaments hypertrophy and stretch

(2) Management

(a) Rule out appendicitis, gallbladder disease, peptic ulcer, and PTL

(b) Warn patient that pain may be intense, and "grabbing," but will resolve after pregnancy

(c) Flex knees onto abdomen

(d) Heating pad, warm baths

(e)   Advise to avoid sudden, twisting movements

(f)   Avoid excessive exercise, standing, or walking

(g)   When side-lying, support uterus with pillow and place pillow between knees

(h)   Acetaminophen

o.   Varicosities

(1)   Etiology

(a)   History of varicosities in mother or grandmother

(b)   Pressure of enlarged uterus causes impaired venous circulation and increased venous pressure in lower extremities

(c)   Progesterone-induced relaxation of vein walls and valves and surrounding smooth muscles

(d)   Increased weight

(2)   Management

(a)   Rule out thrombophlebitis

(b)   Elevate legs frequently

(c)   Supportive or elastic pantyhose

(d)   Avoid crossing legs, standing for long periods, round garters and knee-high hose

(e)   For vulvar varicosities—support vulvar area with sanitary pad supported by belt; frequent elevation of legs and pelvis; cool packs; sitz baths

p.   Fatigue

(1)   Etiology

(a)   Common in early pregnancy, cause undetermined; hypotheses include

i)   Increased metabolic demands of early gestation

ii) Rise in hCG and progesterone

(b)   Sleep deprivation later in pregnancy

        (2) Management

            (a) Rule out iron deficiency, poor diet, depression

            (b) Several rest periods during day

            (c) Increase number of hours sleep at night

            (d) Reassurance that duration is usually no longer than 3-4 months

q. Urinary Frequency

    (1) Etiology

        (a) Occurs early and late in pregnancy

        (b) Early physiological changes in renal system, including increased glomerular filtration rate and hyperemia of bladder lining (may trigger micturition reflex)

        (c) In third trimester, mechanical pressure of uterus as it descends into pelvis prevents filling of bladder

    (2) Management

        (a) Rule out urinary tract infection (UTI)

        (b) Void frequently and when urge is felt

        (c) Maintain adequate fluid intake during day

        (d) Empty bladder every 2 hours during day

        (e) Avoid caffeine, artificial sweeteners

        (f) Limit fluids after 6 p.m. to decrease nocturia

r. Breast Discomfort

    (1) Etiology: High levels of estrogen and progesterone trigger breast enlargement and tenderness in early pregnancy

    (2) Management

        (a) Advise wearing well-fitting, supportive brassiere

        (b) May find it more comfortable to wear a soft brassiere for sleep

5. Guidance for Health Promotion

a. Avoidance of teratogens or other harmful agents

    (1) No alcohol intake

    (2) No medications (prescribed or over-the- counter) or herbal teas without approval of health care provider

    (3) No smoking; avoid exposure to secondhand smoke

    (4) Assess potential for chemical exposure at work and at home

    (5) Avoid exposure to infectious disease, particularly

        (a) Rubella—if non-immune, report any possible exposure immediately

        (b) Varicella—if non-immune, report any possible exposure immediately

        (c) Toxoplasmosis—do not handle or eat raw meat; avoid handling cat litter

    (6) No prolonged immersion in hot tub or spa—elevated core body temperature may be deleterious to fetal development

b. Travel

    (1) Use shoulder and lap belts in automobile; be sure lap belt fits snugly under abdomen

    (2) Travelling by car—stop every 2 hours and walk for 10 minutes

    (3) Air travel in pressurized cabin is safe; get out of seat every hour and walk for a few minutes; maintain hydration

    (4) Avoid travel during last month of gestation

    (5) Do not go where medical care is unavailable

c. Work

    (1) Most pregnant women can continue to work

    (2) Avoid excessive lifting or fatigue

    (3) Take rest periods every 2 hours; avoid work schedules greater than 8 hours/day

    (4) Consider chemical, x-ray or other toxic exposure

    d. Dental care

       (1) A dental exam should be part of prenatal care

       (2) Most procedures are not contraindicated and problems should be corrected

       (3) Local anesthesia without added epinephrine is recommended

    e. Exercise

       (1) Exercise is recommended during a normal pregnancy

       (2) May continue with accustomed exercise regimen but should not initiate an overly rigorous program; avoid back-lying exercises after 20 weeks

       (3) Walking and/or swimming are ideal for those not in good physical condition

       (4) Avoid activities that involve changes of barometric pressure, e.g., sky diving, scuba diving

       (5) Avoid excessive fatigue; keep pulse $\leq$ 120 BPM

       (6) Decrease exercise intensity and duration as pregnancy progresses

       (7) Avoid prolonged overheating

       (8) Wear supportive shoes and brassiere

       (9) Discontinue if short of breath

       (10) If vaginal bleeding or abdominal pain occurs, contact health care provider immediately

    f. Bathing and personal hygiene

       (1) Increased activity of mucous membranes and sweat glands make frequent baths or showers a necessity

       (2) Safety precautions should be taken to prevent falls

       (3) Tub baths contraindicated if rupture of membranes is suspected

       (4) No douching

g. Sexual activity

    (1) Coitus is not contraindicated in a normal pregnancy

    (2) Changes in libido may occur in both partners related to bio-psycho-sociocultural factors

    (3) Changes in position may be required to accommodate enlarged abdomen; encourage couple to be creative

    (4) Woman supine position is contraindicated after 28 weeks

    (5) To prevent rare occurrence of air embolus, do not blow air into vagina during cunnilingus

    (6) Coitus is contraindicated in presence of vaginal bleeding, threatened abortion, PTL, ruptured membranes

    (7) Alternative methods to satisfy male and female sexual needs may need to be explored; when intercourse is contraindicated, usually orgasm by any means is contraindicated for the woman to avoid stimulating uterine contractions

    (8) "Safer" sex still a concern

h. Immunizations

    (1) Live virus vaccines are contraindicated, e.g., measles, mumps, rubella

    (2) Inactivated bacterial vaccines, hyperimmune globulins and DNA-based vaccines are safe when indicated

        (a) Salk polio vaccine

        (b) Hepatitis B vaccine

        (c) Immune globulins for post-exposure prophylaxis

        (d) Tetanus for those who have had no booster in 10 years

i. Warning signs—patients should be instructed to contact provider promptly when any of these occur

    (1) Signs of ectopic pregnancy or threatened abortion

        (a) Pain

        (b) Bleeding

        (c)   Passage of tissue

        (d)   Syncope

    (2) Hyperemesis—severe nausea and vomiting; unable to retain any food or fluids

    (3) Infectious disease

        (a)   Temperature elevation above 100.6°F

        (b)   Dysuria, flank pain

        (c)   Severe or persistent diarrhea; severe abdominal pain

        (d)   Rash or skin lesions

    (4) Signs of PIH

        (a)   Swelling of face; swelling of lower extremities which does not respond to rest or elevation

        (b)   Severe headache, dizziness

        (c)   Blurring of vision, scotomata

        (d)   Epigastric pain

    (5) Signs of PTL

        (a)   Loss of fluid from vagina

        (b)   Lower back pain or lower abdominal cramping

        (c)   Frequent, palpable uterine contractions with or without pain

        (d)   Increase in vaginal discharge, especially if mucoid or blood-tinged

        (e)   Heaviness or pressure

        (f)   Nausea and vomiting, diarrhea

    (6) Signs related to fetal well-being—decreased or absent fetal movement

Assessment of Fetal Well Being

- Amniocentesis
    1. Definition: Transabdominal removal of a sample of amniotic fluid

2. Indications

   a. Genetic screening—for chromosomal disorders, congenital abnormalities, and inborn errors of metabolism

   b. Rh sensitization—spectrophotometric examination predictive of hemolytic disease ($\Delta 0D_{450} > 0.15$)

   c. Fetal lung maturity

      (1) Lecithin/sphingomyelin (L/S) ratio $\geq 2:1$ = lung maturity

      (2) Phosphatidylglycerol (PG)—present if lungs are mature

3. Basic principles

   a. Performed at 15-18 weeks ("Early amnio" 11-14 weeks)

   b. Ultrasound performed immediately prior, or concurrently

4. Risks—less than 1 in 300 due to infection, premature rupture of membranes (PROM), abruption, fetal bleeding or injury

- Chorionic Villus Sampling (CVS)

1. Definition

   a. Removal of a small sample of chorionic tissue via transcervical, transabdominal, or transvaginal means for prenatal genetic diagnosis

   b. Optimal time is 9-11 weeks gestation

   c. Allows earlier screening/diagnosis

2. Indications

   a. Family history of genetic abnormality

   b. Advanced maternal age

   c. Mother is carrier for X-linked disease

   d. Parents known carriers of autosomal recessive disorders

   e. History ≥ 3 successive spontaneous abortions

3. Basic principles

   a. Transcervical or transabdominal recovery between 9-11 weeks

   b. Performed under ultrasound examination

4. Risks

    a. Fetal loss 4/100

    b. May obtain maternal decidua rather than chorionic villi

    c. Rare damage to fetus (limb anomalies), placenta, or cord

- Maternal Serum Alphafetoprotein (MSAFP) and Multiple Marker Screening

  1. Definition: A screening test for certain congenital malformations and genetic defects

  2. Basic principles

    a. Elevated levels of AFP associated with open neural tube defects (NTD), abdominal wall defects, congenital nephrosis, other congenital anomalies, multiple gestation

    b. Low levels of AFP plus changes in hCG and unconjugated estriol (UE_3) associated with Down syndrome (Trisomy 21)

    c. Value is adjusted for maternal characteristics, e.g., age, weight, smoking, diabetes, medications and gestational age

  3. Management

    a. Draw maternal serum at 15 completed weeks gestation (16-18 weeks is optimal)

    b. Positive MSAFP or multiple marker

      (1) Refer for ultrasound (often associated with incorrect dates)

      (2) Repeat and/or consider confirmation via amniocentesis

      (3) If gestational age is changed, re-calculate AFP data using corrected dates

    c. Be supportive of decision to continue or terminate the pregnancy

- Ultrasound

  1. Definition: Sound wave echoes reflected from tissues of varying densities and converted into sequenced images

  2. Indications

    a. Determination of gestational age

    b. Evaluation of fetal growth pattern and weight

    c. Significant size/date discrepancy

    d. Suspected ectopic pregnancy

    e. Fetal presentation

    f. Suspected fetal disease process, anomalies, or fetal demise

    g. Hydramnios/oligohydramnios

    h. Placental location/integrity/maturity, e.g., suspected placenta previa

    i. Aid in diagnostic procedures, e.g., amniocentesis, CVS, biophysical profile (BPP)

    j. Identify number of fetuses

3. Basic principles

    a. Accuracy depends on skill of sonographer, position and gestational age of fetus, maternal habitus

    b. Procedure takes 30-60 minutes

    c. Transabdominal imaging requires a full bladder for optimal visualization (except in third trimester)

    d. Transvaginal technique allows early identification and dating of pregnancy, identification of ectopic pregnancy, and better imaging in obese women

- Electronic Fetal Monitoring (EFM)

1. Definition: Use of an electronic device to correlate the fetal heart rate with the contraction pattern and produce a written record

2. Indications

    a. Test for fetal well-being in third trimester high-risk pregnancies, e.g., decreased fetal movement, intrauterine growth retardation (IUGR), multiple gestation, maternal disorders including diabetes and hypertension

    b. Monitor fetal response to stress of labor; may be used routinely

3. Basic principles

    a. Types of monitoring—external (indirect) and internal (direct)

    b. Fetal heart rate (FHR) patterns

        (1) Rate

            (a) Normal FHR: 120-160 beats per minute (BPM)

(b) Marked bradycardia: < 100 BPM

(c) Marked tachycardia: > 180 BPM

(2) Variability—normal heart rate fluctuations caused by interplay of sympathetic and parasympathetic nervous system

(a) Good variability (fluctuations of 11-25 BPM) indicate fetal well-being

(b) Absent or minimal variability after 28 weeks gestation must be investigated

(3) Decelerations

(a) Early decelerations are usually related to pressure on fetal head from normal contractions—usually normal; rule out prolapsed cord, position mother on side

(b) Late decelerations are a sign of utero-placental insufficiency—abnormal; prompt delivery indicated with repetitive late decelerations

(c) Variable decelerations are usually a sign of cord compression—rule out prolapsed cord, position mother on side

- Diagnostic Tests

  1. Nonstress test (NST)—detects fetal heart rate acceleration in response to fetal movement

     a. External monitoring for approximately 20 minutes

     b. If no FHR accelerations occur, can extend to 40 minutes

     c. Interpretation

        (1) Reactive NST—appropriate fetal heart rate accelerations (repeat weekly)

        (2) Nonreactive NST—insufficient heart rate accelerations over a 40 minute period (repeat in 12-24 hours or refer for workup)

  2. Contraction stress test (CST)

     a. Baseline tracing obtained—if 3 or more uterine contractions (UC) of 40 seconds duration are present in a 10 minute period, uterine stimulation unnecessary; if < 3 UC in 10 minutes, uterine stimulation instituted

 (1) Breast or nipple self-stimulation test

 (2) Oxytocin challenge test (OCT)

  (a) Low-dose IV. oxytocin infusion

  (b) Rate increased until adequate UC develop

 b. Results

  (1) Negative—no late decelerations (repeat in 1 week)

  (2) Positive—late decelerations following 50% or more of UC (delivery recommended)

  (3) Suspicious (equivocal)—intermittent late or significant variable decelerations (repeat in 12-24 hours)

- Biophysical Profile (BPP)

 1. Definition: Assessment of fetal health by combined use of 5 fetal biophysical variables

 2. Indications

  a. Postdate pregnancy

  b. Decreased fetal movement

  c. Chronic maternal disease state

  d. Suspected oligohydramnios

  e. IUGR

  f. Isoimmunization

  g. Premature rupture of membranes (PROM)

  h. Previous stillbirth

 3. Basic principles

  a. BPP consists of NST with the addition of 4 observations made by real time ultrasound; components are

   (1) NST

   (2) Fetal breathing movements

   (3) Gross fetal body movements

    (4) Fetal tone

    (5) Quantitation of amniotic fluid volume (amniotic fluid index-AFI)

   b. Each component is scored as 2 (normal) or 0 (abnormal); total score of 10 is possible

    (1) 8-10 is normal

    (2) 6 is equivocal (retest in 12-24 hours)

    (3) ≤ 4 is abnormal (consider delivery)

- Fetal Movement Counts

 1. Definition: Maternal record keeping of fetal activity

 2. Indications

   a. Fetal surveillance in high and low-risk patients

   b. Monitoring by all pregnant women starting at 28 weeks

 3. Basic principles

   a. Fetal movements decrease in response to hypoxia

   b. Woman assumes lateral recumbent position and counts distinct fetal movements

   c. Perception of 10 distinct movements within 2-hour period is considered reassuring (other regimens possible)

   d. In the absence of reassuring count, NST or BPP may be performed

   e. Maternal perception of relative decrease in fetal activity compared to previous level is important indication for further evaluation

- Percutaneous Umbilical Blood Sampling (PUBS)

 1. Definition: Direct access to fetal circulation via umbilical cord blood sampling for evaluation or treatment

 2. Indications

   a. Prenatal diagnosis of blood disorders

   b. Isoimmunization

    c. Metabolic disorders

    d. Fetal infection

    e. Evaluation of fetal hypoxia

    f. Fetal therapy

        (1) Red cell and platelet transfusion

        (2) Monitor fetal drug therapy

3. Basic principles—under ultrasound, a needle is inserted into umbilical artery or vein; may be performed from 16-40 weeks gestation

4. Risks—bleeding, chorioamnionitis, premature labor, PROM

Complications of Pregnancy

- Weight and Risk

  1. Inadequate weight gain

    a. Definition: Less than standard weight gain recommended for pre-pregnancy height and weight

    b. Etiology/Incidence

        (1) Inadequate or poor nutrition

        (2) Excessive nausea and vomiting (hyperemesis gravidarum)

        (3) Maternal disorders or diseases

    c. Signs and Symptoms/Physical Findings

        (1) 1st trimester loss $\geq$ 5 pounds

        (2) 2nd or 3rd trimester gain < 2.2 pounds per month

        (3) Any weight loss in 2nd or 3rd trimester

    d. Differential Diagnosis

        (1) Hyperemesis gravidarum

        (2) Anorexia, bulimia

        (3) Substance abuse

        (4) Psychosocial issues, e.g., battering

        (5) Infections or other medical conditions

e. Diagnostic Tests/Findings

  (1) Accurate pre-pregnancy and serial weight measurements

  (2) Urine dipstick for ketones at each visit (ketosis indicates inadequate carbohydrate and/or caloric intake)

f. Management/Treatment

  (1) Evaluation of diet per food diary or 24-hour diet recall

  (2) Instruct client in use of daily food guide

  (3) Supplementation

  (4) Referral to dietician and social worker as needed

  (5) Referral to physician (hydration and possible hyperalimentation) as needed

2. Excessive weight gain

  a. Definition: Greater than standard weight gain recommended for pre-pregnancy height and weight

  b. Etiology/Incidence

  (1) Overeating

  (2) Lack of exercise

  (3) Fluid retention

  (4) Preeclampsia (PIH)

  c. Signs and Symptoms/Physical Findings

  (1) 1st trimester gain > 10 pounds

  (2) 2nd and 3rd trimester gain > 2 pounds per week

  (3) Edema, especially in 2nd and 3rd trimesters

  d. Differential Diagnosis

  (1) Diabetes

  (2) Hypothyroid

  (3) Preeclampsia (PIH)

  e. Diagnostic Tests/Findings

  (1) Accurate pre-pregnancy and serial weight measurements

(2) Urine dipstick for albumin and glucose

   f. Management/Treatment

      (1) Nutrition counseling

         (a) Evaluation of diet via food diary

         (b) Referral to dietician and social worker as needed

      (2) Evaluate for preeclampsia when sudden, sharp weight gain occurs

- Anemia

  1. Definition: A deficiency in the amount of hemoglobin necessary to maintain normal tissue requirements for oxygen; usually defined as Hgb < 11 g/dL or Hct < 33%

  2. Types and Etiology

     a. Nutritional

        (1) Iron deficiency—occurs in almost 50% of pregnant women due to lack of iron stores, poor diet, and fetal demands for iron

        (2) Folic acid deficiency—seen in 0.5-15% of U.S. populations studied; may be due to insufficient dietary intake of folic acid, impaired folic acid absorption and/or metabolism

     b. Hemolytic—Glucose-6-phosphatase dehydrogenase (G6PD) deficiency which occurs in approximately 3% of African-American women; ingestion of oxidant drugs, e.g., antipyretics, sulfonamides and nitrofurans leads to hemolysis of maternal and fetal red blood cells within 24-48 hours; severity of hemolysis varies with amount and type of drug ingested and spontaneous recovery begins within 1 week

     c. Hemoglobinopathies

        (1) Sickle cell (see Non-Gynecologic Disorders chapter)

           (a) Sickle cell trait—woman is not anemic and usually has no problems except under conditions of hypoxia; increased risk of asymptomatic bacteriuria in pregnancy; gene is inherited as autosomal recessive;

if both parents are carriers, 1 in 4 chance that child will have sickle cell disease

(b) Sickle cell disease (homozygous for hemoglobin S)—have chronic hemolytic anemia with intermittent crises; pregnancy can be precipitating factor for occurrence of crises; increased maternal morbidity and mortality, and increased rates of spontaneous abortion, stillbirth, preterm delivery and intrauterine growth retardation; care should be undertaken by team of specialists

(c) Women who are heterozygous for hemoglobin S and another abnormal hemoglobin, i.e., C or beta Thalassemia—may have a variety of complications depending on concentration of particular hemoglobins

(2) Thalassemias—group of hypochromic anemias associated with defective synthesis of one of polypeptide chains of hemoglobin molecule; inherited as autosomal recessive trait, and involve abnormal synthesis of hemoglobin A in either alpha or beta chain; seen primarily in persons of Mediterranean, southeast Asian and central African descent

(a) Thalassemia minor (heterozygous thalassemia of beta chain)—a mild hypochromic, microcytic anemia; hemoglobin levels 2-3 g/dL below normal values; elevation of Hemoglobin A_2 levels (> 3.5%) is diagnostic; no therapy is effective or necessary; may be diagnosed when patient fails to respond to iron therapy

(b) Thalassemia major (homozygous beta- thalassemia or Cooley's Anemia)—produces profound anemia usually requiring regular transfusions and iron chelation therapy; affected individuals often die in teen or young adult years; during pregnancy, fetus is protected from severe disease because fetal hemoglobin has no beta chain

(c) Alpha thalassemias—prevalent in southeast Asians; trait is seen in 5% of African-Americans

        i)   Alpha trait produces microcytic anemia that is unresponsive to iron; diagnosis is made by excluding other forms of anemia; hemoglobin electrophoresis helpful only in neonates; patients are asymptomatic and should not have iron prescribed

      ii) Hemoglobin H disease—three genes are deleted; seen primarily in Asians, produces moderately severe anemia similar to thalassemia major

3. Signs and Symptoms/Physical Findings—(note: management discussed will include only nutritional anemias; all others should be referred to physician)

   a. Usually asymptomatic until hemoglobin falls below 6-7 g/dL

   b. Fatigue, headache, dizziness, vertigo, palpations, flow murmur

   c. Iron deficiency—skin pallor, cheilosis, brittle hair or nails

   d. Folacin deficiency—nausea and vomiting, pallor, soreness of tongue

4. Differential Diagnosis

   a. Hemoglobinopathies

   b. G6PD deficiency

   c. Blood loss

5. Diagnostic Tests/Findings

   a. Hgb and Hct decreased

   b. Mean corpuscular volume (MCV)—decreased in iron deficiency anemia; increased in folate deficiency (megaloblastic anemia); normal value 80-94

   c. Serum iron decreased

   d. Total iron binding capacity (TIBC) increased

   e. Ferritin < 10 ng/mL in iron deficiency

   f. Serum folate < 165 ng/mL in folate deficiency

g. Quantitative hemoglobin electrophoresis— normal findings: Hgb $A_1 = 95\%$; Hgb $A_2 = 3\%$; Hgb F = < 2%

6. Management/Treatment

    a. Iron supplementation, e.g., ferrous sulfate or ferrous gluconate 2-3 times daily with vitamin C rich foods to enhance absorption; if iron is not well tolerated

        (1) Take after meals

        (2) Try different iron compound, or use timed-release or liquid formulations

        (3) Use stool softener if constipation occurs

    b. Folacin supplementation of 1 mg daily (included in all standard prenatal vitamin supplements)

        (1) Up to 4 mg may be prescribed prophylactically for women with history of baby with NTD

        (2) Daily supplementation of 0.4-0.8 mg is recommended for all women of reproductive age

    c. Nutritional assessment and counseling to include foods rich in iron and folacin

    d. Repeat Hgb and Hct in 2-4 weeks; Hgb should increase 2 points within 1 month of therapy

    e. Consult with physician if

        (1) Anemia is severe (Hgb < 9 g/dL)

        (2) Hgb not improved after 4 weeks supplementation

        (3) MCV < 70 or > 110

        (4) Underlying pathology suspected

            (a) Hemoglobinopathy

            (b) Clotting disorder

            (c) G6PD deficiency

- Rh Isoimmunization

    1. Definition

a. Sensitization of Rh- mother to D antigen after exposure to Rh+ blood through transfusion or fetomaternal hemorrhage from incompatible (Rh+) fetus; following exposure, Rh- mother produces antibodies against Rh+ red blood cells of fetus

b. Isoimmunization of mother carries risk for hemolytic disease of the fetus or newborn; occurs when fetal red blood cells are destroyed by circulating maternal antibodies, causing fetal anemia and elevated heme and bilirubin; if anemia is severe, heart failure and ascites may develop; known as hydrops fetalis; high risk of fetal mortality and morbidity

2. Etiology/Incidence

   a. Prevalence of Rh negative varies in different ethnic groups—Caucasian: 15%; African-American: 8%; Native American: 1%; Asian: 0%

   b. Isoimmunization may be initiated with any leakage of Rh+ red blood cells into the circulatory system of an Rh- mother

      (1) Transfusion with Rh+ blood

      (2) Leakage of fetal Rh+ red blood cells during delivery, abortion, amniocentesis, or fetal-maternal bleeding during pregnancy

   c. In normal pregnancies, fetal red blood cells have been detected in maternal bloodstream in 25-30% of women during 3rd trimester

   d. Sensitization may be caused by 0.1 ml of Rh+ cells, but 30% of Rh- women never produce Rh antibodies; coexisting presence of ABO and Rh incompatibility reduces risk by 50% or more

3. Signs and Symptoms

   a. Asymptomatic

   b. History of previous child with hemolytic disease of the newborn (hydrops fetalis)

4. Differential Diagnosis—nonimmune hemolytic disease

5. Physical Findings—within normal limits

6. Diagnostic Tests/Findings

   a. Blood type, Rh and antibody screen

  b. Antibody titers to determine if mother is sensitized

 7. Management/Treatment

  a. Rh- mother who is antibody negative at the initial visit

   (1) Screen father for Rh status; if paternity is certain and father is Rh-, no further follow-up needed

   (2) If father is Rh+ or type undetermined, repeat maternal antibody screen at 28 weeks

   (3) If 28 week antibody screen is negative, give a 300 μg dose of Rh immune globulin (RhoGAM)

   (4) At delivery, infant's blood type is determined and if Rh+, another 300 μg dose is given within 72 hours of delivery

   (5) Other indications for RhoGAM administration

    (a) Following amniocentesis, CVS, PUBS

    (b) Following spontaneous or induced abortion

    (c) Following any incident in which fetomaternal hemorrhage is suspected

  b. Rh- mother who is antibody positive at initial visit

   (1) Further screening for specific antigen; if father is negative for specific antigen, no further management needed

   (2) If father is specific antigen positive, mother should be monitored in high-risk obstetrical facility; monitoring will include

    (a) Serial antibody titers; if titers remain < 1:16 in initially unimmunized pregnancy, fetus is probably not in jeopardy

    (b) Serial studies of fetal well-being

    (c) Amniotic fluid analysis for

     i) Amount of pigment from degrading red blood cells

     ii) Reported in delta optical density zones 1, 2, or 3; zone 3 indicates severely affected infant/fetus

(d) Treatment for affected infant may include

      i) Early delivery

      ii) Intrauterine transfusion

- ABO Incompatibility

  1. Definition: Major blood group incompatibility which may develop when type O mother is carrying a type A, B, or AB fetus

  2. Etiology/Incidence

    a. Type O mother has naturally occurring anti-A and anti-B antibodies in her system

    b. Fetus is A, B, or AB

    c. Less than 10% of ABO incompatible pregnancies develop hemolytic disease; most do not develop significant hemolysis until after birth

  3. Signs and Symptoms

    a. Mother is asymptomatic

    b. Onset of fetal jaundice within 24 hours following delivery

    c. Varying degrees of fetal anemia, reticulocytosis, and erythroblastosis; usually less severe than effects of Rh hemolytic disease

  4. Differential Diagnosis—nonimmune hemolytic disease

  5. Physical Findings—within normal limits

  6. Diagnostic Tests/Findings

    a. No adequate method of antenatal diagnosis; titers and amniocentesis during pregnancy not required

    b. Coombs antiglobulin test usually positive

  7. Management/Treatment

    a. Infant treatment begins after delivery

      (1) Monitoring of bilirubin and hemoglobin levels

      (2) Phototherapy for jaundice

      (3) Transfusion occasionally required

    b. No treatment indicated for mother

      c. Implications

          (1) May occur with any pregnancy, including first

          (2) Unlike Rh disease, no relationship between occurrence in one pregnancy and recurrence in subsequent pregnancies

- Endocrine Conditions

    1. Diabetes Mellitus

      a. Definition: A chronic familial disease characterized by inadequate production or utilization of insulin with alterations in carbohydrate, protein and fat metabolism

          (1) Type I: Insulin dependent diabetes (IDDM)

              (a) Usual onset in childhood or young adulthood

              (b) Lack of insulin production by pancreas probably due to autoimmune process

              (c) Ketosis prone

          (2) Type II: Non-insulin dependent diabetes (NIDDM)

              (a) Usual onset after age 30

              (b) Associated with obesity

              (c) Produce insulin, but functions abnormally

          (3) Type III: Gestational Diabetes Mellitus (GDM)

              (a) Onset during pregnancy

                   i) Class A_1—diet controlled

                  ii) Class A_2—requires insulin

              (b) Usually resolves after pregnancy, but woman has increased lifetime risk of Type II diabetes

      b. Etiology/Incidence

          (1) Approximately 2-3% of pregnant women are diabetic, with 90% of them having GDM

          (2) GDM is precipitated by hormonal changes of pregnancy and increased glucose demand for fetal growth

              (a) Estrogen acts as insulin antagonist

(b) Human placental lactogen (hPL) causes increase in insulin resistance and mobilizes free fatty acids which increase likelihood of ketosis

(c) Progesterone decreases peripheral effectiveness of insulin

(d) Insulin demand peaks at 20-30 weeks gestation; in the woman with suboptimal production of insulin, deficiency will become apparent at or before that time

(3) Maternal/fetal risks increased

(a) Congenital anomalies more prevalent in pregnancies where diabetes is poorly controlled during 1st trimester

(b) Influence of pregnancy on diabetes

    i) Insulin requirements change—decrease during 1st trimester; rise in 2nd trimester; may double or quadruple by term

    ii) Increased risk of ketoacidosis, insulin shock, coma

(c) Increased incidence of stillbirths after 36 weeks

(d) Fetal macrosomia/dystocia/cesarean section

(e) Hydramnios

(f) PIH occurs in 12-13% of diabetics

(g) Maternal hyperglycemia/hypoglycemia and/or ketoacidosis

c. Signs and Symptoms of GDM

(1) Classic triad of polyuria, polydipsia and polyphagia may be present in previously undiagnosed Type II diabetics

(2) Usually asymptomatic

d. Physical Findings

(1) Obesity

(2) Hypertension

(3) Fundal height > 2 cm above that expected for dates after 20 weeks gestation

(4) Hydramnios

e. Diagnostic Tests/Findings

    (1) 1 hour post 50 gram glucose screen (1 hr PG) at initial visit for women with risk factors, and at 24-28 weeks for all patients

        (a) Risk factors include—prior history of GDM; prior delivery of macrosomic infant; previous unexplained stillbirth or spontaneous abortions; obesity; first degree relative with diabetes; glucosuria of > 2+; maternal age > 35 years

        (b) If 1 hr PG is 140-199 mg/dL, order 3 hour 100 gram glucose tolerance test (3 hr GTT); if 2 or more values are abnormal, a diagnosis of GDM is made

            i) Class A_1—normal fasting blood sugar (FBS)

            ii) Class A_2—elevated FBS

        (c) If 1 hr PG is > 200 mg/dL, order FBS; if FBS > 130 mg/dL, can omit GTT and refer immediately for treatment

    (2) Glycosylated hemoglobin A_{1C}—reflects glucose levels over previous 4-6 weeks; levels above 7.5% indicate prolonged hyperglycemia; may be useful in estimating duration of GDM diagnosed at first prenatal visit

f. Management/Treatment

    (1) Type I and Type II diabetes

        (a) Ideally, known diabetics should consult provider preconception to establish euglycemia and substitute insulin for oral hypoglycemics which may be teratogenic

        (b) Close management by specialist team throughout pregnancy

            i) Perinatal mortality not increased with good diabetic control and prenatal care

        ii) Maintain euglycemia with more frequent injections of insulin in response to home blood glucose monitoring

        iii) Diet counseling

        iv) Serial ultrasound for macrosomia

        v) Fetal movement counts beginning at 28 weeks

        vi) Antenatal fetal surveillance beginning at 32-36 weeks (NST, BPP, CST as indicated)

        vii) Avoid postterm delivery

  (2) GDM

    (a) Class A_1

      i) Diet control

      ii) FBS and 2 hour postprandial blood sugar every 2 weeks (may progress to insulin dependence during pregnancy)

      iii) Begin antepartal testing at term

      iv) Encourage regular exercise unless contraindicated

    (b) Class A_2—management is the same as for other insulin dependent diabetes; client usually needs extensive education regarding diet and insulin regimen

    (c) All GDM

      i) Screen for persistent diabetes with GTT at postpartum examination

      ii) Counsel regarding diet and importance of achieving and maintaining normal weight to reduce future risk

2. Thyroid Disorder

  a. Definition: "Euthyroid of pregnancy"—term used to describe physiologic hyperthyroid state occurring during pregnancy

   b. Etiology/Incidence

   (1) Hyperthyroid state due to increase in estrogen and other physiologic changes

   (2) Hypothyroidism and thyrotoxicosis may occur during pregnancy but are rare

   c. Signs and Symptoms/Physical Findings

   (1) Modest, diffuse enlargement of thyroid gland is normal

   (2) Asymptomatic unless hypo or hyperthyroidism present

   d. Differential Diagnosis

   (1) Hypothyroidism

   (2) Thyrotoxicosis

   (3) Thyroid cancer

   (4) Grave's disease

   e. Diagnostic Tests/Findings (for euthyroid of pregnancy)

   (1) Thyroid binding globulin (TBG) increased

   (2) TSH is within normal limits (WNL)

   (3) Total T_4 increased

   (4) Resin T_3 uptake (RT_3U) decreased

   f. Management/Treatment

   (1) No treatment indicated for euthyroid

   (2) Refer to physician if suspect hypo or hyperthyroid, thyroid is nodular or asymmetrical, or if symptoms occur

• Hypertensive Disorders

   1. Definition

   a. Pregnancy induced hypertension (PIH)

   (1) Hypertension (HTN)—blood pressure (B/P) $\geq$ 140/90, or rise in systolic $\geq$ 30 or diastolic $\geq$ 15mm Hg above baseline on at least two occasions, 6 hours apart

   (2) Preeclampsia—HTN plus generalized edema and/or proteinuria after 20 weeks gestation

        (3)   HELLP Syndrome—life threatening complication of preeclampsia involving **H**emolysis, **E**levated **L**iver enzymes, and **L**ow **P**latelets

        (4)   Eclampsia—the convulsive phase following preeclampsia

   b. Chronic hypertensive disease

        (1)   Persistent hypertension before 20 weeks gestation

        (2)   Hypertension beyond 6 weeks postpartum

   c. Chronic hypertension with superimposed PIH

2. Etiology/Incidence

   a. PIH occurs in 12% of pregnancies

   b. Predisposing factors

        (1)   Primarily in primigravidas

        (2)   Maternal age < 20 and > 35

        (3)   Preexisting hypertensive, vascular, autoimmune, or renal disease

        (4)   Family or personal history of preeclampsia

        (5)   Multiple gestation

        (6)   Gestational trophoblastic disease

        (7)   Lupus erythematosus

3. Signs and Symptoms

   a. PIH without proteinuria and edema—elevated B/P only

   b. Mild preeclampsia

        (1)   Sudden weight gain

        (2)   Edema of fingers or face

        (3)   Absence of significant proteinuria

   c. Severe preeclampsia

        (1)   Sudden excessive weight gain

        (2)   Generalized edema

        (3)   Frontal or occipital headaches

(4) Visual disturbances, e.g., blurred vision, spots of light (scotomata)

(5) Hyperreflexia

(6) Epigastric or right upper quadrant (RUQ) pain

(7) Oliguria: < 500 mL/24 hours

(8) Decreased fetal movement

   d. HELLP syndrome

(1) Signs and symptoms of preeclampsia

(2) Severe fatigue

(3) Nausea with or without vomiting

(4) Jaundice

   e. Eclampsia—occurs in 5% of women with preeclampsia

(1) Relatives describe a seizure or "fit"

(2) Drowsiness or coma following seizure

4. Differential Diagnosis

   a. Chronic HTN

   b. Brain tumor

   c. Renal failure

5. Physical findings

   a. Mild preeclampsia

(1) HTN (2 readings ≥ 6 hours apart)

   (a) Diastolic ≥ 90 mm Hg

   (b) Systolic ≥ 140 mm Hg

   (c) Diastolic rise ≥ 15 mm Hg

   (d) Systolic rise ≥ 30 mm Hg

(2) Weight gain > 2 lbs/week or > 6 lbs/month

(3) Nondependent edema ≥ 1+

(4) Reflexes WNL

b. Severe preeclampsia

   (1) HTN > 160/100 (2 readings ≥ 6 hours apart)

   (2) Weight gain > 2 lbs/week or > 6 lbs/month

   (3) Pretibial edema ≥ 3-4+

   (4) Urinary output ≤ 400-500 mL/24 hours (oliguria)

   (5) Size small for dates (S<D)

   (6) Hyperreflexia 3-4+ with or without clonus

   (7) Possible retinal changes, tachypnea, dyspnea

   (8) Proteinuria levels ≥ 5 g in a 24° urine collection (or 3+ to 4+ based on semiquantitative assay)

c. HELLP Syndrome—above plus

   (1) Tenderness to palpation in epigastric or RUQ area

   (2) Enlarged, firm liver

   (3) Jaundice (in 40% of cases)

   (4) Ascites may be present

d. Eclampsia—severe preeclampsia plus

   (1) Tonic-clonic seizure followed by coma

   (2) Cyanosis and tachypnea (with pulmonary edema)

   (3) Oliguric, may be anuric

   (4) Decreased or absent FHT

6. Diagnostic Tests/Findings

   a. Mild preeclampsia

      (1) Proteinuria ≤ 1+

      (2) CBC—hemoconcentration, low platelets

      (3) AST, serum creatinine, uric acid—elevated

      (4) Ultrasonography—may find mild IUGR

      (5) Serial 24° urine for protein > 300 mg < 5 g/24°

      (6) Edema > 1+ after 12 hours of bed rest

      b. Severe preeclampsia and eclampsia

         (1) Proteinuria $\geq$ 3+, or $\geq$ 5 g/24° urine collection

         (2) CBC—hemoconcentration, platelets < 100,000

         (3) AST, LDH, serum creatinine, uric acid— elevated

         (4) Ultrasonography—may find IUGR

         (5) Coagulation studies—decreased clotting factors and platelets, and increased fibrin

      c. HELLP syndrome—as above plus

         (1) Decreased clotting factors and very low platelets (< 50,000)

         (2) Serum glucose may be significantly decreased

         (3) Severe hemoconcentration

   7. Management/Treatment

      a. Bedrest—left lateral recumbent position for mild to moderate preeclampsia

      b. Adequate nutrition

      c. Antenatal fetal surveillance, including fetal movement counts

      d. Physician consultation

      e. Anticipate hospitalization if condition worsens

- Bleeding Conditions

   1. Spontaneous Abortion (SAB)

      a. Definition: Termination of pregnancy prior to 20 weeks gestation

      b. Etiology/Incidence

         (1) Blighted ovum or chromosomal abnormality

         (2) Faulty implantation or exposure

         (3) Teratogen exposure

         (4) Maternal diseases, infections, or endocrine imbalance

         (5) Immune factors

      c. Signs and Symptoms/Physical Findings

(1) Threatened abortion (50% progress to complete SAB)

    (a) Vaginal bleeding with or without cramping

    (b) No cervical changes

(2) Inevitable abortion (irreversible)

    (a) Vaginal bleeding with cramping

    (b) Cervical changes and rupture of membranes

(3) Missed abortion

    (a) Products of conception (POC) retained 4-8 weeks after fetal death

    (b) Loss of pregnancy symptoms

    (c) Decrease in uterine size and brownish vaginal discharge

    (d) Cervix closed, firm

(4) Incomplete abortion (D&C usually needed)

    (a) Cramping, bleeding

    (b) Incomplete expulsion of POC

(5) Complete abortion

    (a) Spontaneous expulsion of all POC

    (b) Usually occurs < 6 weeks or > 14 weeks gestation

(6) Habitual abortion—SAB in ≥ 3 consecutive pregnancies

d. Differential Diagnosis

(1) Ectopic pregnancy

(2) Implantation bleeding

(3) Molar pregnancy

(4) Vaginal infection

(5) Cervical polyp

(6) Incompetent cervix

e. Diagnostic Tests/Findings

(1) Ultrasound for gestational size/evidence of fetal heart action

(2) Serial human chorionic gonadotropin (hCG) levels

(3) Pelvic exam—size, cervical dilation, bleeding characteristics

f. Management/Treatment

(1) Bedrest may be indicated

(2) Abstain from intercourse

(3) If bleeding persists and/or abortion is incomplete may need:

　(a) D&C

　(b) Transfusion

　(c) Immunoprophylaxis with RhoGAM for all Rh-women

(4) Counsel regarding signs of infection

(5) Offer reassurance and support for grief/loss

(6) Provide diabetic screening

2. Incompetent Cervix

a. Definition: Painless dilatation of the cervix in the 2nd trimester, with ballooning of the membranes into the vagina, and expulsion of the fetus

b. Etiology/Incidence

(1) Associated with

　(a) Cervical trauma or surgeries

　(b) Abnormal cervical development, e.g., DES exposure in utero

(2) Usually occurs between 16 and 20 weeks

(3) Tends to recur

c. Signs and Symptoms

(1) Pressure sensation in vagina

(2) Leaking of fluid

d. Differential Diagnosis

(1) Uterine infection

(2) Premature labor

e. Physical Findings

(1) Speculum exam shows membranes bulging through the cervical os

(2) Fetal parts in vagina

f. Diagnostic Tests/Findings—ultrasound shows short cervix

g. Management/Treatment

(1) Placement of a cervical cerclage

(2) Bedrest

(3) Pelvic rest

(4) Observe for PROM or chorioamnionitis

3. Ectopic Pregnancy

a. Definition: Implantation of fertilized ovum outside the endometrial cavity

b. Etiology/Incidence

(1) Most (95%) occur in fallopian tubes, primarily in ampulla or isthmus

(2) Incidence 1/100 pregnancies; causes 12% of maternal deaths

(3) Risk factors—pregnancy that occurs in woman with history of

(a) Prior bilateral tubal ligation (BTL)

(b) PID, STD

(c) Tubal surgery

(d) IUD in situ

(e) Previous ectopic pregnancy

(f) Progestin-only contraceptive use

   c. Signs and Symptoms/Physical Findings

      (1) Before rupture

         (a) History of early pregnancy symptoms

         (b) May be asymptomatic

         (c) Amenorrhea followed by vaginal spotting/bleeding

         (d) Lower abdominal pain, usually one-sided

         (e) Normal or slightly enlarged uterus

      (2) After rupture

         (a) Sharp, one-sided abdominal pain; may radiate to shoulder

         (b) Vertigo/fainting/shock

         (c) Vaginal spotting/bleeding

         (d) Adnexal tenderness, fullness/possible mass

         (e) Pronounced cervical motion tenderness

         (f) Posterior fornix may bulge secondary to blood in cul-de-sac

   d. Differential Diagnosis

      (1) SAB

      (2) Appendicitis

   e. Diagnostic Tests/Findings

      (1) Ultrasound—adnexal mass without intrauterine pregnancy

      (2) CBC—may show leukocytosis with decreased Hgb/Hct

      (3) Serum Beta hCG—positive, but lower hCG level than expected for gestation

      (4) Serial Beta hCG—abnormal doubling time

   f. Management/Treatment

      (1) Hospitalization

      (2) Surgical repair or removal of damaged tube

      (3) Replacement of blood/fluid loss

(4) RhoGAM administration for Rh- woman

(5) Methotrexate therapy may be considered if gestation < 6 weeks, tubal mass < 3.5 cm diameter, and no fetal heart activity

4. Placenta Previa

a. Definition: Placenta improperly implanted in lower uterine segment

b. Etiology/Incidence

(1) Unknown, may have defective blood vessels in decidua

(2) Associated with multiparity, previous cesarean birth, breech or transverse lie, multiple gestation, previous uterine surgery

c. Signs and Symptoms/Physical Findings

(1) Painless vaginal bleeding with onset at end of 2nd trimester or into 3rd trimester

(2) Uterus soft, relaxed, nontender

(3) No evidence of fetal distress unless hypovolemic shock, abruption, or cord accident

(4) Persistent abnormal fetal presentation

d. Differential Diagnosis

(1) Abruptio placentae

(2) Severe cervicitis

(3) Cervical lesions

(4) Nonvaginal bleeding

e. Diagnostic Tests/Findings

(1) Ultrasound demonstrates low-lying placenta

(2) Hgb/Hct may indicate need for transfusion

(3) Electronic fetal monitoring may indicate fetal distress

f. Management/Treatment

   (1) Prior to 37 weeks with minimal bleeding—expectant management

    (a) Usually requires hospitalization and bedrest

    (b) Fetal surveillance

    (c) Observation of mother for increased bleeding

    (d) Address psychosocial issues associated with bedrest and pregnancy complication

   (2) After 37 weeks, or with maternal hemorrhage or fetal distress, anticipate delivery

   (3) Vaginal or rectal digital examination is contraindicated

 5. Abruptio Placentae

  a. Definition: Premature separation of normally implanted placenta from uterine wall (usually partial, may be complete)

  b. Etiology/Incidence

   (1) Unknown

   (2) Contributing factors

    (a) Trauma

    (b) Decreased blood flow to placenta

    (c) PIH or chronic hypertension

    (d) Uterine anomaly or tumor

    (e) Alcohol consumption, smoking, cocaine use

    (f) Increased maternal age or parity

    (g) Short umbilical cord

   (3) Complications

    (a) Fetal death

    (b) Maternal death from hemorrhage or irreversible shock

    (c) Disseminated Intravascular Coagulation (DIC)

  c. Signs and Symptoms/Physical Findings

   (1) Accompanied by severe, unremitting abdominal pain

      (2) Bright red vaginal bleeding may be:

         (a) Very large in amount, or

         (b) Minimal, secondary to concealed hemorrhage

      (3) Rigid, irritable, hypertonic uterus

      (4) Shock

      (5) Fetal distress

   d. Differential Diagnosis

      (1) Placenta Previa

      (2) Appendicitis

      (3) Hematoma of rectus muscle

      (4) Ovarian cyst

   e. Diagnostic Tests/Findings

      (1) Ultrasound—for placental location/integrity

      (2) Hgb/Hct may indicate need for transfusion

      (3) Electronic fetal monitoring may indicate fetal distress

      (4) Vaginal or rectal digital examination is contraindicated

   f. Management/Treatment

      (1) Immediate transport for emergency care

      (2) Treatment varies according to maternal/fetal status

         (a) Maternal hemorrhage, fetal distress—immediate delivery

         (b) Immature fetus, absence of fetal distress, maternal hypovolemia or anemia—expectant management

6. Gestational Trophoblastic Neoplasia (GTN)

   a. Definition: A disease process caused by abnormal development of the trophoblast resulting in a benign or malignant tumor

      (1) Hydatidiform mole—chorionic villi are converted into a mass of clear vesicles which vary in size; may be complete or partial; most common form of GTN

    (2) Invasive mole—trophoblastic tissue overgrowth may invade the uterus, adjacent structures, or distant sites

    (3) Choriocarcinoma—rare, highly malignant form of trophoblastic mole with rapid local or distant spread

  b. Etiology/Incidence

    (1) Higher incidence in women from Mexico and southeast Asia

    (2) Associated with advanced maternal age, especially > 40

  c. Signs and Symptoms

    (1) Severe nausea and vomiting extending beyond 12 weeks gestation

    (2) Persistent dark-red or brownish vaginal discharge

    (3) Absence of quickening

    (4) Passage of grape-like vesicles

    (5) Symptoms of preeclampsia prior to 20 weeks

  d. Differential Diagnosis

    (1) SAB

    (2) Hyperemesis gravidarum

    (3) Multiple gestation

  e. Physical Findings

    (1) Size large for dates until 2nd trimester, then decreases

    (2) Signs of preeclampsia prior to 20 weeks

    (3) No fetal heart tones or fetal movement

  f. Diagnostic Tests/Findings

    (1) Ultrasound—"snow storm" pattern

    (2) Beta hCG—abnormally elevated 100 days or more after LMP

    (3) Hgb/Hct—decreased

  g. Management/Treatment

    (1) If GTN suspected—ultrasound, beta hCG, CBC

      (2) Consult with physician—anticipate evacuation of mole

      (3) Chemotherapy if serum beta hCG fails to fall, plateaus, or rises after evacuation

      (4) Chemotherapy may be given prophylactically for invasive mole

      (5) Beta hCG weekly until 3 consecutive negative results after procedure completed, then monthly beta hCG for 6 months; if still negative, beta hCG every 2 months for 6 months

      (6) Pregnancy contraindicated for 1 year

          (a) Recommend reliable contraception

          (b) Oral contraceptives not contraindicated

- Dermatologic Conditions

   1. Dermatitis of Pregnancy

      a. Definition: Pruritic condition over entire body that can occur any time in pregnancy

      b. Etiology/Incidence—unknown, but resolves following delivery

      c. Signs and Symptoms

         (1) Severe itching

         (2) Papular rash

      d. Differential Diagnosis

         (1) Allergic rash

         (2) Contact dermatitis

         (3) Pruritic urticarial papules and plaques of pregnancy (PUPPP)

         (4) Pruritus gravidarum

         (5) Varicella

         (6) Scabies

      e. Physical Findings

         (1) Discrete erythematous papules with or without excoriation

(2) Hyperpigmented areas where papules have healed

f. Diagnostic Tests/Findings—not significant

g. Management/Treatment

(1) Oatmeal baths/Aveeno Solution

(2) Loose fitting clothing; no skin irritants

(3) Systemic corticosteroids in severe cases per physician

2. Pruritic Urticarial Papules and Plaques of Pregnancy (PUPPP)

a. Definition: A pruritic condition characterized by discrete erythematous papules, plaques and hive-like patches over the abdomen, thighs, occasionally buttocks, legs and arms (rarely seen above mid-thorax, and never on the face)

b. Etiology/Incidence—unknown; more common in primiparas, rarely recurs, has no adverse effects

c. Signs and Symptoms

(1) Itching of lesions

(2) Hive-like or vesicular rash

d. Differential Diagnosis—same as Dermatitis of Pregnancy

e. Physical Findings

(1) Discrete erythematous papules, plaques, and hive-like patches on the abdomen, thighs, buttocks, arms, legs

(2) May observe thin, pale halo surrounding papules

(3) Face, neck and upper trunk are free from lesions

f. Diagnostic Tests/Findings—none indicated

g. Management/Treatment

(1) Soothing baths, e.g., oatmeal, Aveeno, Domeboro

(2) Avoid scratching affected areas

(3) Wear loose clothing

(4) Topical antipruritic, e.g., Calamine lotion, corticosteroid cream

(5) Antihistamine, e.g., Diphenhydramine (Benadryl)

3. Pruritus Gravidarum—Cholestasis of Pregnancy, Jaundice of Pregnancy

   a. Definition: A dermatologic condition characterized by general pruritus resulting from intrahepatic cholestasis

   b. Etiology/Incidence

      (1) Cause is unknown, but may be stimulated by high levels of estrogen in those with dominant inherited trait

      (2) Usually occurs in 3rd trimester, but has been reported earlier

      (3) Pruritus caused by elevated serum bile acids

      (4) Adverse pregnancy outcomes may include—preterm labor/birth, intrapartum fetal distress, postpartum hemorrhage

   c. Signs and Symptoms

      (1) Mild to severe itching on hands, soles of feet, and torso

      (2) Itching is worse at night

      (3) May report jaundice

   d. Differential Diagnosis—hepatitis; scabies; varicella; contact dermatitis; allergic rash; PUPPP; pruritus gravidarum; dermatitis of pregnancy

   e. Physical Findings

      (1) Absence of skin lesions except scratch marks in affected areas

      (2) Jaundice of skin and sclera may be seen in about 20% of cases

   f. Diagnostic Tests/Findings

      (1) Alkaline phosphatase—increased 2-4 times

      (2) Total bile acids—increased 50-100 fold

      (3) Total bilirubin—may be increased

      (4) Ultrasound WNL—no cholelithiasis

   g. Management/Treatment

      (1)   Soothing baths, e.g., oatmeal, Aveeno, Domeboro

      (2)   Avoid scratching affected area

      (3)   Wear loose clothing

      (4)   Topical anti-pruritic, e.g., Calamine lotion or corticosteroid cream (1% Hydrocortisone)

      (5)   Antihistamine, e.g., Diphenhydramine (Benadryl)

      (6)   Cholestyramine with or without sedative, e.g., phenobarbital

      (7)   Vitamin K supplementation for mother/newborn

      (8)   Fetal surveillance

- Infections

   1. Urinary Tract Infections (UTI)

      a. Asymptomatic Bacteriuria (ASB)

         (1)   Definition: The presence of actively multiplying bacteria in the urinary tract without accompanying symptoms

         (2)   Etiology/Incidence

            (a)   Incidence in pregnancy 2-10%; if untreated, 25% will progress to acute infection

            (b)   Predisposing factors

               i)   Diabetes, sickle trait/disease, immunosuppression

              ii)   Increased age and parity

             iii) Economically disadvantaged

            (c)   Causative organisms

               i)   *Escherichia coli* (80-90% of asymptomatic infections)

              ii)   *Klebsiella* and *Proteus*

         (3)   Signs and Symptoms—none

         (4)   Physical Findings—within normal limits

            (a)   Afebrile

(b) Absence of suprapubic tenderness

(c) Absence of costovertebral angle tenderness (CVAT)

(5) Diagnostic Tests/Findings

    (a) Urinalysis (UA) may be positive for leukocyte esterase or nitrites

    (b) Over 10 WBC/HPF on UA

    (c) Urine culture >100,000 colony forming units per mL (cfu/mL) of same bacteria on clean-catch specimen

(6) Management/Treatment

    (a) UA at first prenatal visit

    (b) Culture and sensitivity as indicated; treat according to sensitivities on urine culture

        i) Amoxicillin

        ii) Nitrofurantoin (Macrodantin)

        iii) Cephalosporin (Keflex)

    (c) Repeat UA, culture and sensitivities following completion of therapy

    (d) Physician consult for recurrence, failure to respond, or suspected pyelonephritis

b. Cystitis

(1) Definition: The presence of >100,000 colonies of the same species of bacteria in the bladder of a person with urinary tract symptomatology

(2) Etiology/Incidence

    (a) Urinary tract infections are the most common bacterial infections encountered during pregnancy

    (b) Usually uncomplicated, but may progress to kidney infection (pyelonephritis) if untreated or not successfully treated

    (c) Causative organisms—usually *E. coli, Klebsiella,* and *Proteus*

(3) Signs and Symptoms

    (a) Frequency

    (b) Urgency

    (c) Dysuria

    (d) Hematuria

    (e) Pyuria

    (f) Suprapubic discomfort

(4) Differential Diagnosis

    (a) Pyelonephritis

    (b) Vaginal infection

(5) Physical findings

    (a) May be WNL

    (b) Erythema/edema at urinary meatus

    (c) Suprapubic tenderness

    (d) CVAT, fever are suspicious for pyelonephritis

(6) Diagnostic Tests/Findings

    (a) Urine culture >100,000 of a single pathogenic bacteria on a clean-catch, midstream specimen

    (b) Microscopic exam may reveal WBCs, RBCs, or bacteria

(7) Management/Treatment

    (a) Treat according to sensitivities on urine culture

        i) Amoxicillin

        ii) Nitrofurantoin (Macrodantin)

        iii) Cephalosporin (Keflex)

    (b) Urinary analgesic as needed—Phenazopyridine (Pyridium)

    (c) Repeat culture following completion of therapy

      (d)   Increase oral fluids (use urinary acidifier, e.g., cranberry juice)

      (e)   Prophylaxis—void before and after intercourse, frequent voiding to keep bladder empty, proper hygiene, avoid bladder irritants, e.g., caffeine, smoking, alcohol

      (f)   Physician consult for recurrence, failure to respond, or suspected pyelonephritis

c. Pyelonephritis

    (1) Definition: Kidney infection with positive urine culture and systemic symptoms of fever, flank tenderness, chills

    (2) Etiology/Incidence

      (a)   A common serious medical complication, occurs in 1-2.5% of pregnancies

      (b)   Women with UTI history prior to pregnancy and ASB at first prenatal visit are 10 times more likely to develop active UTI

      (c)   Unilateral, right-sided in > 50% of cases; bilateral in 25%

    (3) Signs and symptoms

      (a)   Abrupt onset of fever, chills, and CVA discomfort

      (b)   May complain of

          i) Dysuria, urgency, frequency

          ii) Anorexia, nausea, vomiting

    (4) Differential Diagnosis

      (a)   Appendicitis

      (b)   Ectopic pregnancy

      (c)   PID

    (5) Physical Findings

      (a)   Fever

      (b)   Unilateral or bilateral CVAT

(6) Diagnostic Tests/Findings

    (a) Clean-catch, midstream urine culture with >100,000 cfu/mL of bacteria (usually *E. Coli, Klebsiella,* or *Proteus*)

    (b) Additional labs may include CBC, sedimentation rate and blood cultures

(7) Management/Treatment

    (a) Prompt hospital treatment indicated

    (b) IV hydration

    (c) Broad spectrum IV antibiotics

    (d) Urine cultures every 2-4 weeks for remainder of pregnancy, with antibiotic therapy if bacteriuria returns; prophylactic antibiotic therapy may be necessary for remainder of pregnancy after second recurrence of bacteriuria

2. Vulvovaginitis

  a. Definition: Inflammation of vagina and vulva usually caused by *Candida albicans, Trichomonas vaginalis,* or mixed bacterial flora (bacterial vaginosis)

  b. Etiology/Incidence

    (1) Interference with normal physiology, nutritional status, or protective mechanisms of vaginal epithelium

    (2) Vulvovaginal Candidiasis (VVC or Monilia)—fungi growing as budding yeast cells and chains or hyphae; very common in pregnancy; increased incidence in HIV positive women and with diabetes mellitus

    (3) Trichomoniasis—presence of motile protozoan with undulating membrane and 4 flagella; usually sexually transmitted

    (4) Bacterial vaginosis (BV)—increase of several species of anaerobic bacteria

  c. Signs and Symptoms—may include complaints of pruritus, irritation, burning, abnormal discharge, strong odor, spotting, dyspareunia, dysuria

d. Differential Diagnosis—gonorrhea; chlamydia; leukorrhea of pregnancy

e. Physical Findings

   (1) Monilia—thick, curdy white discharge; possible erythematous/excoriated vulva

   (2) Trichomoniasis—frothy, greenish-white discharge; reddened vaginal mucosa; possible friable and/or "strawberry" cervix; possible edema and erythema of vulva

   (3) Bacterial vaginosis—thin, grayish-white discharge with strong "fishy" odor (usually without vulvar involvement)

f. Diagnostic Tests/Findings

   (1) Monilia

      (a) Wet mount with saline and KOH to identify mycelia (hyphae and spores)

      (b) pH = 3.8-4.2

   (2) Trichomoniasis

      (a) Wet mount with saline to identify motile or non-motile trichomonads

      (b) pH ≥ 5

   (3) Bacterial vaginosis

      (a) Wet mount with saline to identify clue cells (stippling of epithelium) and with KOH for +amine odor (whiff test)

      (b) pH ≥ 4.5

   (4) When indicated, test for STDs including HIV

   (5) Diabetic screen for recurrent monilia

g. Management/Treatment

   (1) Monilia

      (a) Antifungal vaginal cream or tablet, e.g., miconazole, clotrimazole, terconazole

           (b) Seven day therapy, as opposed to 1 or 3 day therapy, more effective during pregnancy

           (c) Infant born through infected vagina may develop thrush

      (2) Trichomoniasis

           (a) Metronidazole (Flagyl) is drug of choice, but is contraindicated in 1st trimester

               i) If used for severe infection in 2nd or 3rd trimester, administer 2 g single dose

               ii) Avoid alcohol during treatment (can cause abdominal cramping and severe nausea and vomiting)

           (b) In early pregnancy, clotrimazole may be used to alleviate symptoms

           (c) Refer sexual partner for treatment and STD/HIV testing

      (3) Bacterial vaginosis

           (a) Clindamycin—vaginal gel preferred during pregnancy

           (b) Amoxicillin

           (c) Metronidazole—not in 1st trimester

      (4) General considerations

           (a) Good hygiene

           (b) Cotton underwear

           (c) Loose clothing

  3. Sexually Transmitted Diseases (STDs)

    a. Chlamydia—see Gynecologic Disorders Chapter

      (1) Pregnancy Implications

           (a) In utero transmission has not been demonstrated

           (b) Treatment of chlamydial infection during pregnancy has been reported to improve obstetric outcome;

may be associated with premature rupture of membranes

    (c) Infant

        i) Conjunctivitis will develop in 20-50% without prophylaxis; develops 7-15 days after birth

        ii) Pneumonia will develop in up to 10% of exposed infants; develops within 1-3 months after birth

  (2) Management/Treatment in Pregnancy

    (a) Ideally, screen all pregnant women for chlamydia at first prenatal visit and repeat testing at 36 weeks and as indicated by symptoms or history of exposure

    (b) Treatment in pregnancy

        i) Erythromycin base (see CDC Guidelines for current recommendations)

        ii) If erythromycin not tolerated, use amoxicillin (limited data regarding efficacy)

        iii) Tetracycline contraindicated in pregnancy due to teratogenic effect on fetal bone and tooth formation

    (c) Refer sexual partners for treatment—treat all sexual partners (contacts within 30 days of symptom onset)

    (d) Abstain from intercourse until patient *and* partner have completed treatment

    (e) Test-of-cure not required if erythromycin is used

    (f) Notify delivery room personnel of positive culture if patient in labor at time of diagnosis

 b. Gonorrhea—see Gynecologic Disorders Chapter

  (1) Pregnancy Implications

    (a) Incidence in pregnancy is estimated at 0.5-7%

    (b) In utero transmission has not been shown to occur

   (c) Gonorrhea infection during pregnancy may lead to premature rupture of membranes, chorioamnionitis, preterm delivery, IUGR, and maternal postpartum sepsis

   (d) Infants born through a gonococcal-infected birth canal are at high risk for ophthalmic infection and possible disseminated gonococcal infection

  (2) Management/Treatment in Pregnancy

   (a) Ideally, screen all pregnant women at first prenatal visit, and repeat testing at 36 weeks if previously positive or at high risk for STD

   (b) Treatment in pregnancy—see CDC Guidelines

    i) Cefixime plus erythromycin (to cover coexisting chlamydia)

    ii) If allergic, substitute spectinomycin plus erythromycin

   (c) Treat all sexual partners

   (d) Abstain from intercourse until patient and partner have completed treatment

   (e) Test-of-cure not routinely recommended

 c. Herpes Genitalis (HSV)—see Gynecologic Disorders Chapter

  (1) Pregnancy Implications

   (a) Neonatal infections may be acquired at delivery via contact with infected secretions

   (b) Transplacental transmission to fetus is rare but incidence increased with primary infection

   (c) Infants may be born vaginally to asymptomatic mothers

  (2) Management/Treatment in Pregnancy

   (a) Acetaminophen

   (b) Topical anesthetic

   (c) Keep lesions dry and clean

(d) Acyclovir not recommended in pregnancy unless disseminated infection occurs

(e) If no genital lesions present at onset of labor, vaginal delivery indicated (cervical cultures done during labor if mother has history of HSV-2)

(f) If lesions present at onset of labor, cesarean delivery is indicated if membranes are intact or have ruptured within specified hours of surgery

d. Human Papillomavirus (HPV)—see Gynecologic Disorders Chapter

(1) Pregnancy Implications

(a) Condylomata acuminata may increase during pregnancy due to relative immunosuppressed state

(b) Lesions may be so large as to impede delivery

(c) Fetus rarely infected, although laryngeal papillomatosis possible

(2) Management/Treatment in Pregnancy (if possible, avoid treatment during pregnancy)

(a) Trichloracetic acid to small vulvar lesions

(b) Cervical evaluation/treatment by trained colposcopist

(c) Podophyllin and 5-fluorouracil (Efudex) contraindicated during pregnancy

(d) Treat co-existent vaginitis or STDs

(e) Refer partner(s) for examination/treatment

(f) Physician consult for cervical lesions or large, extensive growths

e. Syphilis—see Gynecologic Disorders Chapter

(1) Pregnancy Implications

(a) Fetus can acquire infection through placenta; infection may result in SAB, preterm delivery, death, congenital defect or congenital disease

       (b) Forty percent chance of fetal transmission if untreated in primary or secondary stages; 10-30% chance of transmission in latent

   (2) Management/Treatment in Pregnancy—see CDC Guidelines for treatment of choice

       (a) Early syphilis—benzathine penicillin 2.4 million units

       (b) Late syphilis—benzathine penicillin 7.2 million units

       (c) For penicillin allergy, consider desensitization, or erythromycin (does not treat fetus)

       (d) Refer partner for testing and treatment

       (e) Jarisch-Herxheimer reaction possible with treatment during primary or secondary stage (acute febrile response within first 24 hours which could lead to uterine contractions and/or FHR decelerations)

       (f) Treatment prior to 18 weeks will usually prevent fetal infection; treatment after 18 weeks will treat fetal infection and reduce risk of congenital syphilis

  f. Hepatitis B—see Non-Gynecologic Disorders Chapter

   (1) Pregnancy Implications

       (a) Hepatitis B is a serious infection and is threatening to fetus and neonate as it can cause lasting severe sequelae; HB_eAG+ mother (chronic carrier) is associated with high rate of transmission to infant

       (b) Transmitted in semen, vaginal secretions, blood products, saliva, breast milk, and across placenta

       (c) Some adults and many neonates with acute hepatitis B develop chronic carrier state and may develop its sequelae

       (d) Increased rate of preterm delivery

   (2) Management/Treatment in Pregnancy

       (a) Screen all pregnant women

   (b) Prevention—active immunization with hepatitis B vaccine prior to pregnancy, or during pregnancy in high risk clients

   (c) Hepatitis B immunoglobulin (HBIG) plus vaccination upon exposure

   (d) Infant born to HB_sAG positive mother

     i) HBIG within 12 hours of birth

     ii) Hepatitis B vaccine within 12 hours of birth and again at 1 month and at 6 months

 g. Human Immunodeficiency Virus (HIV)—see Non-Gynecologic Disorders Chapter

  (1) Pregnancy Implications

   (a) Transmission to fetus/infant through

     i) Vertical infection (perinatal transmission)

     ii) Breast milk

   (b) Perinatal transmission approximates 20-30% if untreated; increased transmission occurs when mother is severely ill during pregnancy due to multiplying virus; treatment with Zidovudine (AZT) during pregnancy can significantly reduce vertical transmission

  (2) Management/Treatment in Pregnancy—in consultation with physician

   (a) Offer screening to all pregnant women

   (b) If mother is HIV positive

     i) Monitor for progression of disease (CD4 cell count at least in every trimester)

     ii) Counsel regarding perinatal transmission

     iii) Zidovudine (AZT) therapy to treat mother and decrease risk of transmission to fetus

     iv) Screen for other STD (especially those producing ulcerations) and tuberculosis

v) Refer to support systems

vi) Avoid invasive procedures during labor and delivery

vii) Bathe infant prior to injections

viii) Mother should not breastfeed

4. Other Infections—note: TORCH is an acronym for a variety of organisms which can cause harm to the fetus during pregnancy; **T**oxoplasmosis, **O**ther, (an ever expanding and wide range of infections including hepatitis B, streptococcus, gonococcus, treponema, etc.), **R**ubella, **C**ytomegalovirus, and **H**erpes; some of these conditions appear elsewhere in this chapter; others are discussed below

a. Toxoplasmosis

(1) Definition: Protozoan infection which is innocuous in adults but can cause severe fetal damage if contracted during pregnancy

(2) Etiology/incidence

(a) Caused by *Toxoplasma gondii,* an organism found in

i) Raw or poorly cooked meat of infected animal

ii) Cat feces

iii) Contaminated soil

(b) Many women have antibodies prior to pregnancy which protect fetus

(c) With maternal infection, organism crosses placenta

i) Risk of infection increases with duration of pregnancy

ii) Early gestation infection is more virulent but less common

iii) Can cause an increase in SAB, IUGR, preterm birth, stillborn, neonatal anomalies or death

(3) Signs and Symptoms—maternal infection

(a) Usually subclinical

(b) Malaise, fatigue

(c) Headache, sore throat, slight fever

(d) Skin rash

(e) Enlarged nodes

(4) Differential Diagnosis—other viral syndromes

(5) Physical Findings

(a) Lymphadenopathy—posterior cervical nodes

(b) Splenomegaly

(c) Maculopapular rash

(d) Slight temperature elevation

(6) Diagnostic Tests/Findings

(a) Elevated IgG antibodies per serologic testing

(b) Current infection identified by serial titers

(c) Differential may show atypical lymphocytes

(7) Management/Treatment

(a) Primary prevention

i) Avoid close contact with cats and cat feces

ii) Do not eat undercooked meat

iii) Use care in gardening where cats have access; wear gloves

(b) Acute infection of mother

i) No universal agreement on treatment during pregnancy

ii) Refer to physician

b. Rubella

(1) Definition: Highly contagious droplet-spread viral disease usually of minor import in the absence of pregnancy

(2) Etiology/Incidence

      (a) Caused by rubella virus with incubation of 14-21 days

      (b) Ten to fifteen percent of women at risk for infection

      (c) Airborne transmission

      (d) Fetus infected transplacentally

      (e) Highly teratogenic—risks for fetal death or congenital rubella syndrome (CRS):

            i) In first 4 weeks are 50%

            ii) In weeks 5-8 are 25%

            iii) In weeks 9-12 are 10%

            iv) No reported cases of CRS after 20 weeks

      (f) CRS consists of classic symptoms of cataracts, heart defects, deafness, and delayed mental, physical, and motor development

    (3) Signs and Symptoms (of maternal infection)

      (a) May be asymptomatic or have very mild prodrome, e.g., slight fever, malaise, headache, conjunctivitis

      (b) Itchy, red rash starting on face and moving down body to trunk

    (4) Differential Diagnosis

      (a) Rubeola

      (b) Fifth Disease

      (c) Allergic rash

      (d) Contact dermatitis

      (e) Scarlet fever

    (5) Physical Findings

      (a) Afebrile or low grade fever

      (b) Macular rash lasting 3 days

      (c) Posterior auricular, suboccipital and posterior cervical lymphadenopathy frequently present

(6) Diagnostic Tests/Findings

    (a) Screen all pregnant women for immune status

    (b) Serologic rubella titer of ≤ 1:8 indicates non-immune

    (c) Following exposure in a non-immune woman, a 4-fold rise in titer 2 weeks later indicates infection

(7) Management/Treatment

    (a) Discuss prevention with non-immune mother

    (b) With exposure to rubella

        i) Discuss possible risks to fetus

        ii) Support decision regarding continuation of pregnancy

    (c) Treat symptomatically

        i) Acetaminophen for fever and headache

        ii) Diphenhydramine (Benadryl) for pruritus

    (d) Vaccinate in immediate postpartum period

    (e) Immunization during pregnancy is contraindicated, however, no cases of CRS have been documented from immunization

c. Tuberculosis (TB)—see Non-Gynecologic Disorders Chapter

  (1) Pregnancy Implications

    (a) Pregnancy does not alter course of active TB

    (b) Infant commonly infected through postnatal exposure, but also possible through placenta and amniotic fluid

  (2) Management/Treatment in Pregnancy

    (a) Treat active disease with at least 2 tuberculostatic drugs, e.g., isoniazid (INH) plus rifampin or ethambutol

    (b) Streptomycin and Pyrazinamide (PZA) are contraindicated in pregnancy

        (c) Infants born to mothers with active infection need INH prophylaxis and should be isolated from mother until her sputum becomes negative

        (d) Screen household contacts and treat accordingly

- Preterm Labor (PTL)

  1. Definition: Labor that occurs after 20 weeks but before the completion of 37 weeks of gestation; characterized by cervical dilatation of ≥ 2 cm or cervical effacement of $\geq 80\%$; associated contractions may not be painful or apparent to mother

  2. Etiology/Incidence—unknown; risk factors include

     a. Prior preterm delivery

     b. Multiple gestation or hydramnios

     c. Low pre-pregnant weight and/or inadequate weight gain

     d. Cigarette smoking and drug abuse (especially cocaine)

     e. Uterine anomalies and incompetent cervix, cervical trauma

     f. Selected genital and urinary tract infections

     g. Economically disadvantaged

     h. Age < 17 or > 34

  3. Signs and Symptoms/Physical Findings

     a. Change or increase in vaginal discharge, including spotting

     b. Uterine contractions, with or without pain—more than 5 per hour

     c. Cramping in lower abdomen—periodic or constant

     d. Dull, low backache—periodic or constant

     e. Pelvic pressure or fullness

  4. Differential Diagnosis

     a. Incompetent cervix

     b. Braxton Hicks contractions

  5. Diagnostic Tests/Findings—none apply

  6. Management/Treatment

a. Prevention

(1) Preconception counseling to identify/eliminate behavioral risks and identify/treat infections, i.e., UTI, STD

(2) Assess for risk factors at first prenatal visit, reassess at 22-26 weeks and as needed

(3) Modify risk factors whenever possible, e.g., nutrition counseling, stop or reduce smoking or drug use, reduce strenuous activity and prolonged standing, no sexual orgasm after 28 weeks with prior or current PTL

(4) Fetal movement record beginning at 28 weeks gestation

(5) Educate all women about PTL warning signs and symptoms

b. Hospitalization, hydration, fetal monitoring

c. Tocolytic therapy if membranes intact, cervical dilatation is < 4 cm, effacement is < 80% and no fetal distress

d. Commonly used tocolytic agents include ritodrine, terbutaline, magnesium sulfate, nifedipine

e. After PTL is stopped, mother may be on tocolysis (oral or by pump at home, with activity limitations and selected EFM)

f. Fetal assessments, particularly lung maturity as indicated

g. Interval prenatal visits every 2 weeks or as indicated until 36 weeks, and then weekly

- Postterm Pregnancy

  1. Definition: gestation which exceeds 42 weeks from onset of last normal menstrual period

  2. Risks

     a. Macrosomia—can produce shoulder dystocia during delivery, postpartum hemorrhage due to overdistended uterus

     b. Meconium aspiration

     c. Fetal distress due to:

        (1) Oligohydramnios with cord compression accidents

        (2) Placental insufficiency with resultant hypoxia

       d. Increased chance for traumatic or surgical delivery

  3. Assessment

       a. Review accuracy of dating (best if done early in pregnancy)

       b. Monitor fetal movement counts by mother

       c. Weekly cervical assessment from 40 weeks

       d. Ultrasound to determine oligohydramnios, macrosomia, anomalies, placental senescence

  4. Management/Treatment

       a. Beginning at 41 weeks (earlier if indicated)

           (1) Bi-weekly NST

           (2) Weekly biophysical profile (NST and AFI in some practice settings)

       b. Refer for induction as appropriate

       c. Refer to physician for management by 42 weeks (earlier in some practice settings); higher incidence of significant morbidity occurs

- Substance Use/Abuse

  1. Cigarette Smoking

       a. Maternal effects

           (1) CNS stimulation

           (2) Addiction

           (3) Respiratory damage

           (4) Increases risk for certain cancers

           (5) Associated with placenta previa and abruptio placentae, premature and prolonged rupture of membranes

       b. Fetal/infant effects

           (1) Reduced oxygen resulting in fetal distress

           (2) IUGR

           (3) Increased risk for SAB, PTL, and fetal demise

           (4) Increased risk for cleft palate and heart defects

     (5) Abnormal nursing pattern

     (6) May increase risk for sudden infant death syndrome

2. Alcohol

  a. Maternal effects

     (1) Intoxication

     (2) CNS depression

     (3) Withdrawal can be associated with hypertension, tachycardia, and PTL

     (4) At risk for seizures

     (5) End organ damage to stomach, liver, esophagus, heart, CNS

  b. Fetal/infant effects

     (1) Fetal alcohol syndrome (number one cause of mental retardation); characteristics include:

        (a) Growth retardation

        (b) CNS abnormalities

        (c) Structural abnormalities, including facial, skeletal, and organ defects

     (2) Infant may have CNS depression and withdrawal, with irritability and restlessness

     (3) Long-term mental retardation and developmental delays

3. Heroin

  a. Maternal effects

     (1) Tolerance

     (2) CNS depression

     (3) At significant risk for HIV

     (4) Acute, painful withdrawal

     (5) Higher incidence of SAB and PTL

  b. Fetal/infant effects

     (1) IUGR

        (2) Vertically acquired HIV

        (3) Neonatal addiction and narcotic withdrawal syndrome

        (4) Irritable, agitated, tremulous, hyperactive newborn, with increased tonicity and high-pitched cry

        (5) Infant at risk for abnormal sleep and ventilatory patterns, and also for poor feeding

        (6) Possible long-term neurobehavioral deficits

  4. Cocaine/Crack

      a. Maternal effects

        (1) Increased heart rate and blood pressure

        (2) Anorexic and underweight

        (3) Vascular constriction

        (4) Decreased blood flow to placenta

        (5) At significant risk for SAB, abruptio placentae, and PTL

      b. Fetal/infant effects

        (1) IUGR

        (2) Fetal hypertension

        (3) At risk for intrauterine stroke

        (4) Increase in genitourinary abnormalities

        (5) Fetal distress and possible fetal death

        (6) Infant is irritable, agitated, with tremors and jitters, and is inconsolable

        (7) At risk for seizures

        (8) Abnormal sleep and ventilatory patterns

        (9) Long-term developmental delays and deficits in attention and learning

  5. Other Substances—a variety of other substances can be abused, including illicit drugs or prescription drugs, all of which can have deleterious effects on mother and infant

a. Phencyclidine (PCP)—hallucinatory, depressant, and stimulating effects may complicate labor and delivery for mother, and cause fetal CNS damage, including microcephaly

b. Sedative-hypnotics, e.g., Valium, Halcion, Xanax, can cause respiratory and CNS depression in mother and cleft lip, abnormal heart rhythm, and death to the fetus

c. Amphetamines—cause increases in maternal heart rate, blood pressure, and breathing; anorexia and weight loss; fetus is at risk for IUGR and hypoxia

- Genetic Disorders

   1. Definition: An abnormality in number and/or structure of chromosomes or in alteration of genes leading to congenital anomaly or inborn error of metabolism

   2. Etiology/Incidence

      a. Chromosomal abnormalities

         (1) Incidence

            (a) Chromosomal aberrations occur in 1:160 liveborns or 2-3% of deliveries

            (b) Chromosomal abnormalities seen in > 50% of spontaneous abortions and in 5% of stillborns

         (2) Examples

            (a) Trisomy 21—Down Syndrome

            (b) Monosomy, 45,XO—Turner Syndrome

            (c) Polysomy, 47,XXY—Klinefelter Syndrome

      b. Single gene disorders

         (1) One percent of liveborns have single gene mutation

         (2) May be autosomal dominant, autosomal recessive, or sex-linked

         (3) Examples include cystic fibrosis, sickle cell anemia, Tay-Sachs disease, achondroplasia, hemophilia

      c. Polygenic/multifactorial disorders

(1) One percent of liveborns have mutations of multiple genes that in conjunction with environmental factors lead to single organ/structure defects, e.g., neural tube defects, facial clefts, cardiac defects, club foot

(2) Incidence increases for offspring of affected parents

3. Signs and Symptoms/ Physical Findings—depends upon individual circumstance of family or personal history of congenital anomaly

4. Diagnostic Tests/Findings

   a. Maternal serum alphafetoprotein/multiple marker

   b. Ultrasound may show anomaly or IUGR

   c. Genetic studies of cell samples to identify single gene defects may be obtained via:

      (1) CVS

      (2) Amniocentesis

      (3) PUBS

5. Management/Treatment

   a. Preconception counseling for couples with a history of congenital anomalies

   b. Offer referral for genetic counseling to all pregnant women over age 35 and to other high risk couples

   c. Be supportive with decision to terminate or proceed with pregnancy

- Other Conditions

   1. Multiple Gestation

      a. Definition: More than one fetus in utero at the same time

      b. Etiology/Incidence

         (1) Multiple pregnancy in the U.S. approximates 1.5% of live births

            (a) Monozygotic—two or more fetuses develop from same ovum

        (b) Dizygotic—results from fertilization of 2 separate ova

            i) Increases with age and parity of mother

            ii) Is familial

            iii) More common in African-Americans and rare in Asians

            iv) More common with infertility treatment

    (2) Morbidity and mortality are 2-5 times higher than for singleton primarily due to:

        (a) Preterm labor/birth

        (b) Small for gestational age

        (c) Cord accidents

        (d) Malpresentations

        (e) Congenital anomalies

        (f) Twin-to-twin transfusion

    (3) Maternal complications include:

        (a) PIH

        (b) Hyperemesis

        (c) Anemia

        (d) Placenta previa

        (e) Preterm labor

        (f) Postpartum hemorrhage

c. Signs and Symptoms

    (1) Exaggerated or prolonged nausea and vomiting

    (2) Excessive fetal movement

    (3) "Feels" larger than expected

d. Physical Findings

    (1) Fundal height greater than expected

    (2) Two or more fetal heart tones

   (3) Many fetal parts upon abdominal palpation

  e. Diagnostic Tests/Findings

    (1) Ultrasound to demonstrate multiple gestation

    (2) MSAFP level elevated

  f. Management

    (1) Frequent prenatal visits

    (2) Prevention/identification of preterm labor

    (3) Serial ultrasound to assess fetal growth

    (4) Adequate nutrition

      (a) Additional 300 calories per day

      (b) Iron and folic acid supplements based on lab values

      (c) Suggested weight gain of 40-60 pounds

    (5) Reduced activity and extended rest

    (6) Antepartum testing as needed

 2. Oligohydramnios

  a. Definition: Abnormally low volume of amniotic fluid, less than 200 mL

  b. Etiology/Incidence

    (1) Etiology unknown

    (2) Associated with IUGR, congenital anomalies, especially renal, and postdatism

    (3) Occurrence in early pregnancy associated with poor fetal outcome

    (4) Fetal complications

      (a) Pulmonary hypoplasia

      (b) Musculoskeletal malformation or amputation

      (c) Cord compression

      (d) Chronic fetal hypoxia

  c. Signs and Symptoms

      (1)   Small for dates

      (2)   Beyond due date

      (3)   May have fluid slowly leaking from vagina

  d. Differential Diagnosis

      (1)   Premature rupture of membranes (PROM)

      (2)   IUGR

  e. Physical Findings

      (1)   Uterine size smaller than expected for date

      (2)   Fetal outline easily palpated

      (3)   Fetus not ballottable

  f. Diagnostic Tests/Findings

      (1)   Largest pocket of amniotic fluid is < 1 cm by ultrasound

      (2)   Sterile speculum exam—if PROM:

          (a)   Vaginal pooling—positive (amniotic fluid forms pool)

          (b)   Fern test—positive (amniotic fluid applied to slide dries to form "fern-like" crystals on microscopic exam)

          (c)   Nitrazine test—positive (test strip turns dark blue; alkaline pH of 7.0-7.5)

  g. Management/Treatment

      (1)   Antenatal fetal surveillance once or twice per week

      (2)   Rest in left lateral recumbent position

      (3)   Fetal movement counts from 28 weeks

      (4)   Refer to physician

      (5)   Consider amnioinfusion in labor

      (6)   If PROM present evaluation for expectant management vs delivery

3. Hydramnios (Polyhydramnios)

a. Definition: Abnormally high volume of amniotic fluid, over 2000 mL

b. Etiology/Incidence

    (1) Occurs in 0.2-1.6% of pregnancies

    (2) Etiology unknown

        (a) Maternal factors

            i) Multiple gestation

            ii) Rh or other isoimmunization

            iii) Diabetes

        (b) Fetal factors

            i) CNS or neural tube defects

            ii) GI tract anomalies

    (3) Complications

        (a) Maternal discomfort

        (b) Fetal anomalies

        (c) Preterm labor

        (d) Prolapsed cord

        (e) Placental abruption if fluid removed too quickly

        (f) Postpartum hemorrhage

c. Signs and Symptoms

    (1) Rapid abdominal growth

    (2) Dependent edema

    (3) Uterine contractions

    (4) Shortness of breath

d. Differential Diagnosis

    (1) Multiple gestation

    (2) Fetal macrosomia

    (3) Molar pregnancy

e. Physical Findings

    (1) Uterine size larger than expected for dates

    (2) Difficulty hearing fetal heart tones and palpating fetus

f. Diagnostic Tests/Findings—increased amniotic fluid as measured by ultrasound

g. Management/Treatment

    (1) Refer to physician

    (2) Antenatal fetal surveillance

    (3) Modified bedrest

    (4) Fetal movement counts from 28 weeks

    (5) Amniocentesis to remove excess fluid in presence of pain and shortness of breath in mother

Preparation for Childbirth

Although the nurse practitioner does not usually manage labor, a basic level of knowledge is important to enable the NP to provide anticipatory guidance and to answer questions

- Diagnosis of labor

  1. True labor

    a. Contractions—should be timed from beginning of one to the beginning of the next

      (1) Occur at regular intervals which gradually shorten and increase in duration and intensity

      (2) Contractions initially felt in back, then radiate to lower abdomen

      (3) Intensified by walking

      (4) Positive association between strength of contraction and intensity of discomfort

    b. Cervix dilates and effaces

    c. Bloody show usually present (pink tinged mucus from cervix)

      d. Station shows presenting part is descending into pelvis

      e. Sedation does not stop true labor

  2. False labor

      a. Contractions are irregular in frequency, duration, and intensity

      b. Discomfort is felt mainly in abdomen

      c. Walking has no effect on contractions

      d. Cervix does not dilate or efface

      e. Sedation will stop contractions of false labor

  3. Rupture of membranes

      a. Spontaneous rupture of membranes occurs at onset of labor in 50% and during Stage I or II in 50%

      b. Premature rupture of membranes occurs before the onset of labor and places the woman at risk for:

         (1) PTL if before 37 weeks gestation

         (2) Ascending intrauterine infection possible with prolonged rupture (> 24 hours); prophylactic antibiotics instituted

      c. Assessment of membrane status

         (1) Nitrazine test is blue when in contact with amniotic fluid (alkaline pH of 7.0-7.5)

         (2) Fern test—positive in presence of amniotic fluid

- Assessment for vaginal birth after cesarean delivery (VBAC)

  1. Standards

      a. Women with 1 previous lower transverse uterine incision cesarean birth (LTCS) are encouraged to attempt VBAC

      b. With 2 or more previous LTCS, women may attempt VBAC, but need very close monitoring during labor

      c. Women with previous classical incisions are not candidates for VBAC

  2. Contraindications to VBAC

      a. Previous incision into body of uterus, e.g., classical cesarean

      b. Fetal malpresentation or macrosomia

      c. Multiple gestation

      d. If reason for prior cesarean is again present, e.g., dystocia

  3. Risks of VBAC

      a. Complete or incomplete rupture of previous scar in uterus

      b. Need for cesarean birth after trial of labor

- Patient Education Issues

  1. Childbirth education should be available to all pregnant women and their partners; need to identify or advocate for development of classes to meet needs of parents of various cultural and linguistic backgrounds; various types of classes are designed to meet special needs

      a. Preconception counseling provides anticipatory guidance and assures maximum state of health and reduced risk factors prior to conception

      b. Prepared childbirth series may be Lamaze or Bradley, or an eclectic combination of several, with content including

          (1) Prenatal education—nutrition, exercise, rest, self-care measures, sexuality, fetal development, danger signs

          (2) Preparation for labor and delivery—birth process, relaxation and breathing exercises, positioning, analgesia/ anesthesia

          (3) Postpartum care—self-care, feeding methods, infant care, management of common discomforts, nutrition, exercise, danger signs, follow-up, contraception

      c. Special classes—refer as needed

          (1) Cesarean or VBAC classes

          (2) Teen pregnancy classes

          (3) Classes for siblings or grandparents

          (4) Breastfeeding classes

          (5) Parenting classes

      d. Client education remains an important component of prenatal visits

2. Analgesia/Anesthesia

   a. Ideal pain relief alleviates discomfort of labor but is safe for mother and fetus and does not impede labor

   b. Mother cannot be guaranteed specific analgesia/anesthesia because individual situations vary

   c. There is diversity of opinion regarding goal of unmedicated childbirth among professional and lay communities

   d. Types of relief

      (1) Non-pharmacologic, e.g., imagery, hypnosis, massage

      (2) Analgesics, e.g., morphine, meperidine, fentanyl, stadol, nisentil

      (3) Sedative-hypnotics, e.g., secobarbital, pentobarbital

      (4) Ataractics, e.g., hydroxyzine, promethazine (potentiate effects of opiates, have antiemetic properties)

      (5) Regional anesthesia

         (a) Pudendal nerve block

         (b) Spinal blocks—for delivery

         (c) Epidural blocks—continuous or episodic

         (d) Paracervical blocks—rarely used due to fetal brady-cardia

      (6) Local anesthesia

         (a) Viscous lidocaine to introitus during second stage labor

         (b) Perineal infiltration prior to episiotomy or repair

3. Fetal monitoring—to evaluate fetal status during labor

   a. Auscultatory

      (1) With fetoscope or doppler

      (2) Normal range = 120-160 BPM, decreases during contrac-tions

   b. Electronic

      (1) External

      (2) Internal—requires rupture of membranes, allows for electrocardiography

      (3) Assessment in relation to contractions identifies:

          (a) Early decelerations (normal—due to head compression)

          (b) Late decelerations (due to fetal hypoxia)

          (c) Variable (due to cord compression; may occur normally in late labor, or be an indication of fetal distress)

Postpartal Period

- Definition: First 6 weeks following delivery

  1. Immediate—first 24 hours

  2. Early—first 2 weeks

  3. Late—2-6 weeks

- Physiologic Changes

  1. Involution

     a. Uterus approximates pre-pregnant state in 6 weeks

     b. Decidua is cast off as lochia; stages are

        (1) Rubra—red, lasts up to 3 days; persistent lochia rubra may indicate retained placental fragments or subinvolution

        (2) Serosa—pink, 3-10 days

        (3) Alba—yellowish white, 10-21 days

     c. Placental site healed by exfoliation to prevent scar formation

     d. Entire uterus has new endometrium (compact and spongy layers)

     e. Cervix, vaginal walls and perineum may be bruised and lacerated following delivery, but heal within 6 weeks

  2. Perineum—episiotomy should heal without swelling, redness, infection or drainage

3. Cardiovascular/Hematological

   a. Blood loss up to 500 mL considered normal

     (1) Hgb will fall 1-1.5 g/dL and Hct 2-4% for each 500 mL of blood loss

     (2) Hgb and Hct usually rise by 3-7 days unless blood loss excessive

   b. Cardiac output increases 60-80% over pregnancy levels during first 24-48 hours

     (1) Increased venous return

     (2) Decreased systemic vascular resistance due to reduction in uterine size

     (3) Return of interstitial fluids to vascular compartment

   c. Blood volume returns to pre-pregnant levels by 2 weeks postpartum

   d. Compensatory bradycardia (50-70 BPM) from increased cardiac output common for 6-10 days

   e. White blood cell count may be elevated due to granulocytosis

4. Pulmonary

   a. Twenty-five percent increase in chest wall compliance due to decreased pressure on diaphragm

   b. Lower progesterone levels cause rapid return to pre-pregnant tidal and minute volume; sensations of dyspnea disappear

5. Vital Signs

   a. Woman expected to be afebrile after first 24 hours

   b. Puerperal fever—temperature elevation of 100.4°F or greater on any of the first 10 days postpartum, excluding day 1

6. Urinary Tract

   a. Bladder and urethra often bruised and edematous

   b. Hematuria normal immediately postpartum

   c. Diuresis occurs first 12-24 hours

   d. Bladder tone usually restored within 5-7 days

e. Dilated ureters and renal pelves return to normal by 6 weeks

7. Gastrointestinal

a. Hunger is normal post-delivery

b. Peristalsis decreased due to decreased muscle tone and decreased intra-abdominal pressure

c. Constipation is common

d. Large hemorrhoids may have appeared with second stage pushing

8. Hormonal changes

a. Return of menses

(1) Non-nursing mothers—45% in 6-8 weeks; 70% within 12 weeks; 90% by 24 weeks

(2) Nursing mothers—45% within 12 weeks; 90% by 6 months; tends to be longer when mother is exclusively breastfeeding

b. Return of ovulation

(1) Fifty percent of non-nursing mothers ovulate during first cycle

(2) Nursing mothers—one or more anovulatory cycles usually occur before ovulation

c. Nursing mothers have prolonged hypo-estrogenic state

(1) May cause vaginal dryness

(2) Associated with postpartum affective disorders

- Family Integration

1. Maternal psychologic responses

a. Taking-in behaviors

(1) Need for rest and replenishment of energy after work of labor

(2) Need to review labor and delivery experience and deal with questions and disappointments

(3) Need to establish physical intactness and basic functioning

      b. Taking-hold behaviors—ready to assume care of infant and self

  2. Parent-infant interactions

      a. Reciprocal relationship between parents and baby; need baby in alert state

         (1) Exploration of infant

         (2) Identification and claiming behaviors

      b. First-time parents may need reassurance regarding performance of caretaking

  3. Barriers to bonding process

      a. High-risk or complicated birth

      b. Prematurity

      c. Complications which necessitate separation of mother and infant

      d. Poor social support

  4. Sibling relationships

      a. Responses include interest and pride in new sibling as well as jealousy, anger and regression

      b. Intervention

         (1) Sibling visitation in hospital

         (2) Coming home from hospital

            (a) Bring gift from new baby

            (b) Have father carry new baby into home so mother is free to embrace older child

            (c) Plan quality one-on-one time with siblings

            (d) Allow older children to help

- Postpartum assessment—routinely scheduled at 6 weeks postpartum; some providers see clients at 2 weeks postpartum to offer support, and to assess and intervene more promptly with developing problems

  1. History

      a. Review prenatal and intrapartum records

      b. Interval maternal history

(1) General adaptation—rest/sleep, activity/exercise, nutrition

(2) Physical condition—breasts, bowel and bladder elimination, perineum/episiotomy/hemorrhoids, bleeding, pain

(3) Behavioral and psychological responses to childbearing/infant care

(a) Infant feeding

(b) Maternal blues

(c) Response to infant's temperament

2. Physical assessment

a. Two weeks postpartum

(1) Vital signs returned to normal; PIH should be resolving

(2) Uterus no longer palpable above symphysis; external cervical os closed

(3) Vagina

(a) Introitus lacks tone; cystocele/rectocele may be present

(b) Kegel exercises recommended

(4) Episiotomy and/or lacerations healed with no signs of infection

(5) Abdomen

(a) Striae pink/purple and obvious

(b) Diastasis recti abdominis may be present; may respond to abdominal tightening exercises

(6) Breasts

(a) Non-lactating—breast engorgement should be resolved

i) Should be soft and non-tender

ii) Small amount milk may be expressed

(b) Lactating

i) Lactation well-established

ii) Nipples prominent without damage

      b. Six weeks postpartum—all systems returned to pre-pregnant state

- Breastfeeding

  1. Physiology

      a. Following delivery, rapid drop in estrogen and progesterone levels, with rise in prolactin secreted by anterior pituitary

      b. Prolactin stimulates alveolar cells and promotes milk production

      c. Oxytocin is released from posterior pituitary in response to infant suckling, stimulating myoepithelial cells to speed flow of milk from breast (let-down reflex)

      d. Emptying of the breast triggers increased production of milk

  2. Maternal nutritional needs

      a. Caloric demand is increased 200 Kcal over pregnancy or 500 Kcal per day over non-pregnant requirements

      b. Total requirement—2500-2700 Kcal per day

  3. Education for successful breastfeeding

      a. Start as soon as possible after delivery

      b. Position infant with mouth in line with nipple and stimulate rooting reflex until mouth is open wide; infant's jaws should grasp behind the nipple, covering most of the areola

      c. Infant should be fed on demand, every $1\frac{1}{2}$ to 3 hours using both breasts at each feeding

      d. Avoid nipple confusion by not offering bottle or pacifier until nursing is well-established

      e. Avoid supplementary feedings

      f. Check with provider before taking medications; almost all medications enter milk to some degree, but most needs can be met with drugs that do not contraindicate breastfeeding

      g. Six to eight wet diapers per day indicate adequate fluid intake

      h. Inform of community resources such as lactation consultant or La Leche League

      i. Sexual arousal normal with breastfeeding

4. Contraindications to breastfeeding

   a. HIV positive mother

   b. Systemic illness of mother

      (1) Active TB

      (2) Other debilitating illness

      (3) Hepatitis B carrier state is not a contraindication if infant receives prophylaxis and immunization at birth

   c. Maternal medication which would enter milk and harm infant

      (1) Refer to reliable resources for alternative to avoid unnecessary discontinuation of breastfeeding

      (2) Can pump breasts until free of medication

   d. Mother's aversion to breast feeding

5. Common Problems/Interventions

   a. Nipple soreness

      (1) Minimize by correct positioning and attachment of infant; varying positions may help

      (2) Expose nipples to air

      (3) Use of ointments/lanolin controversial

   b. Engorgement

      (1) Frequent feedings with adequate emptying of breasts

      (2) Warm soaks

      (3) Support with brassiere or binder

   c. Plugged duct—localized area of fullness, tenderness, afebrile; can progress to mastitis if not relieved

      (1) Warm soaks

      (2) Frequent nursing with massage over affected area

      (3) Change infant position

6. Complications

   a. Mastitis

(1) Definition: Infection of glandular tissue of breast with potential for abscess formation

(2) Etiology/Incidence

    (a) Occurs in 1-2% of nursing mothers

    (b) Ten percent of these develop abscesses which must be surgically drained

    (c) *Staphylococcus aureus* isolated in about 50% of cases; *E. coli* and various other aerobes and anaerobes may be involved

    (d) Predisposing factors

        i) Trauma—nipple damage

        ii) Poor handwashing or other contamination

        iii) Stasis—infrequent feedings or failure to empty breast

(3) Signs and Symptoms

    (a) Breast tenderness, inflammation

    (b) Fever

    (c) Malaise; flu-like symptoms

(4) Differential Diagnosis

    (a) Clogged duct

    (b) Simple engorgement

    (c) Breast abscess

    (d) Viral syndrome

(5) Physical Findings

    (a) Unilateral involvement—breast swollen, tender, tense and warm

    (b) Mild temperature elevation

    (c) Axillary lymphadenopathy

(6) Diagnostic Tests/Findings

    (a) Usually not necessary

        (b) Periglandular tissue is involved and pus may not be present in milk; therefore, culture is of little value

        (c) Leukocytosis in peripheral blood smear

   (7) Management/Treatment

        (a) Antibiotics—oral semi-synthetic penicillin or cephalosporin; small amount in milk is not harmful to infant

        (b) Rest; emptying of breast by nursing or pump; supportive, non-restrictive brassiere; analgesics for pain 20-40 minutes prior to breastfeeding

- Bottle feeding

  1. Early feedings per hospital protocol

  2. Usual intake $1\frac{1}{2}$ to 3 ounces every 3-4 hours

  3. Clean technique is adequate—sterilization no longer required

  4. Position infant with head slightly elevated and hold bottle so that no air enters nipple

  5. Burp infant carefully midway and after each feeding

  6. Feed-on-demand schedule

  7. Hold for all feedings—never prop bottles

  8. Formula alone is adequate for first 4 months of life

  9. Use formula for first year of life; whole milk is not well-digested, and provides inadequate nutrition for proper growth

- Education for self-care

  1. Care of perineal area/hemorrhoids

     a. Prevent infection and promote healing

     b. Ice and/or heat

     c. Avoid contamination of episiotomy/lacerations with feces

     d. Adequate analgesia

     e. Kegel exercises

     f. Sitz baths

2. Breast care

    a. Non-nursing

        (1) Snug brassiere or binder

        (2) Avoid stimulation in shower or by hand expression

        (3) Ice pack 20 minutes every 2 hours for severe engorgement

        (4) Analgesics if indicated

    b. Breastfeeding

        (1) Well-fitting, supportive brassiere

        (2) Cleanliness—wash hands before touching nipples; avoid soap when bathing which removes natural protective oils

        (3) Frequent emptying to build milk supply and avoid stasis

3. Exercises

    a. In hospital—chin to chest abdominal tightening

    b. Avoid heavy lifting immediately postpartum

    c. Resume vigorous exercise program after postpartum check-up

    d. Post-cesarean section advice similar to that for any abdominal surgery

4. Family planning

    a. Sexual activity may be resumed when episiotomy is healed and lochia stopped

    b. Contraception, i.e., condoms and spermicides should be used with resumption of intercourse for nursing and non-nursing mothers

    c. If breastfeeding, combined hormonal contraception should be delayed, but progestin-only preparations are acceptable

    d. Non-breastfeeding mother may be given Depo-Provera or Norplant prior to discharge, or may begin oral contraceptives 2 weeks postpartum

5. Fatigue and sleep disturbances

    a. Sleep deprivation and resulting fatigue can complicate recovery

    b. Delay return to work for as long as possible

    c. Rest periods should be taken during day

- Complications of the Postpartum Period

  1. Delayed postpartum hemorrhage

    a. Definition: Excessive vaginal bleeding after the first 24 hours postpartum

    b. Etiology/Incidence—overall incidence of hemorrhage is 5-8% of deliveries, with the majority occurring immediately following delivery; late hemorrhage occurs most often between 6-10 days after delivery due to retained placental fragments, infection and/or uterine subinvolution

    c. Signs and Symptoms

      (1) Fatigue, abdominal pain, persistent low backache

      (2) Steady oozing of brownish lochia or brisk bright red bleeding

    d. Differential Diagnosis—coagulopathy, trauma

    e. Physical Findings

      (1) Heavy lochia with foul odor

      (2) Cervical os open after first week

      (3) Uterus soft, boggy, tender

    f. Diagnostic Tests/Findings

      (1) CBC may reveal anemia

      (2) Ultrasound may identify retained placental fragments

    g. Management/Treatment

      (1) Refer to physician for consideration of curettage

      (2) Methylergonovine Maleate (Methergine) 0.2 mg every 6 hours for 2 days

      (3) Antibiotic therapy if infection present

  2. Perineal/vaginal hematoma

a. Definition: Collection of blood in connective tissue of reproductive tract; may occur anywhere in the birth canal; may involve significant amount of concealed hemorrhage

b. Etiology/Incidence—occurs after injury to a blood vessel; blood slowly oozes into the tissue and forms the hematoma; usually recognized while the mother is in the hospital, although with early discharge or delayed formation, this may be seen after patient is discharged; more likely to occur with forceps delivery or difficult, prolonged second stage labor

c. Signs and Symptoms

    (1) Severe pain, pressure, bruising

    (2) Signs of hypovolemic shock if hemorrhage is severe

d. Differential Diagnosis—abscess

e. Physical Findings

    (1) Fluctuant, tender mass felt on vaginal or rectal examination

    (2) Asymmetrical size of vulva or buttocks

f. Management/Treatment

    (1) Ice pack to perineum post-delivery to decrease bleeding

    (2) Monitor for signs and symptoms of shock/infection

    (3) Notify physician for surgical evacuation and repair

3. Thrombophlebitis/thromboembolism

a. Definition: Inflammation of vein with thrombus formation; if thrombus is detached, is called an embolism

    (1) Superficial thrombophlebitis (SVT)—involves the superficial vascular system, and is not life-threatening

    (2) Deep vein thrombophlebitis (DVT)—more dangerous because an embolism can travel directly to heart or lungs

b. Etiology/Incidence

    (1) Less common with early ambulation; occurs in about 0.1-1% of deliveries

    (2) If untreated, up to 24% of DVT will develop pulmonary embolism

    (3) Contributing factors

        (a) Varicosities

        (b) Obesity

        (c) Prolonged inactivity

        (d) Advanced maternal age

        (e) Traumatic delivery or cesarean section

c. Signs and Symptoms—swelling, pain and tenderness in affected leg

d. Differential Diagnosis—SVT or DVT; pain due to muscular strain or injury

e. Physical Findings

    (1) Positive Homan's sign

    (2) Induration along affected vein

f. Diagnostic Tests/Findings—doppler ultrasound, impedance plethysmography to visualize thrombi and measure blood flow

g. Management/Treatment

    (1) SVT—bedrest, elevation, warm soaks

    (2) DVT—rest and anticoagulation

    (3) Observe for signs of embolism

4. Pulmonary Embolism

a. Definition: Clot travels through the venous system and obstructs a portion of the pulmonary circulation; can result in sudden death, and must be treated immediately in hospital; size and location determine severity of symptoms

b. Etiology/Incidence—most commonly preceded by DVT; may also occur in women with pelvic infection when septic pelvic emboli develop

c. Signs and Symptoms

    (1) Dyspnea and shortness of breath

(2) Tachycardia

(3) Chest pain

(4) Cough, hemoptysis

(5) Sweating, pallor

(6) Fear of impending death

    d. Management/Treatment—immediate emergency care

5. Genital Infection—overview

    a. Definition: Puerperal infection has occurred when client has temperature of 38°C (100.4°F) on 2 occasions at least 24 hours apart; types of infection include

        (1) Localized episiotomy/laceration/wound infections

        (2) Endometritis

        (3) Parametritis

        (4) Peritonitis

    b. Etiology/Incidence

        (1) Occurs in 2-8% of postpartum women

        (2) Major risk factors

            (a) Premature rupture of membranes

            (b) Long labor

            (c) Chorioamnionitis during labor

            (d) Operative delivery

        (3) Contributing factors—poor nutritional status; anemia; pre-existing beta streptococcal, chlamydia or mycoplasma infection; diabetes; lacerations of reproductive tract

    c. Signs and Symptoms—depend on location of infection; fever common to all

    d. Management/Treatment

        (1) Identification of infection site

        (2) Identification of organism if possible—usually polymicrobial

        (3) Antibiotic therapy—route is determined by site and severity

        (4) Rest, fluids

        (5) Incision and drainage of any developing abscess

6. Episiotomy Infection

    a. Definition: Localized infection involving skin, subcutaneous tissue and superficial fascia; may spread to deeper tissues

    b. Etiology/Incidence—occurs in 0.5-3% of women; more likely with more extensive incision

    c. Signs and Symptoms—pain, drainage, incontinence of flatus or stool

    d. Differential Diagnosis—rectovaginal fistula; lack of integrity of anal sphincter

    e. Physical Findings—serous, serosanguineous or purulent drainage, possible foul odor; wound disruption with gaping incision which may be covered with necrotic material

    f. Diagnostic Tests/Findings—wound culture (probably not helpful, because area is grossly contaminated); CBC showing elevated WBC with shift to left

    g. Management/Treatment

        (1) Physician consultation

        (2) Warm sitz baths

        (3) Open and debride wound if indicated

        (4) Allow to heal by granulation; if necessary, surgical repair can be performed later

        (5) Oral broad-spectrum antibiotic

7. Endometritis/Parametritis/Peritonitis

    a. Definition: Intrauterine infection initially involving decidua which, if untreated, spreads to myometrium, adjacent pelvic structures, and ultimately to the abdominal cavity via the broad ligament

b. Etiology/Incidence—most common type of postpartum infection; as high as 50% incidence after cesarean section in some studies

c. Differential Diagnosis—extragenital infection; thrombophlebitis

d. Signs and Symptoms/Physical Findings

(1) Fever

(2) Tender, boggy uterus

(3) Cervical motion pain on pelvic exam

e. Management/Treatment

(1) Physician referral

(2) Usually begin with high dose multiple IV. antibiotic regimen with aerobic and anaerobic potency

(3) In some high-risk cases, prophylactic therapy is initiated at delivery

8. Bladder Distention, Urinary Retention and UTI

a. Etiology/Incidence

(1) UTI occurs in 2-4% of postpartum women

(2) Bladder and lower tract somewhat atonic

(3) Trauma from labor and delivery, conduction anesthesia, and rapid filling of bladder from diuresis contribute to occurrence of bladder distention in early postpartum period

(4) Risk of UTI increases with urinary stasis

(5) Intrapartum catheterization and vaginal examinations increase risk of UTI

b. Diagnosis, Management and Treatment—see previous discussion; guidelines are not different from UTI occurring at any other time

9. Perinatal Loss

a. Grief-causing events

(1) Miscarriage/abortion

(2) Stillbirth

(3) Premature birth

(4) Birth of infant with congenital anomaly

(5) Unplanned cesarean section

b. Stages of grief

(1) Shock/denial—may need to have explanations repeated many times

(2) Anger—may be directed at caregivers

(3) Bargaining

(4) Depression

(5) Acceptance/reorganization

c. Interventions

(1) Plan—hospital should have protocol and personnel trained and comfortable in dealing with perinatal grief

(2) Assign patient to primary nurse to provide continuity of care

(3) Mementos—prepare mementos, e.g., photographs, lock of hair, ID bracelet, crib card, etc.

(4) Have appropriate literature available

(5) Encourage client to view fetus/infant

(6) Referrals to social worker, psychologist, or specialized support groups

    (a) Hospital social worker

    (b) Resolve Through Sharing

    (c) Compassionate Friends

    (d) AMEND (Assisting Mothers Experience Neonatal Death)

    (e) Local groups

10. Postpartum Affective Disorders

a. Postpartum Blues

      (1)   Definition: Mild depression, occurs 3-10 days after delivery, usually lasting no more than 2 weeks

      (2)   Etiology/Incidence—occurs in 50-80% of women; possibly related to hormonal changes, fatigue, increased responsibilities

      (3)   Signs and Symptoms—depressed mood, crying spells, irritability, insomnia

      (4)   Differential Diagnosis—major depression, significant physical illness

      (5)   Management/Treatment—usually resolves with social support; discuss normality of postpartum stress; encourage communication with significant others; refer to support group if indicated

b. Postpartum Depression

      (1)   Definition: Meets standards for diagnosis of situational depression at other periods of life; onset 2 weeks to 3 months post delivery; includes sleeping and eating changes, feelings of worthlessness, lack of bonding; risk of child neglect or abuse

      (2)   Etiology/Incidence—reported in 10-26% of women; may progress to chronic depression in 25% of these women; etiology similar to postpartum blues; increased risk in women with family history of depression, previous history of depression, lack of social support

      (3)   Signs and Symptoms—persistent and increasing in severity; tearfulness, despondency, insomnia, loss of appetite, social withdrawal, feelings of inadequacy

      (4)   Differential Diagnosis—postpartum blues, psychosis

      (5)   Management/Treatment—important to evaluate all women for symptomatology; refer for medication, psychotherapy and social support

c. Postpartum Psychosis

      (1)   Definition: Severely impaired functional ability; may include hallucinations, delusions, cognitive impairment,

suicidal or homicidal ideation; acute onset usually 2-4 weeks post-delivery, but may occur up to 3 months

(2) Etiology/Incidence—occurs in 1-2/1000 women; genetic, physiologic and psychosocial factors have been implicated

(3) Signs and Symptoms—may include classic symptoms of depression or bi-polar disorder; inability to care for self and/or infant

(4) Differential Diagnosis—organic brain syndrome; schizophrenia; non-psychotic depression

(5) Management/Treatment—refer for immediate evaluation for hospitalization and therapy

QUESTIONS

Select the best answer.

1. During pregnancy, a common physiologic alteration seen in the CBC is:

    a. Decreased platelet count
    b. Elevated WBC
    c. Decreased mean corpuscular volume

2. The least predictive risk factor for the development of varicose veins during pregnancy is:

    a. Family history
    b. Weight gain in prior pregnancy
    c. Occupation which involves standing

3. A positive sign of pregnancy is:

    a. Positive pregnancy test
    b. Auscultation of fetal heart sounds
    c. Uterine enlargement

4. During pregnancy, sexual relations are contraindicated when:

    a. 36 weeks gestation has been reached
    b. Placenta previa is present
    c. There is a previous history of spontaneous abortion

5. Nausea, vomiting and fatigue usually subside by:

    a. 8-10 weeks
    b. 12-14 weeks
    c. 16-20 weeks

6. Which of the following antibiotics is always contraindicated in pregnancy:

    a. Cephalosporins
    b. Erythromycin
    c. Tetracycline

7. The most common indication for referral for genetic counseling and amniocentesis is:

    a. Elevated serum alphafetoprotein (AFP)
    b. Drug or medication exposure during first trimester
    c. Maternal age

8. The occurrence of bleeding gums for the first time during pregnancy is probably related to:

    a. High progesterone levels
    b. Pre-existing periodontal disease
    c. High estrogen levels

9. An increased risk for preterm labor is associated with:

    a. Congenital fetal anomaly
    b. Excessive weight gain
    c. Previous preterm labor or delivery

10. The most common initial emotional response to the diagnosis of pregnancy is:

    a. Ambivalence
    b. Denial
    c. Fear

11. The recommended weight gain in pregnancy for women of normal weight for height is:

    a. Not more than 20 pounds
    b. Approximately 25 pounds
    c. Over 30 pounds

12. The leading known cause of mental retardation in the U.S. is:

    a. Down Syndrome
    b. Birth injury
    c. Fetal alcohol syndrome

13. The recommended screening test for gestational diabetes is:

    a. Three-hour glucose tolerance test
    b. Blood sugar measurement 1 hour 50 gram glucose screen
    c. Random blood sugar on women with positive urinary glucose

14. The best initial step in counseling about prenatal nutrition is:

   a. Give list of all recommended foods
   b. Assess nutritional adequacy based on 24-hour recall
   c. Stress importance of adequate intake of milk

15. The largest percentage of calories in the prenatal diet should come from:

   a. Meat and milk
   b. Breads and cereals
   c. Fruits and vegetables

16. Which of the following immunizations is contraindicated in pregnancy:

   a. Hepatitis B
   b. Measles
   c. Diphtheria/Tetanus

17. Dietary alterations to reduce the severity of nausea and vomiting of pregnancy include:

   a. Increase iron and vitamin supplements to 2 times per day
   b. Small, frequent low-fat meals
   c. Avoid carbonated beverages

18. When assessment of the pregnant woman reveals a discrepancy between actual uterine size and that expected by dates, which of the following tests would be ordered:

   a. Non-stress test (NST)
   b. Ultrasound
   c. 24-hour urine for creatinine

19. The most significant risk factor for the development of postpartum psychiatric illness is:

   a. Previous perinatal loss
   b. Previous history of psychiatric illness
   c. Unplanned pregnancy

20. A pelvic examination of a pregnant woman at 8 weeks post LMP might find:

   a. Uterus firm, not enlarged
   b. Softening of utero-cervical isthmus, uterus about 9 cm
   c. Uterus soft, approximately 12 by 14 cm

21. One of the elements in the fetal biophysical profile is the:

    a. Amniotic fluid volume
    b. Fetal movement count
    c. Umbilical cord blood sampling

22. Examination of the thyroid in pregnancy may normally find:

    a. Slight enlargement
    b. Increased firmness
    c. Diffuse nodularity

23. Rh antibody testing is performed at 28 weeks when:

    a. The mother is A- and the father is A-
    b. The mother is A- and the father is A+
    c. The mother is A+ and the father is A-

24. Asymptomatic bacteriuria can put the woman at risk for:

    a. Pyelonephritis
    h Abruptio placentae
    c. Intrauterine growth retardation

25. A low-risk mother should initiate fetal movement counts at which gestation:

    a. 28 weeks
    b. 32 weeks
    c. 36 weeks

26. Chadwick sign is positive when:

    a. The cervix is soft
    b. The isthmus is soft
    c. The cervix is blue

27. The infant has the greatest risk of developing hepatitis B if the mother is:

    a. HB_eAG positive
    b. HB_sAG positive
    c. HB_sAG negative

28. Evidence suggests that chlamydial infection during pregnancy may be associated with which of the following:

a. Congenital anomaly of the urinary tract
b. Premature rupture of membranes
c. Transplacental fetal transmission

29. Which of the following is a risk factor for development of gestational diabetes:

    a. Oligohydramnios in previous pregnancy
    b. Prior macrosomic infant
    c. Insulin-dependent diabetes mellitus in first cousin

30. Increasing severity of preeclampsia is evidenced by:

    a. Hemoconcentration with decreased platelets
    b. Patellar hyporeflexia
    c. Significant increase in urinary output

31. Physiologic changes of normal pregnancy increase the risk of developing:

    a. Vulvovaginal candidiasis
    b. Bacterial vaginosis
    c. Trichomoniasis

32. Which of the following best describes preterm labor:

    a. Moderate uterine contractions, 35.2 weeks gestation, 50% cervical effacement
    b. Minimal uterine contractions, 36.1 weeks gestation, 3 cm of cervical dilation
    c. Rhythmic uterine contractions, 37.6 weeks gestation, 1 cm of cervical dilation

33. A 45XO chromosomal karyotype is indicative of:

    a. Klinefelter Syndrome
    b. Marfan Syndrome
    c. Turner Syndrome

34. The most accurate early ultrasound measurement for purposes of dating a pregnancy is:

    a. Crown-rump length
    b. Biparietal diameter
    c. Abdominal circumference

35. A non-nursing postpartum mother can be apprised that the earliest she should anticipate return of menses is:

    a. 3-4 weeks
    b. 6-8 weeks
    c. 10-12 weeks

36. The main risk for a woman undergoing VBAC is:

    a. High level of pain
    b. Unsuccessful delivery and need for forceps
    c. Rupture of previous scar

37. Antenatal fetal surveillance in a woman with a postterm pregnancy would include:

    a. Non-stress test or contraction stress test
    b. In-home fetal monitoring
    c. Hospitalization for 24-hour assessment

38. In a pregnant woman with suspected hyperthyroid, which of the following tests should be ordered?

    a. TBG and AST
    b. T_3 and T_4
    c. TSH and free T_4

39. The appropriate test to determine if an individual is a sickle cell carrier is:

    a. Total iron binding capacity
    b. Hemoglobin electrophoresis
    c. ELISA

40. Which of the following is characteristic of pruritus gravidarum:

    a. Generalized itching in the absence of eruptions
    b. Symmetrical pruritic plaque and urticarial lesions
    c. A fine macular rash over most of the body

41. Most urinary tract infections are caused by which of the following organisms:

    a. *Proteus*
    b. *Klebsiella*
    c. *E. Coli*

42. A woman with a twin gestation is at significant risk for:

    a. Renal failure
    b. Preeclampsia
    c. Third degree laceration

43. Inadequate amount of folic acid during pregnancy is related to:

    a. Cleft lip and palate
    b. Neural tube defects
    c. Cardiovascular anomalies

44. Syphilis is highly sensitive to which of the following drugs:

    a. Erythromycin
    b. Tetracycline
    c. Penicillin

45. A predisposing factor for preterm labor is:

    a. Urinary tract infection
    b. Oligohydramnios
    c. Hypothyroidism

46. Management for postpartum mastitis includes:

    a. Empty the breast via breastfeeding or pump
    b. Binding of the breasts or firm fitting brassiere
    c. Discontinuing breast feeding

47. A possible effect from the use of crack cocaine during pregnancy is:

    a. Abruptio placentae
    b. Postterm pregnancy
    c. Congenital anomalies

48. Cigarette smoking during pregnancy is associated with a higher incidence of:

    a. Intrauterine growth retardation
    b. Hydrocephalus
    c. Cord anomalies

49. The initial management option for a pregnant woman with a positive PPD is:

    a. Refer for genetic counseling

    b. Order a chest x-ray

    c. Begin INH after the fourth month

50. Without treatment, perinatal transmission of HIV occurs in approximately what percent of HIV+ mothers:

    a. 15%

    b. 25%

    c. 40%

ANSWERS

1. b	26. c
2. b	27. a
3. b	28. b
4. b	29. b
5. b	30. a
6. c	31. a
7. c	32. b
8. c	33. c
9. c	34. a
10. a	35. b
11. b	36. c
12. c	37. a
13. b	38. c
14. b	39. b
15. b	40. a
16. b	41. c
17. b	42. b
18. b	43. b
19. b	44. c
20. b	45. a
21. a	46. a
22. a	47. a
23. b	48. a
24. a	49. b
25. a	50. b

Bibliography

American College of Obstetricians and Gynecologists. Technical Bulletin #130 (July, 1989), *Diagnosis and Management of Postterm Pregnancy*. Washington, DC: Author.

American College of Obstetricians and Gynecologists. Technical Bulletin #171 (August, 1992), *Rubella in Pregnancy*. Washington, DC: Author.

American College of Obstetricians and Gynecologists. Technical Bulletin #174 (November, 1992), *Hepatitis in Pregnancy*. Washington, DC: Author.

American College of Obstetricians and Gynecologists. Technical Bulletin #181 (June, 1993), *Thyroid Disease in Pregnancy*. Washington, DC: Author.

American College of Obstetricians and Gynecologists. Technical Bulletin #185 (October, 1993), *Hemoglobinopathies in Pregnancy*. Washington, DC: Author.

American College of Obstetricians and Gynecologists. Technical Bulletin #188 (January, 1994), *Antepartum Fetal Surveillance*. Washington, DC: Author.

American College of Obstetricians and Gynecologists. Technical Bulletin #195 (July, 1994), *Substance Abuse in Pregnancy*. Washington, DC: Author.

American College of Obstetricians and Gynecologists. Technical Bulletin #200 (December, 1994), *Diabetes in Pregnancy*. Washington, DC: Author.

Callister, L. (1995). Cultural means of childbirth. *JOGNN, 24* (4), 327-331.

Cunningham, F.G., MacDonald, P.C., & Grant, N.F. (1993). *Williams obstetrics* (19th ed.). Norwalk: Appleton & Lange.

Dean, C., et al. (May, 1994). STD update '93: STDs in the 90s. ARHP Clinical Proceedings, 1-15.

Gabbe, S.G., Niebyl, J.R., & Simpson, J.L. (Eds.). (1989). *Obstetrics: Normal & problem pregnancies* (2nd ed.). New York: Churchill Livingston..

Hatcher, R.A., Guest, F., Stewart, F., Stewart, G.K., Trussell, J., Kowal, D., Cates, W., & Policar, M. (1994). *Contraceptive technology* (16th ed.). New York: Irvington Publishers.

Hawkins, J.W., Roberta, D., & Stanley-Haney, J.L. (1991). *Protocols for nurse practitioners in gynecologic settings* (3rd ed.). New York: The Tiresia Press.

Centers for Disease Control and Prevention (1993). Sexually transmitted diseases treatment guidelines. *MMWR*, 42(No. RR-14). Atlanta: U.S. Dept. of Health & Human Services.

Olds, S.B., London, M.L., & Ladewig, P.A. (1992). *Maternal newborn nursing* (4th ed.). Menlo Park, CA: Addison Wesley.

Reinhardt, M. (1994). Emergency: Ectopic pregnancy rupture. *AJN, 7* (41).

Scott, J.R., Disaia, P.J., Hammond, C.B., & Spellacy, W.N. (1994). *Danforth's obstetrics and gynecology*. Philadelphia: J.B. Lippincott.

Sherwan, L.N., Scaloveno, M.A., & Weingarten, C.T. (1991). *Nursing care of the childbearing family*. Norwalk: Appleton & Lange.

Sinclair, B.P., Fahey, L., & Yamauchi, N. (Eds.). (1993). *Regional practice guidelines, protocols, and furnishing formulary for nurse practitioners, certified nurse midwives, and physicians assistants*. Los Angeles: Kaiser Permanente, Southern California Region.

Star, W.L., Shannon, M.T., Sammons, L.N., Lommel, L.L., & Gutierrez, Y. (1990). *Ambulatory obstetrics: Protocols for nurse practitioners/nurse-midwives* (2nd ed.). San Francisco: University of California, San Francisco, School of Nursing.

Wright, L. (1994). Prenatal diagnosis in the 1990s. *JOGNN, 23* (6), 506-515.

Professional Issues

Judith A. Grandin

Nursing Research

- Significance of Nursing Research
  1. Goals of nursing research
     a. To develop a scientific knowledge base for nursing practice directed toward improving quality care and patient outcomes
     b. To influence practice, education, and health policy
     c. To provide scientific base for practice
     d. To promote professional accountability to society and individual patients
  2. Information obtained through scientific investigation influences patient outcomes directly and indirectly through
     a. Evaluation of quality of care
     b. Health promotion and disease prevention interventions
     c. Ethical dilemmas
     d. Methods for delivery of health care services
     e. Nursing education curricula
  3. Increased visibility for nursing research achieved in 1985 through creation of The National Center for Nursing Research (NCNR) under the National Institutes of Health (NIH), now the National Institute of Nursing Research; priorities for nursing research in Phase II, 1995–1999 identified as
     a. Community based nursing models
     b. Effectiveness of nursing interventions in HIV/AIDS
     c. Cognitive impairment
     d. Living with chronic illness
     e. Biobehavioral factors related to immunocompetence (L. Cooke, National Institute of Nursing Research, personal communication, June 1995)
- Nurse Research Roles
  1. Participate in evaluation and sharing of research findings for clinical application, incorporation into practice, and identification of researchable problems

2. Conduct research investigations

3. Collaborate in research projects

4. Provide clinical expertise

5. Assist others engaged in research projects

6. Expand nursing knowledge through theory development grounded in practice

- Types of Research—using a scientific method of inquiry that is rigorous, logical, and controlled permits the practitioner to design and conduct various types of research for the purpose of describing, exploring, predicting, controlling, or explaining events (Polit & Hungler, 1991)

    1. Basic research—directed towards generating new knowledge and generating or testing theory

    2. Applied research—influences clinical practice to propose solutions to current problems

- Research Methods and Designs—selection of a method usually determined by type of research problem to be studied in order to answer research questions and collect data; once method has been chosen, the researcher will select research design which guides selection of population, sampling techniques, measurement modes, data collection, and analysis (Polit & Hungler, 1991)

    1. Quantitative research methods—narrowly focused and characterized by use of numerical data to obtain information and perform statistical analyses; instruments are used to collect information under controlled conditions that limit the influence of other factors on the phenomenon under investigation

        a. Descriptive designs—often used to describe characteristics, to determine frequency of events and to categorize relationships as they naturally occur; may be used to study characteristics of a single group or differences between two groups

            (1) Longitudinal design—data is collected over time from the same group of subjects

            (2) Cross-sectional design—collects a single measure of data from various groups or subjects at one point in time

    b. Correlational designs—studies that investigate associations or relationships among variables; sometimes referred to as ex post facto designs, especially when a causal relationship is thought to exist; correlational studies examine relationships between variables in situations that have already occurred or are currently happening

        (1) Retrospective studies—ex post facto investigations in which the investigator is interested in linking some presently occurring event with other events that occurred in the past; e.g., past events are examined in a study of women with heart disease to identify factors that occurred in the past that might explain the occurrence of heart disease

        (2) Prospective Studies—variables studied prospectively, beginning with examination of the presumed cause and observing presumed effects in the future; studies undertaken to determine the effects of cigarette smoking over time are prospective studies

    c. Experimental designs—examine cause and effect relationships

        (1) The controlled experiment offers the most powerful evidence concerning the effects of one variable on another

        (2) The researcher manipulates the independent variable and randomly assigns subjects to different treatment groups

        (3) Essential characteristics

            (a) Manipulation of an independent variable believed to cause or influence the dependent variable (the outcome of interest)

            (b) Random sampling

            (c) A control group

    d. Quasi-experiments—unlike experimental research, lack either randomization or a control group but require manipulation of the independent variable

  2. Qualitative research

    a. Seeks to understand human beings by discovering the meaning of their thoughts and interactions with their environment

b. Focuses on non-numerical observations and analysis of more subjective information in narrative format to discover patterns of relationships

c. Thought to be less appropriate for establishing cause and effect relationships, studying large populations, and testing research hypotheses

d. Types of approaches to qualitative research

    (1) Phenomenological—the holistic study of experiences as they are lived emphasizing the complexity of human experience

    (2) Grounded theory—the observation of real-world experiences with the aim of developing theories that explain the event studied in these observations

    (3) Ethnographic—a method of investigating cultures or sub-cultures to develop a theory of cultural behavior

    (4) Historical—a narrative description of past events

    (5) Philosophical inquiry—includes analysis of theories, conceptual meanings and intellectual analysis of morality

    (6) Critical social theory research—analyzes thought and communication processes which have societal meaning

- Steps in the Research Process

1. Problem Statement—the statement that identifies and defines the topic to be researched; in the declarative, the problem is stated as the purpose of the study; the problem statement might also be posed as a question; the decision to use a specific type of research method and design plan is determined by the type of problem

2. Review of Literature—summary of what is known about the topic; information is gathered from primary sources (those written by the originator of the study) and secondary sources (information written by someone other than the original researcher); purpose is to identify studies for replication, and to distinguish areas where additional research is needed; this review is often done before the problem is clarified

3. Placing Study within a Framework—the use of a guiding structure such as a theory, conceptual scheme, or model that permits the

researcher to link and integrate findings to current knowledge for the purpose of advancing knowledge

4. Hypothesis—a prediction of the expected relationship between two or more variables; hypotheses translate the problem and purpose into a statement of the relationship(s) to be tested to confirm or disprove the prediction; a hypothesis contains a dependent and an independent variable

   a. Dependent variable—the outcome or effect that is predicted or explained by the research and is presumed to be produced by the independent variable

   b. Independent variable—the treatment or cause of the outcome or effect, and the variable that is manipulated in experimental designs

5. Selecting a Research Design—a methodological plan to answer the research question(s) as described previously in Research Methods and Designs

6. Defining a Population and Sampling—accurately selecting a representative sample which allows generalization of the findings beyond the specific sample being studied

   a. Population—all members of a group who have some common attribute

   b. Sample—a subset of the population selected to represent the population

      (1) Random sampling—every member of the population has the possibility of being included in the sample; studies that use random sampling based on probability reduce sampling error and increase the usefulness and generalizibility of the findings

      (2) Simple random sample—elements are selected at random from a sampling frame for inclusion in a study; most common is the use of a table of random numbers until the desired sample size is obtained

      (3) Stratified random sample—division of the sample into various strata according to certain characteristics such as age, sex, income, and diagnosis

(4) Cluster samples—a subsampling of smaller units from a comprehensive larger group representative of all states, cities, institutions, or organizations under study

(5) Nonrandom samples—e.g., convenience samples, use people who are available and agree to participate; do not give all members of the population an equal chance of being included in the sample; cannot generalize findings to the population from which this sample is taken

7. Data Collection—steps used to collect data; measurement of data requires the use of instruments such as questionnaires, rating scales, and interviews; the choice of instrument influences the significance of the study

8. Analyzing the Data—qualitative and statistical applications used to interpret data; instruments are evaluated for reliability and validity

   a. Reliability—measures of how consistently the instrument measures the item of interest

   b. Validity—the extent to which the instrument measures what it is intended to measure

   c. Level of significance—data are analyzed for significance or meaning of the statistical test to determine the probability that the observed relationship could be caused by chance rather than a response to manipulation of the variables; a statistically significant test means that the findings are unlikely to have been the result of chance at some level of probability

      (1) Level of significance most frequently used is the alpha .05 ($p < .05$); using this criteria, of 100 samples, the probability that the observed relationship would be found by chance is five times in 100; if the researcher selects alpha .01 as the level of significance the probability of the observed relationship occurring by chance would be once in a sample of 100

      (2) Type I Error—data analysis indicates the results are significant and the researcher rejects the null hypothesis concluding that there is a relationship when actually no relationship exists

(3) Type II Error—a decision to accept the null hypothesis concluding that no relationship exists when in fact a relationship does exist

d. Statistical tests

(1) Measures of central tendency

(a) Mean—the arithmetic average obtained by adding all the values and dividing by the number of values

(b) Median—the middle value of a set of numbers or the point above and below which 50% of the distribution falls (also known as the 50th percentile)

(c) Mode—the most frequent value or category

(d) Standard Deviation—the most commonly used measure of variability around the mean

(2) Non-Parametric Tests—used when there is no assumption about the distribution of the variable in the population for nominal and ordinal data

(a) Chi-Square—used with one or more groups; compares the actual frequency in each group with the expected frequency

(b) Spearman's Rho—correlation

(3) Parametric Tests—estimate at least one population parameter from the sample statistics

(a) t-tests—Pooled, Separate, and Paired t-tests; measures of the differences between two groups; compare two means in relation to the distribution of the differences between pairs of means drawn from a random sample; interpret the significance of differences between groups and require interval or ratio measurement of the variable on which the groups are being compared

(b) Analysis of variance (ANOVA)—more than two groups are compared for the differences among the set of groups considering the variance across all groups at once to determine if group means differ from each other

9. Dissemination of the Results—preparing a research report for publication, dissertation, thesis, or presentation at professional conferences is necessary to communicate the findings, the final step in the research process

- Utilization of Research in Nursing Practice—understanding and using research is a professional responsibility at all levels of clinical practice to gain knowledge, solve problems, and influence change; application of research in practice is vital to improve patient outcomes and contain health care costs; activities or skills that demonstrate various aspects of the utilization of research are:

  1. Significance of the research—can refer to both clinical relevance and statistical significance (Burns & Grove, 1993); in general, research should be critiqued for clinical application, scientific merit, and feasibility of implementing the research project (Polit & Hungler, 1991); statistical levels of significance make inferences from analysis of the data that the results were unlikely to have been caused by chance at some specified level of probability

  2. Generalization—the ability to generalize or apply research findings to other groups or the general population is enhanced by research that is statistically significant, uses random sampling, and is methodologically sound (Munro & Page, 1993; Polit & Hungler, 1991; Burns & Grove, 1993)

  3. Replication—repeating a study to determine if earlier results can be duplicated; replicated studies provide evidence to support earlier findings leading to conclusions or statements of fact

  4. Incorporating research into practice—conducting and using research findings can improve clinical outcomes and service delivery; reading professional journals, attending professional conferences, identifying and studying clinical problems and communicating research findings are other methods to incorporate research into practice

Ethical and Legal Issues

- Ethics in health care is concerned with the rights, duties, and obligations of professionals, institutions of care, and clients. Ethical principles guide the practitioner in numerous practice situations in which there is reason to reflect, judge or decide whether a course of action is morally acceptable. Ethical dilemmas arise when there are strong moral reasons supporting equally satisfactory or unsatisfactory alternatives or courses of action (Beauchamp & Walters, 1994; Kelly, 1992)

- Role of the Nurse in Decisions on Ethical Issues—practitioners in women's health rely on ethical principles to

    1. Arrive at moral judgements

    2. Resolve ethical dilemmas

    3. Evaluate policies regarding controversial and private issues

        a. Abortion

        b. Surrogate parenting

        c. End of life decisions

        d. Genetic testing

        e. Allocation of scarce resources

- Professional Codes of Ethics—rules that offer specific application of ethical principles

    1. Professional organizations have professional codes or practice committees on ethics which offer ethical guidelines to practitioners; interpretive statements on various issues are available from the National Association of Nurse Practitioners in Reproductive Health (NANPRH), the Association of Women's Health, Obstetrics, Neonatal Nurses (AWHONN), and the American Nurses' Association

    2. According to AWHONN, the role of the nurse in ethical decision making involves responsibilities and rights to care for the whole person and includes the right to play a critical role in ethical decision making, thereby integrating ethics into practice (AWHONN, 1994)

    3. Some rules defined in nurse practice acts

    4. Ethical Violations—the nurse who identifies incompetent, unethical, or illegal practice is obligated to report these violations, first through appropriate institutional channels and then to the State Board of Nursing (ANA Code for Nurses, 1985, 3.2)

- Ethical Principles and the Law

    1. Informed Consent—implies that the client is given the knowledge and opportunity to evaluate the options and risks associated with each option; is used as basis for practitioner authorization to either imple-

ment a plan of care for the client or to involve the client in research; informed consent assumes that the client receives full disclosure about the options, understands the disclosure, voluntarily agrees, is competent to act, and consents to the intervention

a. Legal Implications of Informed Consent—informed consent requires adherence to institutional legal requirements for consent; e.g., the Patient Self-Determination Act of 1990 focuses on advance directives and the rights of patients to refuse life-sustaining treatment. At the time of admission, institutions that receive Medicare/Medicaid funds are required to provide written policies and information that describe the patient's legal rights to make decisions, to refuse treatment, and to give advance directives (Living Will, Durable Power of Attorney for Health Care Decisions). Directives instruct the health care provider, family and friends to withhold life-sustaining treatment and/or refuse treatments such as mechanical respiration, tube feedings and resuscitation

(1) Refusal of treatment—the U.S. Supreme Court's 1990 Cruzan decision in Missouri affirms the premise that competent individuals have a constitutional right to refuse life-sustaining treatment (Cruzan v. Director, Missouri Dept. of Health); nurse's role in refusal of treatment includes:

(a) Support patient in achieving a dignified death by directing care toward the prevention and relief of suffering

(b) In situations where a presently competent patient or previously competent patient who has issued advance directives refuses food and fluid, the nurse is permitted to honor the decision (ANA Committee on Ethics, 1985)

(2) Confidentiality—rules derived from the ethical principle of justice which includes the right to privacy. Informed consent to share information is provided through patient authorization for release of information to insurance companies and employers. Confidentiality protects the subjects' rights to privacy in research projects. In some instances, such as in cases of certain STDs, state statutes

require the disclosure of otherwise confidential information for the public's protection

    (3) Veracity—the duty to tell the truth is supported by the ethical principles of autonomy, beneficence, and justice; frequently cited in ethical dilemmas about disclosing health conditions to patients when the patient's right to know conflicts with the principle of "do no harm"

    (4) Withdrawal of treatment—in instances where the patient has never been competent (infants, children, mentally disabled, etc.), the withdrawal of treatment such as food and fluids is rarely condoned. The practitioner is obliged to continue to provide food and fluids considered to provide nurture and comfort. Treatment may be withdrawn in most states in cases where competent individuals have made their wishes known through issuance of advance directives (ANA,1988). Once life-sustaining measures have been instituted, a court order must be obtained in some states that do not have a natural death act in order to withdraw treatment. The nurse is obligated to provide supportive care in cases where life-sustaining treatment is withdrawn or refused (The Hastings Center, 1987)

  b. Informed Consent for Children and Adolescents—consent for treatment and/or research, and protection against abuse are primary issues related to the rights of children and adolescents. Although parents or guardians are generally required to give consent for medical or surgical interventions for minors (except in emergency situations), emancipated and mature minors are considered competent to consent to treatment under most circumstances. Exceptions that may not require parental consent include treatment for sexually transmitted disease (STD), pregnancy related care, contraception, rape, incest, sexual abuse and drug abuse. The practitioner should be aware of state laws that specify ages and situations in which parental permission is required for consent to treat. Practitioners have no legal requirement to report such treatment to a parent or guardian in most states (Greydanus & Patel, 1991)

2. Beneficence—the obligation to do good. Codes for nurses assert a commitment to protect the client from harm (a principle of nonmalefi-

cence) and to promote the client's welfare and support action to meet the health and social needs of the public (beneficence). Beneficence assumes that the practitioner will weigh the benefits against harm

3. Justice—the formal principle of equality in which each individual is accorded a fair share, due, or owed treatment. Under this principle all people should be accorded equal access to care

Health Policy and Legislative Issues for Nurse Practitioners

- Role of the Nurse Practitioner: Nurse practitioners (NPs) provide direct client care, and assume indirect roles including those of educator, administrator, clinical supervisor, consultant, and researcher. As nurses, NPs are responsible for leadership toward redistribution of health care resources, and for the provision of an adequate quantity of care achieved at the lowest cost compatible with quality

- Evolution of the Role—occurred in response to a lack of health care services and the need for better access to services, especially in inner-city and rural areas. The practitioner movement has its roots in the Frontier Nursing Services begun in 1925. Public health nurses in California in the early 1960s expanded the role to include history taking and increased responsibility for pediatric health maintenance visits. The first NP program (pediatrics) was established by Loretta Ford and Henry Silver in 1965. Currently there are over 20,000 employed NPs (Safriet, 1992; DeAngelis, 1994)

- NP Scope of Practice: Determined by state licensure laws that define nursing under the Nurse Practice Act and/or through additional state licensure requirements for advanced practice nurses

  1. State licensure laws establish requirements for education, and licensing, and stipulate the functions of the nurse (Mezy & McGivern, 1993)

  2. Nurses are professionally accountable and legally mandated in many states to practice only within the scope of practice for which they have been educated

  3. Regulatory authority is given to administrative agencies responsible for enforcement of the Nurse Practice Act; state agencies authorized to regulate nurse practitioner practice vary and include state Boards of Nursing, Boards of Medicine, Joint Committees (Boards of Medicine and Nursing), and Pharmacy Boards

- Standards of Practice—declarations that outline educational preparation and minimum levels of acceptable performance that attempt to provide the consumer with a way to measure the quality of care they receive. Standards are found in state Nurse Practice Acts and in statements of professional organizations such as AWHONN, NANPRH, ANA, and the American Academy of Nurse Practitioners (AANP). Standards and scope of practice are further delineated in collaborative agreements and protocols between NPs and physicians

- Legislative Barriers To Nurse Practitioner Practice

  1. State legislative statutes reflect a trend to increase NP authority and autonomy. By 1994, 20 states gave exclusive authority to Boards of Nursing (BON) to regulate practice and allow independent practice without physician supervision or collaboration (Pearson, 1995). Written agreements, protocols and review procedures provide "contract" guidelines for supervision and collaboration arrangements

  2. Prescriptive authority

     a. Has been an issue over the past 15 years with legal authority to prescribe trailing behind efforts to recognize the role of NPs (Henry, 1994)

     b. Legal authority to prescribe drugs or devices is contained within the state Nurse Practice Act or separate statutes for prescriptive authority

     c. In some states the Board of Medicine or other agencies must approve prescriptive authority

     d. Provisions required by some states include a physician co-signature, collaborative agreement or written protocols

     e. The Medical Practice Act and Pharmacy Acts in some states have statutes that conflict with the Nurse Practice Act thereby indirectly restricting NP prescribing authority

     f. Currently, NPs have some degree of prescriptive authority in over 35 states

  3. Reimbursement—traditionally, limits have been placed on NP scope of practice through legislative requirements that prevent direct reimbursement for NP services and conditions under which NPs can be reimbursed. NPs have made progress in acquiring reimbursement from state and federal programs and some third-party payers, however, inequities remain in achieving full economic recognition (Timmons & Ridenour, 1994)

Legal Aspects of Nurse Practitioner Practice

- Credentialing—one of two legal mechanisms whose purpose is to protect patients from negligence, substandard care and inappropriate care. Each state has an administrative system that determines competence, oversees the quality of care and disciplines professionals (Hadley, 1993)

    1. Licensure: "The process by which an agency of the government grants permission to persons to engage in a given profession or occupation by certifying that those licensed have attained the minimal degree of competency necessary to ensure that the public health, safety, and welfare will be reasonably well protected" (U.S. DHEW, 1971)

    2. Certification: "The process by which a nongovernmental agency or association grants recognition to an individual who has met certain predetermined qualifications specified by that agency or association" (U.S. DHEW, 1971)

        a. Certification is an adjunct to licensure and a method to identify specialists and protect the public

        b. Many states require certification by a professional organization as a requirement for advanced nursing practice

- Tort litigation—the second mechanism to protect patients which enables the patient to sue the health care professional, e.g., malpractice suits

    1. Standard of Care—determines nurse's liability for any negligent act; requires the NP to perform the same as any discerning person of ordinary prudence with comparable education, skills, and training under similar circumstances

    2. Adherence to the standard of care determined by comparing documentation of care with

        a. Standards and scope of practice statements

        b. Written protocols

        c. Current practice guidelines found in the literature

        d. Procedure manuals

        e. Agency policies

        f. Community practices

3. Litigation—may involve suits based on negligence or malpractice claims

    a. Negligence—failing to conduct oneself in a specific manner with due care thereby doing harm to another, or failing to do something that another prudent person would do in the same situation

    b. Malpractice—implies professional misconduct, lack of skill or lack of faithfulness or honesty in the conduct of professional responsibilities

    c. Proof of liability—requires that the NP entered into a professional relationship with the patient and violated the standard of care; specific elements must be present to prove violation of standard of care

        (1) The NP breached the established duty to perform in a reasonable manner

        (2) The patient was injured or damaged in some way

        (3) The injury was caused directly by the NP's negligence (Hadley, 1993)

- Malpractice (Professional Liability) Insurance

    1. It is recommended that all nurse practitioners carry professional liability insurance coverage

    2. Malpractice coverage is a requirement to obtain prescriptive authority in several states

    3. Types of liability policies

        a. Occurrence based coverage—includes protection for incidents that occurred at the time of coverage even if the insurance policy is not renewed

        b. Claims made coverage—effective only if claims filed during policy coverage period; optional "tail" coverage extends coverage of a claims made policy into the future to cover all claims filed after the basic claims made coverage period

    4. Statute of limitations—the legal limit of time a person has to file a civil suit; in the case of an infant or minor, the statute does not begin until the child has reached age 18; "tail" coverage is an important consideration for NPs whose practice includes these groups

QUESTIONS

Select the best answer:

1. The process whereby a client is given the knowledge and opportunity to evaluate treatment or research options and risks associated with each option is best described as:

   a. Informed consent
   b. Partial disclosure
   c. Liability protection
   d. Censure

2. Ethical dilemmas are best described as conflicts in which alternatives are:

   a. Totally appropriate
   b. Marginally acceptable
   c. Equally satisfactory or unsatisfactory
   d. Partially inappropriate

3. Research that is rigorous, logical, and controlled is best described as a:

   a. Scientific method of inquiry
   b. Nursing process
   c. Problem-oriented approach
   d. Theoretical construct

4. Quasi-experiments lack either:

   a. Randomization or a control group
   b. Manipulation of a variable or validity
   c. Control or manipulation
   d. A sample or population

5. Selection of a research sample whose characteristics resemble the entire population enhances the ability to :

   a. Capture the target population
   b. Rationalize the findings
   c. Generalize the findings beyond the sample
   d. Determine a level of significance

6. In a research study involving 200 subjects, the researcher used alpha .05($p < .05$)

as the level of significance. According to probability, rejection of a true null hypotheses in this sample might occur:

    a. Five times
    b. Ten times
    c. Two hundred times
    d. .05 times

7. A 15 year old female is not required to have parental permission for treatment under most circumstances if:

    a. She is emancipated or mature to consent
    b. Care is provided by a licensed practitioner
    c. She is a Medicaid recipient
    d. The problem is chronic

8. Participation in public policy forums to discuss the allocation of biotechnological resources is an example of applying the principle of:

    a. Beneficence
    b. Justice
    c. Nonmaleficence
    d. Morality

9. Of the following ethical principles, promoting goodness, kindness, and charity best describe:

    a. Justice
    b. Autonomy
    c. Nonmaleficence
    d. Beneficence

10. A nurse practitioner who seeks employment in a new state is interested in obtaining a description of her authorized role. This information is available from:

    a. Her collaborating physician
    b. The Board of Medicine
    c. The Board of Nursing
    d. Her NP program

11. The mechanism by which a nurse practitioner is recognized as a specialist by meeting educational criteria and demonstrating mastery of a body of knowledge is best described as:

a. Licensure
b. Accreditation
c. Certification
d. Continuing education

12. The scope of practice for nurse practitioners is best described in:

a. Nurse Practice Acts
b. Federal legislation
c. Certification guidelines
d. Beneficence programs

13. Standards of practice are best described as:

a. Community practices that determine how health services are delivered
b. Educational requirements established by schools of nursing
c. Licensure and accreditation processes for institutions
d. Statements by which educational qualifications and the process of care are judged

14. A nurse practitioner is asked to serve as an expert witness. She reviews documentation of the care, compliance with the scope of practice, written protocols, current literature, and community practice in order to evaluate :

a. Standard of care
b. Nurse's rights
c. Legal statutes
d. The physician

15. A nurse practitioner obtains professional liability insurance that covers incidents during the period of coverage and if the policy lapses. This type of policy is described as:

a. Occurrence
b. Incident
c. Tail
d. Group

Answers

1. a
2. c
3. a
4. a
5. c
6. b
7. a
8. b
9. d
10. c
11. c
12. a
13. d
14. a
15. a

BIBLIOGRAPHY

American Nurses' Association. (1994). *The scope of practice of the primary health care nurse practitioner.* Washington, DC: Author.

American Nurses' Association. (1988). *Ethics in nursing: Position statements and guidelines.* Kansas City, MO: Author.

American Nurses' Association. (1985). *Ethical dilemmas confronting nurses.* Committee on Ethics. Kansas City, MO: Author.

American Nurses' Association. (1985). *Code for nurses.* Kansas City, MO: Author.

AWOHNN. (1994). *Committee on Ethics and Committee on Practice Statements.* Washington, DC: Author

Beauchamp, T.L. (1994). Third party interests in bioethics. In T. Beauchamp & A. Walters (Eds.), *Contemporary issues in bioethics* (pp. 75–83). California: Wadsworth.

Beauchamp, T.L,, & Walters, A. (Eds.). (1994). *Contemporary issues in bioethics* (4th ed.). California: Wadsworth.

Brockopp, D.Y., & Hastings-Tolsma, M.T. (1995). *Contemporary issues in bioethics* (4th ed.). California; Wadsworth.

Brockopp, D.Y., & Hastings-Tolsma, M.T. (1995). *Fundamentals of nursing research* (2nd ed.). Boston: Jones and Bartlett.

Burns, N., & Grove, S.K. (1993). *The practice of nursing research: Conduct, critique & utilization* (2nd ed.). Philadelphia: W.B. Saunders.

Caplan, A. (1994). The ethics of in vitro fertilization. In T. Beauchamp & A. Walters (Eds.). *Contemporary issues in bioethics* (4th ed., pp. 216–223). California: Wadsworth.

Clark, F.I. (1994). Intensive care treatment decisions: The roots of our confusion. *Pediatrics, 94* (1), 98–101.

Cruzan v. Director, Missouri Department of Health, 110 *Supreme Court Reporter* (1990), 110 S. Ct. 2841.

DeAngelis, C. (1994). Nurse practitioner redux. *Journal of the American Medical Association, 271,* 868–871.

Freel, M.I. (1985). Truth telling. In J.C. McClosky & H.K. Grace (Eds.), *Current issues in nursing* (2nd ed., pp.1008–1025). Boston: Blackwell Scientific Publications.

Greydanus, D.E., & Patel, D.R. (1991). Consent and confidentiality in adolescent health care. *Pediatric Annals, 20* (2), 80–84.

Hadley, E.H. (1993). Marketing and management: Distinguishing between licensure proceedings and malpractice suits. *Journal of the American Academy of Nurse Practitioners, 5* (3), 135–137.

Henry, P.F. (1994). Seeking legal authority to prescribe. *Nurse Practitioner Forum, 5* (4), 203–204.

Kelly, L.Y. (1992). *The nursing experience, trends, challenges, and transitions.* New York: McGraw-Hill, Inc.

McLaughlin, F.E., & Marascuilo, L.A. (1990). *Advanced nursing and health care research.* Philadelphia: W.B. Saunders Company.

Mezy, M.D., & McGivern, D.O. (1993). *Nurses, nurse practitioners: Evolution to advanced practice.* New York: Springer Publishing Co.

Munro, B.H., & Page, E.B. (1993). *Statistical methods for health care research* (2nd ed.). Philadelphia: J.B. Lippincott Company.

NANPRH. (1994). *Standards of practice and education for the Women's Health Care Nurse Practitioner.* Washington, DC: Author.

National Institutes of Health. (1994). *Summary of conclusions and recommendations of NIH human embryo research panel.* Bethesda, Maryland

Office of Technology Assessment, U.S. Congress. (1986). *Nurse practitioners, physician assistants and certified nurse midwives: A policy analysis.* Washington, DC: U.S. Government Printing Office.

Pearson, L.J. (1995). Annual update of how each state stands on legislative issues affecting advanced nursing practice. *The Nurse Practitioner, 20* (1), 13–51.

Polit, D.F., & Hungler, B.P. (1991). *Nursing research: Principles and practice* (4th ed.). Philadelphia: J.B. Lippincott.

Safriet, B.J. (1992). Health care dollars and regulatory sense: The role of advanced practice nursing. *Yale Journal on Regulation, 9* (2), 419–487.

Sebas, M.B. (1994). Developing a collaborative practice agreement for the primary care setting. *Nurse Practitioner, 19* (3), 49–51.

The Hastings Center. (1987). *Guidelines on the termination of life-sustaining treatment and the care of the dying.* Briarcliff Manor, NY: Indiana University Press.

Timmons, G., & Ridenour, N. (1994). Legal approaches to the restraint of trade of nurse practitioners: Disparate reimbursement patterns. *Journal of the American Academy of Nurse Practitioners, 6* (2), 55–59.

Titler, M.G., Goode, C.J., & Mathis, S. (1992). What happens to nursing research in times of economic cut-backs. *Series on Nursing Administration. IV*, 324–330.

U.S. Department of Health, Education and Welfare, (U.S. DHEW). Public Health Service (1971). *Report on licensure and related health personnel credentialling.* Washington, DC: DHEW Publication No. (HSM) 72–11.

Warren, M.A. (1994). On the moral and legal status of abortion. In T. L. Beauchamp & A. Walters (Eds.). *Contemporary issues in bioethics* (4th ed., pp. 302–316). California: Wadsworth.

INDEX

For information on Certification Review Courses, Home Study Programs and Review Books contact:

Health Leadership Associates, Inc.
Post Office Box 59153
Potomac, Maryland 20859

1-800-435-4775

REVIEW BOOK/AUDIO CASSETTE ORDER FORM
HEALTH LEADERSHIP ASSOCIATES, INC.

PLEASE PRINT OR TYPE

NAME: _____

ADDRESS: Street _____ Apt. # _____ City _____ State _____ Zip Code _____

TELEPHONE: _____ (HOME) _____ (WORK)

Section 1: AUDIO CASSETTES

Professional "live" audio recordings of Review Courses are approximately 15 hours in length unless otherwise noted and include detailed course handouts. Continuing Education contact hours are available for these audio cassette Home Study Programs.

QTY	REVIEW COURSE TITLE	PRICE	
____	Adult Nurse Practitioner	$150.00	_____
____	Ambulatory Women's Health Care Nursing	$150.00	_____
____	Clinical Specialist in Adult Psychiatric and Mental Health Nursing	$150.00	_____
____	Family Nurse Practitioner	$330.00	_____
	(Consists of ANP, PNP & Childbearing Management courses)		
____	* Generalist Gerontological Nurse	$ 75.00	_____
____	Generalist Medical-Surgical Nurse	$150.00	_____
____	* Generalist Pediatric Nurse	$ 75.00	_____
____	* Generalist Psychiatric and Mental Health Nurse	$ 75.00	_____
____	Gerontological Nurse Practitioner	$150.00	_____
____	Home Health Nurse	$150.00	_____
____	Inpatient Obstetric/Maternal Newborn/Low Risk Neonatal/Perinatal Nurse	$150.00	_____
____	** Obstetrics/Childbearing Management	$ 45.00	_____
____	Pediatric Nurse Practitioner	$150.00	_____
____	** Test Taking Strategies and Techniques	$ 30.00	_____
____	Women's Health Care Nurse Practitioner (Formerly Ob/Gyn Nurse Practitioner)	$150.00	_____

* 8 Hour Course, ** 2-4 Hour Course

SUB TOTAL:		_____
Maryland Residents add 5% sales tax:		_____
CEU FEE ($10/course):		_____
Shipping: 2-4 Hour Course	$ 4.00	_____
All other Courses	$10.00	_____
TOTAL:		_____

PAYMENT DUE METHOD OF PAYMENT

☐ Check or money order (US funds, payable to Health Leadership Associates, Inc.) A $25 fee will be charged on returned checks.

☐ Purchase Order is attached. P.O. # _____

☐ Please charge my ☐ MasterCard ☐ Visa

Credit Card# _____ Exp. date _____

Signature _____

Print Name _____

REVIEW GUIDES & AUDIO CASSETTES

1) **Section 1 Total** $ _____
2) **Section 2 Total** $ _____
3) **Section 3 Total** $ _____
TOTAL PAYMENT DUE $ _____

Section 2: REVIEW BOOKS

QTY	BOOK TITLE	PRICE	
____	Adult Nurse Practitioner Certification Review Guide (second edition)	$ 47.75	
____	Family Nurse Practitioner Certification Review Guide Set (Includes ANP,PNP, and Women's Health Care NP Guides)	$123.25	_____
____	Generalist Pediatric Nurse Certification Review Guide (second edition)	$ 47.75	
____	Gerontological Nursing Certification Review Guide for the Generalist, Clinical Specialist, and Nurse Practitioner (revised edition)	$ 47.75	
____	Pediatric Nurse Practitioner Certification Review Guide (second edition)	$ 47.75	
____	Psychiatric Certification Review Guide for the Generalist and Clinical Specialist in Adult, Child, and Adolescent Psychiatric and Mental Health Nursing	$ 47.75	
____	Women's Health Care Nurse Practitioner Certification Review Guide (Formerly Ob/Gyn Nurse Practitioner)	$ 47.75	_____

SPECIAL OFFERING

____	TODAY and TOMORROW'S WOMAN - MENOPAUSE: BEFORE AND AFTER (Girls of 16 to Women of 99) (Author: Virginia Layng Millonig)	$ 19.95

SUB TOTAL:	_____
Maryland Residents add 5% sales tax:	_____
CEU FEE ($10.00)	_____
Shipping $5.00 for one book:	_____
$2.00 for each additional book: (Except $1.00 for each add'l. *Today and Tomorrow's Woman*)	_____
TOTAL:	_____

For orders of 10 or greater call 1-800-435-4775.
(All prices subject to change without notice)

Section 3: REVIEW BOOK/AUDIO CASSETTE DISCOUNT PACKAGES

A discounted rate is available when purchasing Review Book(s) and Audio Cassettes together. When purchasing packages, indicate Book/Audio Cassette selections in sections 1 and 2. Calculate amount due in this section.

QTY	PACKAGE SELECTION	PRICE	
____	8 Hour Course / 1 Review Guide	$120.00	_____
____	15 Hour Course / 1 Review Guide	$190.00	_____
____	FNP Package	$415.00	_____

FNP Package consists of Adult NP, Pediatric NP, Women's Health Care NP Guides & Audio Cassettes of the ANP, PNP, and Childbearing Management Courses.

SUB TOTAL:	_____
Maryland Residents add 5% sales tax:	_____
CEU Fee ($10)	_____
TOTAL:	_____
(Shipping charge included in package rate)	

RETURN POLICY
Due to the nature of the material contained in the review books and audio cassettes, returns on books ONLY will be accepted one week post delivery. No returns on audio cassettes except for defective audio cassettes which will be replaced.

MAIL TO:	Health Leadership Associates, Inc. P.O. Box 59153 Potomac, MD 20859
OR PHONE:	(800) 435-4775; (301) 983-2405
OR FAX:	(301) 983-2693